Neurodevelopmental Disorders

DEVELOPMENTAL PERSPECTIVES IN PSYCHIATRY

Series Editor
James C. Harris, M.D., Johns Hopkins University

Tuberous Sclerosis Complex, Third Edition
Manual Gomez, M.D., Julian Sampson, M.D., and
Vicky Whittemore, PH.D.

Neurodevelopmental Disorders: Diagnosis and Treatment
Randi Jenssen Hagerman, M.D.

Neurodevelopmental Disorders

Diagnosis and Treatment

Randi Jenssen Hagerman

New York   Oxford • Oxford University Press   1999

Oxford University Press

Oxford   New York

Athens   Auckland   Bangkok   Bogotá   Buenos Aires   Calcutta
Cape Town   Chennai   Dar es Salaam   Delhi   Florence   Hong Kong   Istanbul
Karachi   Kuala Lumpur   Madrid   Melbourne   Mexico City   Mumbai
Nairobi   Paris   São Paulo   Singapore   Taipei   Tokyo   Toronto   Warsaw

and associated companies in
Berlin   Ibadan

Copyright © 1999 by Oxford University Press, Inc.

Published by Oxford University Press, Inc.
198 Madison Avenue, New York, New York 10016

Oxford is a registered trademark of Oxford University Press

Library of Congress Cataloging-in-Publication Data
Hagerman, Randi Jenssen, 1949–
    Neurodevelopmental disorders : diagnosis and treatment / Randi Jenssen Hagerman.
        p.   cm.—(Developmental perspectives in psychiatry)
    Includes bibliographical references and index.
    ISBN 0-19-512314-X
    1. Developmental disabilities.   2. Pediatric neuropsychology.   3. Developmental neurobiology
    4. Cognitive neuroscience.   I. Title.   II. Series.
    [DNLM: 1. Mental Retardation.   2. Developmental Disabilities.   WM 300 H144n 1999]
RJ506.D47H34   1999
618.92′8—dc21   98-54687
DNLM/DLC
for Library of Congress

9 8 7 6 5 4 3 2

Printed in the United States of America
on acid-free paper

This book is dedicated to
my husband, Paul,
my daughters, Karin and Hillary,
and my mother, Helen Kalantar.

Their tolerance, support, love,
and sense of adventure
have made all things possible.

PREFACE

This book includes nine chapters that review selected syndromes that I have seen in my clinical and research experience over the last 20 years. Some of these syndromes are common, such as fetal alcohol syndrome and Tourette syndrome, and others are rare, such as Smith-Magenis syndrome. Each of these disorders has an interesting cognitive and behavioral phenotype that necessitates a unique treatment approach, and yet common themes are seen in almost all of the chapters, such as the treatment for hyperactivity or attention deficits. The commonalities and differences in each of these disorders have been fascinating to me and, I hope, to the reader of this book. We can learn treatment approaches to one disorder that may be beneficial to several others.

I have had the good fortune to work with an outstanding clinical team of professionals who have taught me about a global approach to treatment in which interventions can work synergistically to push for the most optimal outcome possible. We have also worked closely with the schools to utilize medical intervention to enhance educational endeavors. The separation of medical and educational professionals is institutional in our society, but we can learn so much from each other. This book highlights a global approach to treatment that includes medications to improve cognitive and behavior problems, language and motor therapy, educational interventions, vocational approaches, and computer technology to enhance the functioning of children and adults with these syndromes. A wide variety of professionals in the medical and educational field should find this book useful, and parents who are interested in more detailed information about their child's syndrome will also benefit from reading this book.

I find the fast-moving field of genetics fascinating, and I have tried to document the latest molecular findings in each of these disorders. Although the information is somewhat technical at times, the benefits of understanding the underlying molecular mechanisms for specific behavioral or cognitive phenotypes are worthwhile from an intellectual viewpoint and from a treatment perspective now and in the future of molecular interventions.

Our clinical team is best known for our research and writings regarding fragile X syndrome, but what we have learned from this disorder we have applied to the other syndromes discussed here. Much of the treatment information for these disorders is anecdotal, with the exception of Tourette syndrome, for which controlled studies of psychopharmacological interventions exist. Hopefully our efforts in compiling treatment information will stimulate further research and controlled trials of a variety of interventions.

This book was written because so much good information passes my way on a daily basis that I could not keep track of it, or even remember it, unless I wrote it down in a cognitive framework for myself and for my students and team members. I began this book during my sabbatical in Australia, and Danuta Loesch of LaTrobe University in Melbourne and Bogden Mdzewski provided the academic environment, intellectual stimulation, and gracious hospitality of their home which made this writing possible. I am deeply grateful to them.

Our clinical and research team provides a daily learning environment for me, and the innovative ideas of team members can be found throughout this book. I am very thankful to Tracy Kovach, Kristen Gray, Cathy Bodine, and Lisa Noble for all they have taught me regarding computers and assistive technology; to Marcia Braden, Rebecca O'Connor, Jennifer Hills, Nancy Mann, Craig Knippenberg, and Bill Sobesky, for their expertise in educational and psychological interventions; to Tracy Stackhouse, Clare Summers, and Lucy Miller for their expertise in sensory integration occupational therapy; to Sarah Scharfenaker for her expertise in speech and language interventions; and to Louise Gane for her expertise in genetic counseling. The physicians who work with me, including Edward Goldson, Sheila Tunnell, and Pamela McKenzie, have been a constant source of support and feedback for new ideas and issues. Most important, our students, residents, and fellows, some of whom are supported by the MCH Training Grant no. MCJ089413, have provided great support, intellectual stimulation, and review of the information in this book. These individuals include Karen Riley, Dick Taylor, Sheila Tunnell, Jason Coe, Jeff Sidders, Matt Holden, Susan Endres, Brenda Sanger, Wade Heinrichs, Rhoda Amaria, Aaron Jodeh, Kathryn Farrow and Kurt Weaver. Kurt did an exceptional job of compiling the appendices; he was funded by the William Rosen Fund of the National Fragile X Foundation. The support staff of the Child Development Unit at The Children's Hospital, including Barbara Wheeler, Mela Barrios, and Jacque Woods, have been invaluable to me and provided the time and opportunity to complete this book. I am also deeply grateful to the patients and families who have taught me about their children. Many parents have reviewed these chapters and provided valuable insight and they are acknowledged at the end of each chapter. Permission was obtained from each patient and parent for use of the pictures included in this book.

Each chapter was reviewed by experts in each field, and I am thankful for the time of these gracious professionals, including Mary Linden, Edward Riley, Sarah Mattson, Heather Carmichael Olson, William McMahon, Bruce Bender,

Arthur Robinson, Jim Salbenblatt, Michele Mazzocco, Ron Rosenfeld, Merlin Butler, Suzanne Cassidy, Joseph Wagstaff, Janet Thomas, David Manchester, Paul Wang, Ursula Bellugi, Ann C. M. Smith, and A. J. Allen. Their critiques improved this book immensely.

Most important, this book was possible because of the dedicated and intense effort of two women, Susan Wood and Megan Lampe, who each spent 6 months of almost full-time effort to complete this book. Their creativity in Internet and library searches, their word processing expertise, and their knowledge of English pulled this book together. If I didn't have a family, I would dedicate this book to Susan and Megan. Their friendship and support have been wonderful.

Finally, financial support for both clinical work and research has been essential. Louise Gane and Sandy Morrison have done a tremendous amount to organize both foundation support and private family support, and I am greatly indebted to them. I thank the Kenneth Kendal King Foundation, the Denver Foundation, the Comprecare Foundation, the Wallace Genetic Foundation, and the Janssen Research Foundation for their support of our clinical work and research. I am very thankful for the efforts of Felix de la Cruz, National Institute of Child Health and Development, the National Fragile X Foundation, and the FRAXA Foundation for promoting fragile X research both at our center and elsewhere. NICHD grant no. HD36071 supports some of the fragile X research reported here. I am greatly indebted to the support of families who have donated money and carried out fund raisers to support both clinical work and research regarding fragile X syndrome at our center. Jim and Vicky Mulvey, Margaret Israel, Eric and Elissa Boory, Shannon Geis, Pam and James Vershbow, and Lori and Chris Beesley stand out remarkably in this regard, and I am deeply grateful.

I continue to learn on a daily basis from the families and patients that I evaluate and treat. I hope this book gives these well-deserving families something in return.

Denver, Colorado   R. J. H.
February 1999

Contents

Neurodevelopmental Disorders

Fetal Alcohol Syndrome

Although Lemoine et al. (1968) reported the teratogenic effects in humans of alcohol use during pregnancy in the French literature, this association was not well recognized until 1973, when Jones et al. (1973) and Jones and Smith (1973) reported the dysmorphic features and introduced the term *fetal alcohol syndrome* in an international and widely read journal, the *Lancet.* Jones and Smith (1973) review ancient literature and find in Roman and Greek writings a warning to bridal couples not to drink wine in order that defective children not be conceived. There are also several admonitions in the Bible regarding the avoidance of wine or drink during pregnancy, but these appear to be related to the customs of the Nazarites and not necessarily to concern for defective offspring (Abel, 1997).

After the ancient writings, it was not until 1726 that documentation of the problems of prenatal alcohol exposure occurred. A report by the College of Physicians to the British Parliament stated that parental drinking is a cause of weak, feeble, and distempered children. Subsequently, in 1834 a select committee to the House of Commons reported on drunkenness and said that infants born to alcoholic mothers had a starved, shriveled, and imperfect look. In 1899, Sullivan published a report on 120 alcoholic women in the Liverpool prison and found just over a twofold increase in stillbirths and deaths in their infants compared to those of nonalcoholic prisoners. He warned people about the damaging effects of alcohol on the fetus, and in 1901, in France, Ladrague also reported problems in the infants of alcoholic mothers, including death, poor development, epilepsy, and mental retardation. As Streissguth (1997) pointed out in her historical review of the field, these reports were unheeded for decades. Even the Kallikak pedigree, which was first reported by Goddard (1912), was considered a prime example of

Neurodevelopmental Disorders: Diagnosis and Treatment, by Randi Jenssen Hagerman. New York: Oxford University Press, 1999. © Oxford University Press, Inc.

hereditary causes of mental retardation and helped to fuel the eugenics movement. It was not until 1995 that Karp and colleagues carefully reviewed the medical reports of the many retarded individuals in this family and documented that they almost certainly had fetal alcohol syndrome (FAS) and fetal alcohol effects (FAE).

Animal research was being carried out, but it was largely ignored and not related to the work with humans until after recognition of FAS (Streissguth, 1997). Papara-Nicholson and Telford (1957) reported that prenatal alcohol exposure in guinea pigs caused low birth weights and motor and feeding problems in their offspring. In 1968, Sandor and colleagues carried out work on chick and rat dysmorphogenesis secondary to alcohol exposure and warned that there was a serious risk to humans with ethanol exposure in utero (Sandor and Elias, 1968).

Work in the human area was carried out in France, but it was not well disseminated because it was written only in French. Rouquette (1957) studied 100 children born to alcoholic mothers for her medical thesis and reported on their malformations, which were typical for what is now recognized as FAS (Streissguth, 1997). Subsequently, Lemoine et al. (1968), in Nantes, France, reported on 127 children of alcoholic mothers who had dysmorphic features, growth retardation, and behavioral problems. Ulleland, a pediatric resident in Seattle, noted low birth weights, failure to thrive, and delayed development in 12 infants born to alcoholic mothers (Ulleland, 1972; Ulleland et al., 1970). These previous reports, however, did not bring recognition to the problem. It took a world-renowned geneticist, David Smith, who had great credibility, to carefully document the dysmorphic features in multiple patients, blame it on alcohol, and then name it *fetal alcohol syndrome* in an international journal before the professional community would pay attention (Jones and Smith, 1973; Jones et al., 1973). Having a specific name or a label for a disorder, as we will see many times in this book in relation to other disorders, makes a dramatic difference in recognizing the syndrome and in facilitating public education.

After 1973, reports of patients with fetal alcohol syndrome flooded the medical literature from all over the world (reviewed by Streissguth, 1997). The important issue was that fetal alcohol syndrome could be completely prevented, and the focus over the last two decades has been on lay and professional education regarding diagnosis and prevention efforts. By the late 1970s there was validation of FAS through comparison studies of FAS patients and controls, follow-up studies involving varying levels of alcohol consumption, and experimental animal research (Streissguth, 1997). In 1977, the secretary of the U.S. Department of Health, Education and Welfare issued a warning to pregnant women that six or more drinks per day was a clear risk to the fetus. The surgeon general realized the importance of this message and publicly announced in 1981 that women should avoid alcohol during pregnancy because of the risk of birth defects. However, more pressure and time was needed before policy was changed. Finally, in 1988, Congress passed the Federal Beverage Labeling Act, which required that all containers of alcoholic beverages display a warning stating that women should not drink alcoholic beverages during pregnancy because of the risk of birth defects.

Studies regarding the prevalence rates of FAS have been carried out in a number of countries (May, 1995). In Europe and Scandinavia, rates have varied from 1.4 to 4.8 children with FAS per 1,000, although if patients with alcohol-related problems are included, the rate is as high as 9.1 per 1,000 (Sampson et al., 1997). Local studies in the United States have yielded a range of from 0.33 to 4.6 children with FAS per 1,000 (reviewed by Abel and Sokol, 1991) and Sampson et al., 1997.

DIAGNOSTIC FEATURES

After the initial case reports and the name of fetal alcohol syndrome were established in 1973, clinicians from all over the world began reporting patients with FAS. In 1978 Clarren and Smith summarized the world's experience regarding the diagnosis of FAS. They emphasized four categories of involvement:

1. Central nervous system dysfunction, including mental retardation seen in 85% of patients reported so far; microcephaly; central nervous system (CNS) malformations, including cerebellar dysplasias and cerebral heterotopias; irritability and poor suck in the newborn period; hypotonicity; hypertonicity; seizures; and hyperactivity.
2. Growth deficiency of height and weight parameters with usually greater deficits in weight than in length; in general, patients remained more than 2 standard deviations (SD) below the norm, although some patients demonstrated postnatal catch-up growth.
3. Characteristic facial features, including short palpebral fissures (small opening of the eye), seen in 91% of their patients; hypoplastic (small) upper lip; flat philtrum; and midfacial and mandibular growth deficiency (Figure 1.1). Additional features of midface hypoplasia included a short nose, low nasal bridge, epicanthal folds, and anteverted nostrils. The authors also mentioned the occasional occurrence of microophthalmia, cleft lip, and cleft palate.
4. Variable major and minor malformations, including cardiac anomalies, cutaneous hemangiomas, hirsuitism in infancy, aberrant palmar creases, radioulnar synostosis, scoliosis, hernias, hypospadius, hypoplastic kidneys, and hydronephrosis. Clarren and Smith (1978) emphasized the variability in FAS but felt that involvement in brain function, growth, and facial appearance was needed before a person could be considered affected prenatally by alcohol.

In 1980, the following criteria for a diagnosis of FAS were spelled out by a study group of the Research Society on Alcoholism (Rosett, 1980):

1. Prenatal and/or postnatal growth retardation (weight, length, and/or head circumference below the 10th percentile).
2. Characteristic facial dysmorphology with at least two of these three signs: microcephaly (head circumference below the 3rd percentile), microophthal-

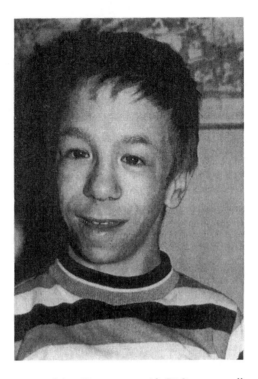

FIGURE 1.1:   Young man with FAS; note small palpebral fissures, flat philtrum, thin upper lip, and broad nasal bridge.

mia and/or short palpebral fissures, and poorly developed philtrum, thin upper lip, and flattening of the maxillary area.

3. Central nervous system involvement (signs of neurological abnormality, developmental delay, or intellectual impairment).

The 1980 report of the Fetal Alcohol Study Group utilized the term *possible fetal alcohol effects* to describe individuals who had some but not all of the criteria for FAS and a documented significant prenatal alcohol exposure. This term has been helpful in understanding and describing the gradations of involvement from alcohol exposure in utero. However, as Aase et al. (1995) point out, the term has perhaps been overused. Individuals who present with just behavioral problems and only questionable exposure to alcohol have been labeled as FAE. This presumes that the prenatal alcohol exposure is the cause of the child's problems, which may not be the case. Aase et al. (1995) recommended elimination of the term FAE. Subsequently, the Institute of Medicine (IOM) stepped in with a detailed study and report on new terminology to be utilized in the clinical diagnosis of children prenatally affected by alcohol. This system preserves the best features of the old criteria but clarifies the FAE controversy (Stratton et al., 1996). They also understood that at times, such as in a foster care situation, it is impossible to document or confirm maternal alcohol exposure, particularly if the biological mother has passed away. Their categories are outlined in Table 1.1.

To clarify the muddy waters of FAE when there are no typical facial features, the IOM (Stratton et al., 1996) added a section of categories called Alcohol Related Effects. This includes Alcohol Related Birth Defects (ARBD) and Alcohol Related Neurodevelopmental Disorder (ARND), because the clinical and animal

TABLE 1.1:   Diagnostic Categories from the Institute of Medicine Report

1. FAS with Confirmed Maternal Alcohol Exposure
   A. Confirmed maternal alcohol exposure
   B. Evidence of a characteristic pattern of facial anomalies that include:
      short palpebral fissures
      abnormalities in the premaxillary zone e.g. flat upper lip, flattened philtrum, and flat
         midface
   C. Evidence of growth retardation, as in at least one of the following:
      low birth weight for gestational age
      decelerating weight over time not due to nutrition
      disproportional low weight to height
   D. Evidence of CNS neurodevelopment abnormalities, as in at least one of the following:
      decreased cranial size at birth
      structural brain abnormalities e.g. microcephaly, partial or complete agenesis of the corpus
         collosom, cerebellar hypoplasia
      neurological hard or soft signs (as age appropriate), such as:
         impaired fine motor skills
         neurosensory hearing loss
         poor tandem gait
         poor eye-hand coordination
2. FAS without Confirmed Maternal Alcohol Exposure
   B, C, and D as above
3. Partial FAS with Confirmed Maternal Alcohol Exposure
   A. Confirmed maternal alcohol exposure
   B. Evidence of some components of the pattern of characteristic facial anomalies as described
      above and either C, D, or E.
   C. as above
   D. as above
   E. Evidence of a complex pattern of behavior or cognitive abnormalities that are inconsistent
      with development level and cannot be explained by familial background or environment
      alone, such as:
      learning difficulties
      deficits in school performance
      poor impulse control
      problems in social perception
      deficits in higher-level receptive and expressive language
      poor capacity for abstraction or metacognition
      specific deficits in mathematical skills
      problems in memory, attention, or judgment

(*continued*)

4. Alcohol-Related Birth Defects (ARBD)

The presence of these congenital anomalies, including malformations and dysplasias:

A. Cardiac

atrial septal defects

ventricular septal defects

aberrant great vessels

Tetralogy of Fallot

B. Skeletal

hypoplastic nails

shortened fifth digits

radioulnar synostosis

flexion contractures

camptodactaly

clinodactaly

pectus excavatum and carinatum

Klippel-Feil syndrome

hemivertebrae

scoliosis

C. Renal

aplastic

dysplastic

hypoplastic kidneys

horseshoe kidneys

ureteral duplications

hydronephrosis

D. Ocular

strabismus

retinal vascular anomalies

refractive problems secondary to small globes

E. Auditory

conductive hearing loss

neurosensory hearing loss

5. Alcohol-Related Neurodevelopmental Disorder (ARND)

Presence of:

A. Evidence of CNS neurodevelopmental abnormalities, as in any one of the following:

decreased cranial size at birth

structural brain abnormalities

microcephaly

partial or complete agenesis of the corpus callosum

cerebellar hypoplasia

neurological hard and soft signs (as age appropriate), such as:

impaired fine motor skills

neurosensory hearing loss

poor tandem gait

poor eye-hand coordination

and/or:

B. Evidence of a complex pattern of behavior or cognitive abnormalities that are inconsistent with development level and cannot be explained by familial background or environment alone, such as:

learning difficulties

deficits in school performance

poor impulse control

problems in social perception

deficits in higher-level receptive and expressive language

poor capacity for abstraction or metacognition

specific deficits in mathematical skills

problems in memory, attention, or judgment

Reprinted with permission from Stratton, Kathleen; Howe, Cynthia; Battaglia, Frederick (1996), Fetal alcohol syndrome: Diagnosis, epidemiology, prevention, and treatment. Institute of Medicine, National Academy Press, Washington, D.C.

literature has linked maternal alcohol ingestion to neurodevelopmental problems and birth defects, even when the growth retardation and the typical facial features are not present (Mattson et al., 1997). These additional conditions can co-occur, but there must be a history of maternal alcohol exposure (see Table 1.1). ARND is defined relatively broadly, and no doubt future research will try to separate learning, behavioral, and motor coordination problems that are genetic or related to other factors from the effects of alcohol exposure in utero. At the present time the combined incidence rate of FAS and ARND is 9.1 per 1,000, which is nearly 1 per 100 live births (Sampson et al., 1997).

PHYSICAL FEATURES

Not all offspring of alcoholic mothers will have the full manifestations of FAS. Streissguth (1997) estimates from existing data that 25 to 45% of women with chronic alcoholism will give birth to children with FAS if they continue to drink during their pregnancies. In Sweden, Aronson and Olegard (1987) evaluated 99 children of alcoholic mothers; 15% had a low birth weight, 10% had malformations, 50% had cognitive deficits, and 49% were neuropsychologically atypical, usually with attention and concentration problems. Both Aronson's group and Streissguth et al. (1978) found a significant association between the number and severity of physical malformations and the degree of cognitive impairment. The stage of the mother's alcoholism is also an important consideration. Although women of all ages are at risk to have children with FAS, older alcoholic mothers will have more severely affected children. A spectrum of FAS involvement can be seen in siblings, with the most severely affected born last (Spohr, 1996).

Alcoholism takes a greater physical toll on women than on men. Women are more susceptible to alcoholic liver disease, heart muscle damage, and brain damage with excessive alcohol use than are men (Frezza et al., 1990). This difference is related to the fact that women, compared with men, have lower activity of the enzyme alcohol dehydrogenase, which metabolizes alcohol in the stomach so that more alcohol reaches the blood. Long-term follow-up 15 years after the diagnosis of FAS was made has shown that 69% of the biological mothers have died (Streissguth et al., 1991).

There is a wide degree of involvement in FAS, in addition to partial fetal alcohol syndrome (PFAS) and ARND. This means that giving tables of percentages of involvement for each manifestation is difficult. In the most severely involved patients, such as the 11 patients originally described in 1973 (Jones et al., 1973; Jones and Smith, 1973), microcephaly occurred in 80%. In the literature from throughout the world that was reviewed by Clarren and Smith (1978), 85% of the 126 patients with FAS who had IQ testing were mentally retarded. In follow-up of the patients originally described by Lemoine in France, 5 of 50 with severe FAS died in childhood from cardiac or respiratory problems (Lemoine and Lemoine, 1992). In 28 patients with mild FAS, two had died from suicide, and five others had attempted suicide. They also found many patients institutionalized and concluded that mental health problems constituted the most severe manifestations of FAS (Lemoine and Lemoine, 1992).

The facial features in the diagnostic criteria for FAS through all of the revisions remain very specific and include features that are reflective of hypoplasia, or a lack of appropriate growth in the facial structures. At the present time there is no single metabolic marker that is diagnostic for alcohol exposure in utero although the presence of multiple positive markers in the mother, including carbohydrate-deficient transferin, γ-glutamyltranspeptidase, and whole blood–associated acetaldehyde, are reflective of significant alcohol use and are predictive of dysmorphic features in the newborn (Stoler et al., 1998). The facial dysmorphology represents the physical evidence of alcohol's teratogenic effect in an individual. The specificity and reliability of the facial dysmorphology has been carefully studied by Astley and Clarren (1995). In a discriminate function analysis, they found that among multiple facial characteristics, the features of a smooth philtrum, thin upper lip, and short palpebral features best differentiated children with FAS from controls. In 194 patients, the sensitivity of these features in identifying children with FAS (true positives) was 100%, whereas the specificity (identification of true negatives) was 89% (Astley and Clarren, 1995). They recommend using these features as a screening tool in the identification of children with FAS. For the clinicians and health care professionals without experience in diagnosing FAS and related conditions, these authors have published a manual (Astley and Clarren, 1997) which reviews diagnostic features and provides a medical history form, an examination form, and a visual Likert scale for degrees of upper-lip thinness and philtrum elongation and smoothness. This manual also provides a complete descriptive diagnostic system with operational definitions of growth retardation, CNS dysfunction, and prenatal and postnatal comorbidities.

Follow-Up Studies

Case reports and follow-up studies have documented the changing physical phenotype of individuals with FAS. In childhood, the weight deficiency is usually more pronounced than the height deficiency, and mothers frequently complain that they cannot get their children to put on any weight no matter how much they eat. In adolescence and adulthood, the height deficiency usually becomes more pronounced. In a follow-up study by Streissguth and colleagues (1991) of 61 patients with FAS (70%) or FAE (30%), only 16% of the patients with FAS were in the normal range for height, whereas 25% were in the normal range for weight (Figure 1.2). The decrement in weight growth was 1.4 SD below the mean in FAS and 0.4 SD below the mean in FAE. The decrement in height growth was 2.1 SD below the mean in patients with FAS and 1.7 below the mean in patients with FAE. The timing of puberty in these patients was usually normal. The decrement in head growth was 1.86 SD below the mean, but 28% had normal head sizes. The facial phenotype of FAS changed with age because of continued growth in the height of the nasal bridge, the length of the nose, the chin, and the midfacial region, which corrected the hypoplasia, and improved soft tissue

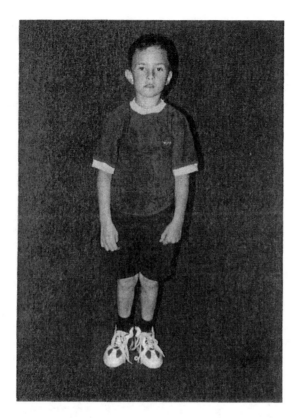

FIGURE 1.2:   Nine-year-old boy with FAS; he has a
height, weight, and head circumference that are far below the 5th percentile. Also note small palpebral fissures, flat philtrum, and thin upper lip.

modeling of the philtrum and upper lip (Streissguth et al., 1991). However, small
palpebral fissures often persisted, and the mean palpebral fissure length for the
patients with FAS was 2.3 cm compared with the mean of 3.1 cm for normal 16-
year-olds. The mean innercanthal distance was also wider than the mean palpebral
fissure length in patients with FAS in adolescence and adulthood. The majority
of patients also continued to demonstrate abnormalities of the philtrum (smooth,
long, or short), abnormal lips, and malformed or misaligned teeth. If the classical
phenotype is not present in adolescence or adulthood, a review of childhood
photos can be helpful in revealing typical features.

Spohr et al. (1993) carried out a 10-year longitudinal follow-up study of 60
patients diagnosed with FAS in infancy and childhood. At the time of original
diagnosis, 88% had microcephaly, and in follow-up 65% were still microcephalic.
Although most of the children with a normal head circumference had an IQ

greater than 70, the presence or persistence of microcephaly does not significantly predict mental retardation. The IQ was relatively stable over time without significant improvements. Eighty-four percent of their sample had low birth weights, and 71% had severe feeding problems in the first few months of life that often required hospitalization. Regarding the growth parameters, girls were consistently less affected than boys, most dramatically in weight but also in height and head circumference measurements.

Alcohol exposure in utero does not affect only the face and brain. Other malformations are also consistently seen, including finger joint abnormalities (clinodactaly, incurving of the 5th finger, or camptodactaly, flexion deformity of the finger) in 68%, palmar crease abnormalities in 56%, and incomplete rotation at the elbow in 24% (Streissguth et al., 1991). In the follow-up study of 60 children with FAS by Spohr and colleagues (Spohr and Steinhausen, 1987; Spohr et al., 1993), renal anomalies were seen in 5%, cleft palate in 7%, cardiac defects in 31% initially and 8% in follow-up, minor external genital anomalies in 27% initially and 18% in follow-up, and hernias in 20% initially and 3% in follow-up.

A remarkable finding in the Streissguth et al. (1991) follow-up study was the instability of the family environments. The patients had lived in five different principal homes on average, not counting temporary placements. One-third of the patients never spent any time with their biological mothers, and 69% of the biological mothers were dead at follow-up. These women died from direct effects of alcoholism, such as cirrhosis, and indirect effects, such as suicide and homicide.

In the largest follow-up study to date, Streissguth and colleagues (1996a) documented both the primary and secondary disabilities in over 400 individuals with FAS and FAE. The mean IQ on the Wechsler Intelligence Scales for the 178 patients with FAS was 79, with 27% of patients scoring at 70 or below, whereas the mean IQ for the 209 patients with FAE was 90, with only 9% scoring at 70 or below. In both populations, the Performance IQ (PIQ) was usually greater than the Verbal IQ (VIQ), with a 5-point discrepancy on average. The highest subtest scores on the Wechsler scales were those for Object Assembly and Picture Completion, which is reflective of strengths in nonverbal skills. The lowest-scoring subtests were Arithmetic, Digit Span, and Information. This is reflective of attentional problems, distractibility, and difficulties with working memory, which interferes with taking in and remembering information about the world. Achievement testing with the Wide Range Achievement Test (WRAT) and Adaptive Behavior scores from the Vineland Adaptive Behavior Scales (VABS) revealed even more striking deficits than the IQ testing did. Both groups demonstrated lower scores in reading and spelling than the IQ predicted, but math scored almost a full standard deviation below what was expected from the IQ. Grade equivalent means ranged from the second to the fourth grade in most academic areas. Even lower were scores from the VABS, with Communication and Socialization subtests as the lowest and the overall Adaptive Behavior Composite typically in the 60s for IQ scores in the 80s. Although the individuals with FAE had, on average, an IQ that was 11 points higher than the individuals with FAS, the discrepancy between IQ and Achievement or IQ and Adaptive Behavior scores was more severe for the individuals with FAE than for those with FAS (Streissguth et al., 1996a). The same is true for the secondary disabilities described later in this chapter.

This study was the first natural history follow-up of cases with FAS and FAE. It is important to remember that a comparison group with developmental disabilities was not used, nor was the group with FAE well defined, but the dramatic results point out the need for further research in this area.

CNS Malformations

At the time of this writing, there are 25 cases of autopsies reported in the medical literature (reviewed by Mattson and Riley, 1996); the first was in one of the original reports of FAS, with diffuse brain damage seen, in addition to severe microcephaly and heterotopias (pockets of arrested migration of groups of cells; Jones and Smith, 1973). The autopsy cases usually represent the severest form of FAS because the patients have died from the physical problems caused by alcohol. The brain abnormalities described in these cases are legion, including anencephaly, holoprosencephaly, microcephaly, enlarged ventricles, agenesis of the corpus callosum (the bundle of fibers that connects the right and left sides of the brain), cerebellar anomalies, cerebral dysgenesis from abnormal neural and glial migration, and neural tube defects (Mattson et al., 1996c).

Brain imaging techniques, on the other hand, allow one to see less severe CNS abnormalities in patients who are still living and suffering from less severe forms of FAS. Brain imaging research has been quite productive in showing more consistent trends in CNS abnormalities related to prenatal alcohol exposure. First of all, microencephaly (small brain) is consistently seen, but certain areas of the brain are more sensitive to alcohol's impact. When the overall brain size is controlled for, the basal ganglia, specifically the caudate, is significantly reduced in size in patients with FAS compared to controls and compared to patients with Down syndrome who had comparable levels of mental retardation and microcephaly (Mattson and Riley, 1995; Mattson et al., 1996c). The caudate is important for memory and cognition, especially executive function abilities including attention and working memory. The cerebellum is also smaller in patients with FAS, particularly the anterior cerebellar vermis (vermal lobules I through V) compared to controls (Sowell et al., 1996). This is consistent with animal data which shows regionally specific Purkinje cell death in the cerebellum with prenatal alcohol exposure (Goodlett and West, 1992). The corpus callosum is also especially sensitive to alcohol's effect (Figure 1.3). In a study of patients with FAS but without agenesis of the corpus callosum there was a significant decrease in the size of this structure compared to controls (Riley et al., 1995). The anterior region was most severely affected. This region carries the fibers that connect the right and left frontal lobes and appears to be the most important region of the corpus for sustaining attention and alertness (Rueckert and Levy,

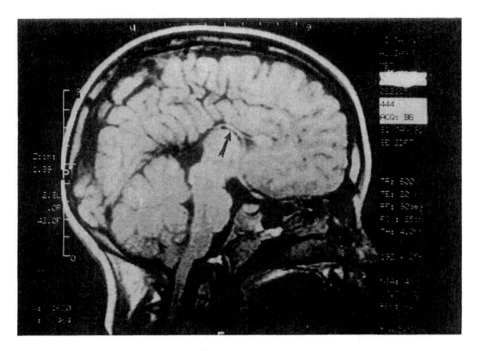

FIGURE 1.3:   MRI study of the patient depicted in Figure 1.1. Note almost complete agenesis of the corpus callosum where the arrow is pointing.

1996). A smaller corpus callosum has also been seen in individuals with ADHD but without prenatal alcohol exposure in utero (Giedd et al., 1994).

Swayze et al. (1997) found midline anomalies in MRI studies (usually hypoplasia or partial to complete agenesis of the corpus callosum) in 6 of 10 patients with FAS and also found that these abnormalities correlated with the number of facial dysmorphological features. The authors postulate that alcohol disrupts the glial migration, which subsequently guides the commissural fibers that make up the corpus. In addition, alcohol can cause excessive or premature cell death which can lead to many of the abnormalities that were described here. Mattson and colleagues (1996c) propose that the callosal agenesis is related to the holoprosencephalic malformation complex spectrum, which is also seen in animal studies of prenatal exposure. The most severe form of this spectrum is holoprosencephaly, in which the prosencephalon or the anterior part of the brain fails to cleave and there is a single anterior ventricle.

Brain imaging studies may turn out to be more sensitive in detecting the teratogenic effects of alcohol than the classical dysmorphic features. MRI studies have shown abnormalities, particularly reductions in the volume of the basal ganglia, in patients with a history of alcohol exposure in utero but without facial diagnostic features of FAS (Mattson et al., 1996c). New PET scanning studies found abnormalities of metabolism in patients prenatally exposed to alcohol when the CNS structure on MRI was normal (reviewed by Mattson et al., 1996c). These abnormalities included hypometabolism of the caudate and cerebellum. Much more research remains to be done using neuroimaging of brain structure and function. It is important to remember that alcohol causes diffuse brain damage, although the evidence supports the concept that some regions of the brain are more sensitive or vulnerable to alcohol's impact.

The earliest reports of FAS have described an association with seizures (Jones et al., 1973; Clarren and Smith, 1978), but this association has not been well studied. A recent report by O'Malley and Barr (1998) evaluated sleep-deprived EEGs in 33 patients with alcohol spectrum disorders. Twenty-one percent were abnormal with temporal lobe dysrhythmia, and all patients with this finding had a complex partial seizure disorder with varying degrees of impaired consciousness, brief explosive moods, and visual or auditory hallucinations. Complex partial seizures are probably underdiagnosed at the present time in this population, and a more aggressive medical workup including an EEG is warrented in patients who present with the above symptoms.

There are likely many mechanisms of alcohol's damaging effect. One recently reported by Ramanathan et al. (1996) is alcohol's inhibition of the activity of L1, an immunoglobulin cell adhesion molecule that is essential for normal human brain development because it promotes cell-cell adhesion, neurite outgrowth, cell migration axon targeting, and synaptic plasticity. Mutation in the L1 gene located at Xq28 causes mental retardation, hydrocephalus, agenesis of the corpus callosum, and cerebellar dysplasia, all of which are reminiscent of the CNS abnormalities seen in some patients with FAS. These authors found that the inhibition of the activity of L1 in mouse fibroblasts transfected with human L1 was very sensitive even to low levels of alcohol (Ramanathan et al., 1996). Although the alcohol effect on L1 prenatally is only transient, during prolonged exposure with heavy drinking, the changes in brain structure can be significant and similar to the genetic condition in which loss of L1 is permanent. The L1 effect may also lead to some of the cognitive defects in adult alcoholics because of disruption of neural plasticity in the adult brain (Ramanathan et al., 1996).

Hearing Deficits

Hearing problems are common in children with FAS and can arise from damage to the eighth nerve or the hearing structures in the middle and inner ear, from chronic fluid in the middle ear that causes a conductive hearing loss, and from damage to the brain that causes central deficits (Church et al., 1996). All of these problems have been reported in children and adults with FAS. Church and Gerkin (1988) were the first to systematically assess for sensory-neural hearing deficits and found that 4 of 14 children with FAS, or 29%, had such a loss. A subsequent study of hearing and vestibular problems in 22 patients with FAS found that 27% had a sensory neural hearing loss (Church et al., 1997). All of these patients had a bilateral and symmetrical mild loss ranging from 15 to 30 db with a variable pattern across frequencies. In addition, 52% had cleft palates, 18% had a cleft lip, and 77% had a conductive hearing loss secondary to recurrent serous otitis media which continued into adolescence and adulthood. Recurrent serous otitis media (SOM) occurred in those with and without a cleft palate in similar frequencies.

All of the patients studied by Church et al. (1997) also had central auditory processing abnormalities which relate to the brain damage in brainstem and cortical areas that process auditory information. Although 50% of these patients were identified as requiring special education support because of cognitive deficits, 82% had receptive language deficits and 76% had expressive language deficits scoring more than 1 SD below the mean for their chronological age. Speech disorders were seen in 90% and included dysfluencies, hypernasality, word formulation problems, and low intelligibility. In addition, dental malocclusions such as misaligned or missing teeth, protrusion of the upper jaw, and protrusion of the lower jaw occurred in all of the patients who were evaluated. These types of problems often require orthodontia and, on occasion, surgery. The hypoplasia of either the maxilla or mandible may improve with age, according to Streissguth et al. (1991). There is a tendency for younger children to have a smaller mandible and for adolescents to have relative prognanthism or prominence of the mandible (Clarren and Smith, 1978; Streissguth et al., 1991).

A final interesting finding from the Church et al. (1997) study is that no significant vestibular abnormalities were seen in the six patients who underwent detailed testing, including a rotary chair and electronystagmography. The authors therefore postulate that the vestibular system is relatively spared and that balance problems which occur in some patients are more likely due to cerebellar deficits. This hypothesis is supported by recent research that demonstrates deficits in postural balance in children with FAS when somatosensory input is manipulated (Roebuck et al., 1998). Postural reactions to the balance difficulties were measured with electromyographic (EMG) studies of the leg muscles, and increased long latency responses were seen in patients with FAS compared to controls (Roebuck et al., 1998). This finding reflects central abnormalities, most likely associated with the cerebellar findings in FAS.

Although the Church et al. (Church and Gerkin, 1988; Church et al., 1997) studies may have utilized a biased patient sample for ENT problems, animal studies have found a similar incidence of sensory neural hearing loss with prenatal alcohol exposure (Church et al., 1996).

Opthalmological Deficits

A wide range of ocular problems occur in individuals with FAS. An epidemiological study of 30 children with FAS demonstrated opthalmological problems in 90%, with visual impairment in 50% and severe problems (less than 20/100 vision) in 12% (Stromland, 1985). Controlled studies in children have shown that the ocular pathology is not simply due to growth retardation or malnutrition in utero but instead is a teratogenic effect of alcohol exposure (Stromland, 1987). Animal studies on fish and chick embryos as early as 1914 demonstrated the teratogenic effects of prenatal alcohol exposure on the eye (Stockard, 1914).

The most common eye abnormality in 25 children with FAS who were followed long term (4 to 19 years in follow-up) was optic nerve hypoplasia (Stromland and Hellstrom, 1996). This was seen in 76% of patients and is caused by a reduced number of axons in the optic nerve. On examination, the optic disc was small with sharp or irregular margins, and a double ring usually surrounded the disc. Strabismus was seen in 52% (Figure 1.4), usually esotropia, and severe tortuosity of the retinal arteries with hairpin-like bends occurred in 36%. Ptosis has also been reported in 20% of patients with FAS. More extensive malformations of the eye were seen in 16% and included one case of severe bilateral microphthalmos and microcornea and another case of severe malformation of both retinas and optic nerves, buphthalmos (ox eye) on one side, and microophthalmia and cataract of the other eye with blindness. On follow-up, those with severe visual impairment did not improve, and the severe eye problems were usually associated

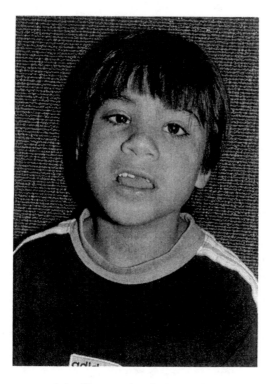

FIGURE 1.4:   Young girl with FAS and strabismus, specifically a right esotropia. Also note flat philtrum and small palpebral fissures.

with mental retardation. Approximately half of those with milder visual impairment (better than 20/70 vision) improved their vision in follow-up, although some of this improvement in acuity may be secondary to better cooperation with the examination as the patient aged (Stromland and Hellstrom, 1996). The opthalmological findings in FAS are varied and are not pathognomonic, but their presence strengthens the diagnosis of FAS. An ophthalmological examination is essential to facilitate treatment of strabismus, refraction errors, or other treatable problems to improve vision and consequently learning.

Renal Abnormalities

Most of the previous papers describing genitourinary or renal abnormalities in children with FAS have been descriptive case reports (reviewed by Taylor et al., 1994). Larger studies have occasionally cited the incidence of renal abnormalities, such as the study by Spohr et al. (1993) which found that 5% of 60 children with FAS had renal anomalies. The largest study supporting the association of renal anomalies and FAS was carried out by Havers et al. (1980). They found genitourinary abnormalities in 12% of 110 patients with FAS, including two patients with malformations of the bladder and one patient with a fistula between the bladder and the vagina. Most of these patients had abnormalities of the external genitalia or were symptomatic.

Taylor et al. (1994) carried out a renal ultrasound screen of 84 patients with prenatal alcohol exposure, including 51 patients with FAS, to determine the frequency of renal abnormalities and the need for routine studies in patients with FAS. They found only three patients (3.6%) who had significant renal abnormalities. One patient had unilateral hydronephrosis secondary to ureteropelvic junction obstruction, one patient had posterior urethral valves with a nonfunctioning right kidney and a left-sided ureteropelvic junction obstruction, and a third patient had hydronephrosis. Although two of these patients required surgery in the newborn period, the detection of renal abnormalities in this screening was not significantly different from the results of newborn screening in general populations (Taylor et al., 1994). However, a higher incidence of small kidneys or some degree of renal hypoplasia was detected in the study patients overall compared to normals and to height–age controls. Small kidneys may have long-term negative consequences, but there were no clinical problems detected in the patients without renal anomalies in this study. Because of the low yield on renal ultrasound screening and because of the lack of clinical findings caused by small kidneys, the authors do not recommend routine ultrasound studies in children with FAS unless they are symptomatic or have visible abnormalities of the genitalia (Taylor et al., 1994).

Moore et al. (1997) demonstrated similar findings in studying 158 infants with renal anomalies compared to two control groups without renal anomalies. Self-reported alcohol consumption to a moderate degree was associated with renal anomalies with an odds ratio of 1.5. Only renal agenesis and hypoplasia were found to be significant, and there were no associations with light alcohol consumption.

BEHAVIORAL AND COGNITIVE FEATURES

Newborns

A newborn withdrawal syndrome caused by the body's physiological withdrawal from alcohol may happen after birth in a baby exposed to chronic alcohol use prior to delivery. The signs are associated with CNS irritability and an enhanced sympathetic release, causing autonomic dysfunction. Hyperarousal, including tremulousness, irritability, feeding difficulties, sleeping problems, tone changes, and even seizures, can occur. Such withdrawal also occurs with other CNS depressants such as barbiturates, benzodiazepines, and heroin. Robe et al. (1981) found that infants with fetal alcohol syndrome were more likely to have problems with seizures, weight loss, and apnea, whereas those infants withdrawing from narcotic exposure were more likely to have gastrointestinal problems and irritability. Broader exposure (i.e., to alcohol, narcotics, cigarettes, marijuana, and cocaine) can lead to more symptoms of newborn withdrawal and more abnormalities on a newborn neurobehavioral assessment than with single agents alone (Coles, 1996; Jacobson et al., 1984). Mothers who stop using alcohol by midpregnancy do not have children who experience neonatal withdrawal (Coles, 1996); therefore, brain damage during the first or second trimesters does not cause the withdrawal syndrome.

Mild or moderate exposure to alcohol has shown more variable results. Walpole et al. (1991) found only subtle effects on motor tone related to mild–moderate alcohol exposure and predicted that this was unlikely to be related to developmental sequelae. However, Streissguth and colleagues (1983) studied more than 400 infants in a prospective study to understand the sequelae of mild to moderate levels of alcohol consumption in middle-class women in Seattle. They found that both habituation abnormalities and low arousal on an infant neurobehavioral scale were related to the level of alcohol use during pregnancy. In their subsequent follow-up work described later in this chapter, problems with learning and attention, in addition to slower reaction time, were associated with the level of alcohol use. Other studies (reviewed by Coles, 1996) have confirmed the findings of Streissguth for newborns and have found problems of decreased arousal with low to moderate alcohol exposure and features of hyperarousal in habituation, startle response, crying, and sleep with heavy alcohol exposure.

Jacobson et al. (1994) carried out important physiological studies measuring reaction time to visual stimuli in 6-month-old infants who had been prenatally exposed to alcohol in the inner city of Detroit. This study controlled well for the mother's emotional status and language ability and quality of the home environment. They found that a slower reaction time and longer visual fixation was strongly associated with prenatal alcohol exposure. The alcohol effect on reaction time was seen even with low alcohol exposure levels of 0.5 ounces of alcohol per day, which represents one drink per day. The slowing down of the reaction time is a reflection of slower central auditory processing, which was seen in the Church study and in the follow-up studies by Streissguth and colleagues.

It may also affect attention and concentration abilities, as described in the next section. A recent study has also shown that alcohol-affected individuals dramatically lose accuracy when they try to do a task too quickly (Sampson et al., 1997).

Hyperactivity and Attention Problems

Although hyperactivity and attentional problems were not mentioned in the original case reports describing FAS, subsequent studies have emphasized these problems. Streissguth et al. (1978, 1980) commented originally on these difficulties, and follow-up studies have found these problems to be persistent and perhaps integral to other long-term psychopathology such as conduct disorder. Steinhausen and colleagues (1993) in Germany found hyperactivity to be the most frequent and persistent form of psychopathology in their follow-up studies of 158 children with FAS. Habbick and colleagues (1996) found similar results in Canada.

Two studies have compared the performance of children with FAS or FAE and children with ADHD without alcohol exposure in utero. The first was carried out by Nanson and Hiscock (1990) with 20 patients in each group, in addition to 20 normal controls. Because IQ was not matched in the study groups, the FAS group was significantly more impaired on intellectual measures compared to the normals and the ADHD group. However, the FAS and ADHD groups were similar in their scores on behavioral measures of ADHD according to parental ratings and in laboratory tests of investment, maintenance, and organization of attention over time, in addition to inhibition of impulsive responses. The children with FAS/FAE performed more slowly in reaction time, and their accuracy degraded faster on multiple trials compared to the other groups, although positive reinforcement enhanced their performance. Although the cognitive deficits were significantly different in children with FAS and ADHD, their attentional problems were similar, and the authors therefore suggested that treatment strategies for patients with ADHD would be helpful for patients with FAS/FAE.

The second study comparing these two populations was carried out by Coles et al. (1997). The 25 children with FAS/FAE were compared to three additional groups with comparable intellectual abilities and socioeconomic status, including controls, patients with ADHD, and patients with alcohol exposure who were not dysmorphic. Although similarities between the ADHD group and the FAS/FAE group included the facts that approximately 50% in each group could not complete the computerized attentional measures and that both groups scored similarly in the attention aspect of behavioral checklists, interesting differences also emerged. The children with ADHD had more problems with focusing and sustaining attention, whereas the children with FAS/FAE had more problems shifting attention (on the Wisconsin Card Sorting Test) and in encoding information. This suggests that children with FAS may not utilize the information they are able to attend to or use new information meaningfully in problem solving (Coles et al., 1997). Therefore, the intervention for children with FAS must not only focus on the attentional components of their disorder but must also include strategies to help with the encoding and problem-solving difficulties.

Longitudinal studies of mild to moderately exposed children have provided helpful information for understanding the attentional components of even limited alcohol exposure. The longitudinal project initiated by Streissguth and her colleagues in Seattle in the 1970s targeted the study of attentional difficulties, among other issues. Their studies in the newborn period showed decreased activity, not hyperactivity, in those exposed to significant alcohol, although arousal problems and habituation difficulties correlated with increased levels of alcohol exposure. The infants were unable to inhibit responding to repetitive stimuli to allow for normal habituation (Carmichael Olson et al., 1994; Streissguth et al., 1983). The same children followed up at 4 years demonstrated deficits on the performance IQ, particularly on the subtests that required sustained attention (Streissguth et al., 1989). On a computerized vigilance task, they had difficulty with attention and inhibiting impulsive responding, which correlated with greater levels of alcohol exposure. Longer reaction times and deficits in motor coordination also correlated with alcohol exposure. The association between attentional deficits and level of alcohol exposure became more pronounced in the 7-year-old follow-up data (Streissguth et al., 1990). Difficulties with distractibility, impulsivity, processing, and organizational skills were documented in the teacher and parent questionnaires and were also seen by the researchers in the clinic. Performance on a computerized vigilance task demonstrated problems with attention and inhibiting impulsive responding. In addition, the Wechsler (WISC-R) IQ subtests which are most sensitive to attentional difficulties, the Arithmetic and Digit Span subtests, correlated best with alcohol exposure. By 11 years of age, the data also showed that alcohol exposure was associated with teacher ratings of distractibility, including restlessness, lack of persistence, and reluctance to meet new challenges (Carmichael Olson et al., 1994; Streissguth et al., 1994). Attentional problems and other behavioral deficits consistent with ADHD persist even at the 14-year follow-up. Alcohol-related deficits were seen in problems with response inhibition on a continuous performance task and in reaction-time measures. Difficulties with response inhibition and with complex problem solving, fluctuating attention, and learning from short-term recall of complex information were all associated with alcohol exposure in utero (Streissguth, 1994). In addition, associations were seen between alcohol exposure in utero and a cluster of problem behaviors, including antisocial behavior, learning problems, and substance abuse as rated by parents, examiners, and the patient (Carmichael Olson et al., 1997).

These longitudinal studies have shown that the most enduring problems associated with prenatal alcohol exposure are neurobehavioral in nature and that they were present from day 1 through the 14-year assessment so far. The main neurobehavioral problems involve attention problems, distractibility, and a slow and/or variable reaction time, which affects complex problem solving. By 7 years of age, the Verbal, Performance, and Full-Scale IQs on the Wechsler Intelligence Scale for Children-Revised (WISC-R) are lowered due to alcohol exposure, and this situation continues into adolescence. A multiple regression analysis demonstrated an average 7-point drop in IQ associated with an average of 1 ounce or more of alcohol per day (Streissguth et al., 1990). In addition, the 14-year, as well as earlier, data show that the prenatal drinking pattern associated with the highest risk to offspring is that in which drinks are clustered (binge drinking) (Streissguth, 1994). These data are supported by work with animals described later in this chapter. Negative effects are also seen in academic performance, specifically in word attack and arithmetic testing. The magnitude of the negative effects is in the range of 1/3 of a standard deviation for each outcome at an average exposure level of 1.5 drinks per occasion (Streissguth, 1994, 1997; Streissguth et al., 1994). It is important to remember that this longitudinal study did not primarily involve heavy drinkers. Instead, this cohort of women included the full range of maternal drinking, in addition to abstainers, and more than 400 children were followed longitudinally with over an 80% follow-up rate. Only two children were found to be diagnosed with FAS at the time of birth. At the 4-year follow-up they were no longer growth deficient, and they were diagnosed as having FAE. For the cohort of patients, there was a significant association between growth parameters, including height, weight, and head circumference and prenatal alcohol exposure at birth. However, after 18 months this association disappears, and there is no relationship between alcohol exposure and growth parameters through the 14-year analysis (Streissguth et al., 1994). Therefore, in mild to moderate exposure conditions, the growth effects of alcohol are not nearly as important as the neurobehavioral and cognitive effects (Streissguth, 1997). Clearly the brain is more vulnerable than the body to alcohol's effects; this finding is supported by the animal research.

The behavioral profile of FAS is associated with significant impulsivity and excessive friendliness at times. As described by one mother:

> No one is a stranger. He will talk to anybody when he is having a problem. He likes male attention, and he will crawl into the lap of a stranger and kiss them and say "I want to live with you." He gets very restless, and he feels he has to move from one activity to another. He is easily overwhelmed by sounds. He is constantly moving and touching things.

Additional Neurocognitive Strengths and Weaknesses

Although the ADHD symptoms combined with response inhibition problems may be the most salient neurocognitive deficits associated with FAS, other learning problems have also been studied. Mattson et al. (1996b) studied verbal learning and memory and found that patients with FAS failed to benefit from repeated verbal exposure to material after the second trial compared to controls. Patients with FAS also demonstrated problems on immediate and long-term recall, with an excessive number of false positive responses; however, their retention for what they learned was as good as that of controls. These data suggest problems in encoding information, in addition to an impairment in response inhibition capabilities. The educational implications include the need to present information in a multimodality format, that is, utilizing both auditory and visual modalities. Once information is learned it appears to be retained fairly well (Mattson et al., 1996b). This also appears to be true for nonverbal information.

In a study of visual spatial processing, Mattson et al. (1996c) utilized the Global Local Test (Bihrle et al., 1989), which includes the use of large letters that are drawn by using small symbols. Previous work has shown that individuals with Down syndrome or left-hemisphere lesions are able to identify the overall outline of the figure but do not identify the small symbols, whereas individuals with Williams syndrome or right-hemisphere deficits are unable to identify the large letters but do well in identifying the small symbols (Bihrle et al., 1989; Wang and Bellugi, 1993). In individuals with FAS, there were significant differences in processing the local, small symbols compared to controls (Mattson et al., 1996a). There was also a tendency to perseverate when drawing the local figures, which likely relates to executive function deficits that are mediated by the frontal–basal ganglia circuits. Patients with FAS would focus on the global figure but be unable to shift focus to the local symbols. The inability to accurately distinguish the local features could have an impact on reading ability. These findings suggest that educational efforts should encourage systematic processing of visual information so that the details in a visual presentation are not neglected. Additional studies by Uecker and Nadel (1996) have shown normal immediate memory for spatial memory but deficits in delayed recall in patients with FAS. Object memory was also much better than spatial memory in patients with FAS. Perhaps the use of concrete objects in the educational process, such as teaching letter recognition by using letters elaborated as objects or people, will utilize this strength in learning and memory.

Among other higher-level cognitive problems, cause and effect issues have been described by clinicians and parents as one area of difficulty for many individuals with FAS. As described by a mother:

> He threw sand in a child's eyes, but when asked if he did it, he said "no" and blamed it on someone else. I had to visually demonstrate to him how sand thrown could end up in someone else's eyes. He just didn't understand the process.

Such problems can lead to significant social difficulties and to the secondary disabilities described in the next section.

SECONDARY DISABILITIES

In 1996, Streissguth and her colleagues published a report describing secondary disabilities in a cohort of 415 individuals in Seattle (between the ages of 6 and 51 years, with a median of 14.2 years) with FAS or FAE who have been followed (Streissguth et al., 1996a). Primary disabilities include physical malformations and direct brain damage, leading to neuropsychological and neurobehavioral deficits caused by prenatal alcohol exposure. Secondary disabilities are those that a person is not born with and that presumably could be ameliorated, either partially or completely, with appropriate interventions (Streissguth et al., 1996a). These authors also assessed protective and risk factors, both environmental issues and intrinsic neurobehavioral or biological characteristics, that relate to secondary disabilities. Their results revealed very high rates of secondary disabilities for individuals with FAS or FAE. Mental health problems characterize 94% of the study group. These included attention deficit problems in 61% of children and adolescents, depression in 42% of adolescents and 52% of adults, suicide attempts in 23% of adults, panic attacks in 24% of adolescents and 34% of adults, and psychotic symptoms in 29% of adults. Other secondary disabilities from childhood into adulthood included inappropriate sexual behavior in 45%, disrupted school experience (expulsion, dropping out, or suspension) in 43%, and trouble with the law in 42%. Violence against these individuals with FAS or FAE, including physical or sexual abuse or domestic violence, was reported in 72% of the sample. Being a victim of violence increased the chance of manifesting inappropriate sexual behavior, including incest, promiscuity, and inappropriate sexual touching, fourfold. Incarceration for a crime occurred in 32% of adolescents and 42% of adults. Alcohol problems occurred in 42% of adults, and 20% were confined in jail or in the hospital for alcohol or drug problems.

A much larger percentage of patients with FAE (70% of adult females and 53% of adult males with FAE) had alcohol and drug problems than did patients with FAS (38% of adult females and 31% of adult males with FAS) (Streissguth et al., 1996a). Similarly, a greater percentage of problems in adolescents and adults with FAE (compared to those with FAS) was demonstrated in confinement rates, inappropriate sexual behavior, and school disruptions. The three intrinsic factors associated with a higher level of secondary disability were (1) having FAE rather than FAS, (2) having a higher rather than a lower score on the Fetal Alcohol Behavior Scale (FABS, Streissguth et al., 1998), and (3) having an IQ above rather than below 70. The authors recommended focusing treatment efforts particularly on clients with these risky characteristics to avoid secondary disabilities. Receiving disability services through social security (SSI) is a strong protective factor for secondary disabilities. However, in our present society it is hard to obtain services if one does not have mental retardation or other obvious disability; and yet the children with FAE who are not retarded and who may not have obvious dysmorphic features are the ones who need intervention the most.

In a study of 25 adults with FAS or FAE who had IQs of 70 or higher, a detailed psychiatric interview was carried out to obtain DSM-IV diagnoses. The results demonstrated a remarkably high rate of psychiatric problems, including 11 (44%) with major depressive disorder, 15 (60%) with alcohol or drug dependence, 10 (40%) with psychotic symptoms (specifically, seven with Brief Psychotic Disorder, one with Schizoaffective Disorder, one with Delusional Disorder, and one with Psychotic Disorder Not Otherwise Specified), 5 (20%) with Bipolar I Disorder, 5 (20%) with anxiety disorders, 4 (16%) with eating disorders, and 1 (4%) with Dysthymic Disorder (Famy et al., 1998).

For the 90 adults who were 21 years of age or older, a study of living circumstances and employment was carried out (Streissguth et al., 1996a). Eighty-three percent were living dependently, and most required help with managing their money and making decisions. In addition, 79% had problems with employment. Holding a job was more difficult than getting a job, and over 50% had problems with easy frustration, poor task comprehension, poor judgment, and social problems while on the job. Both the dependent-living and job difficulties could be helped by developmental disability services, but only 13% of the adults were classified as eligible for such services.

Within this study population of individuals with FAS or FAE, 30 women had given birth to a child, but 40% were drinking during pregnancy. Seventeen percent of the mothers had a child who was diagnosed with FAS or FAE, and 13% had children who were suspected of being fetal-alcohol-affected. Fifty-seven percent of mothers no longer had their children in their care. A top priority for intervention should be special advocacy services regarding child rearing, birth control, and alcohol abuse intervention for these high-risk women, or the cycle of alcohol affectedness will be repeated for another generation (Streissguth et al., 1996a).

For the 473 patients in this natural history study of FAS or FAE, the factors which were universally protective for all of the secondary disabilities evaluated are listed here in order of their strength (Streissguth et al., 1996a). These factors were derived from correlations, so causal implications can only be inferred.

1. Living in a stable nurturing home for over 72% of life.
2. Being diagnosed with FAS or FAE before the age of 6.
3. Never having experienced violence against oneself.
4. Staying in each living situation for an average of more than 2.8 years.
5. Experiencing a good quality home from ages 8 to 12.
6. Having applied for and been found eligible for developmental disabilities services.
7. Having a diagnosis of FAS rather than FAE.
8. Having basic needs met for at least 13% of life.

IMPLICATIONS

As a society we must do a better job regarding early diagnosis and treatment for this group of patients. Their combination of neuropsychological and neurobehavioral deficits puts them at higher risk for secondary disabilities than many of the patient groups described in this book who even have more severe cognitive deficits. The severity of the cognitive involvement is an important point because the data from Streissguth et al. (1996a) show that the nonretarded or more mildly involved patients have more secondary disabilities because they are not recognized for services and perhaps because they are more adventuresome or have more initiative for getting into trouble.

The results of this study have led to a set of recommendations regarding policy, education, and treatment for individuals affected by prenatal alcohol exposure. These recommendations include facilitating an earlier diagnosis of FAS and FAE by educating all professionals who come in contact with affected children. These include educators, mental health therapists, social workers, criminal justice workers, and health care providers. Information regarding prenatal exposures should always be collected during the intake process in the schools, through social services especially during foster or adoptive placements, and in all types of health care, including mental health care. A family support and advocacy program, perhaps modeled on the Seattle Birth to Three program (Grant et al., 1996), for both biological and foster or adoptive homes would encourage stable, long-lasting placements in nurturant homes and would monitor for potential violence or abuse. An advocacy program that works closely with child protective service agencies is essential to reduce exposure to violence or abuse. Recognition of the subgroups of individuals with prenatal exposure who are at highest risk for secondary disabilities is essential for intensification of treatment. These individuals include those with FAE and an IQ above 70, those who have a marked discrepancy between their IQ and their level of adaptive behavior, and those with a high score on the Fetal Alcohol Behavior Scale (Streissguth et al., 1998). It is essential to develop effective vocational training and job support programs, in addition to independent living programs and appropriate mental health support services that are focused on the problems of prenatally exposed individuals.

ANIMAL RESEARCH

Over two decades of animal research has led to significant insights regarding the level and timing of alcohol exposure that leads to the pattern of deficits that we recognize as FAS. The mice studies support the clinical evidence that first-trimester exposure leads to the typical facial dysmorphology features of FAS, although some mice strains are more sensitive to these effects than others (Maier et al., 1996). Sulik et al. (1981) demonstrated how the face of FAS could be produced in the mouse after just two heavy exposures of alcohol on day 7 of gestation. Other animal models, such as primates and beagles, developed facial anomalies after long-term alcohol exposure. In contrast, growth deficits and microencephaly (small brain for body size) are more likely to be caused by exposure in the third trimester (Maier et al., 1996). These animal findings are consistent with human data and support intervention programs during the first part of pregnancy which can prevent at least some of the features of FAS.

Some areas of the brain are more sensitive to the teratogenic effects of alcohol than others. In rats, certain hippocampal pyramidal neurons will die with alcohol exposure, whereas other hippocampal cells are unaffected (West, 1986). In addition, the Purkinje cells of the cerebellum are exquisitely sensitive to alcohol exposure during the third trimester. Exposure for just a few days during this time of differentiation causes significant cell loss and motor deficits in rats (Goodlett et al., 1997; Klintsova et al., 1997). This provides some explanation for the motor problems, including balance difficulties and motor coordination deficits, reported by Streissguth and colleagues in only mild to moderately exposed children. A recent report has demonstrated that rats who have suffered Purkinje cell loss in the cerebellum because of alcohol exposure are able to regain motor function comparable to controls after an intensive motor-skill training program (Klintsova et al., 1997). Therefore significant synaptic plasticity exists in alcohol-exposed rats to allow an increase in parallel fiber synapses in the remaining Purkinje cells after complex motor training. The effect of early motor training in children with FAS has never been studied.

The most common behavioral finding in animal studies of alcohol exposure in utero is an increase in activity level compared to controls. This has been reported in open fields, running wheels, and exploratory chambers (reviewed by Riley, 1990). Although this problem usually improves with age, it worsens when these rats are treated with methylphenidate or amphetamine for their hyperactivity (Hannigan and Pilati, 1991; Riley, 1990), unlike the response in humans with FAS (Snyder et al., 1997). This medication exacerbation occurs in male rats but not in female rats. Females are somehow buffered from this hyperactivity effect, a result which is reminiscent of the human story in that hyperactivity is less common in girls than in boys. Although stimulant medication may decrease appetite in children and cause growth deficits at high doses, this effect was not seen in rats exposed to alcohol prenatally who subsequently were treated with amphetamines. The rats treated with high-dose amphetamine demonstrated better growth than controls, suggesting that amphetamine treatment would probably not exacerbate the growth retardation which occurs with prenatal alcohol exposure in humans (Hannigan et al., 1991).

Animal studies have allowed a detailed look at alcohol's effect on neurotransmitter systems in the CNS. Basically, early alcohol exposure markedly impairs the development of most neurotransmitter systems, including dopaminergic, noradrenergic, serotonergic, cholinergic, glutamatergic, GABAergic, and histaminergic systems (Manteuffel, 1996). Because ADHD symptoms in humans are associated with dopamine and norepinephrine underactivity that is usually improved by stimulants, these neurotransmitter systems are of interest in the child exposed to alcohol prenatally. In prenatally exposed rats, dopamine levels were reduced in the projection areas of the cortex, striatum, and hypothalamus and in the cell body areas located in the substantia nigra and ventral segmental area (Manteuffel, 1996). Because dopamine plays a role in neuronal differentiation and neurite elongation, an early compromise of dopamine levels may have far-reaching effects on neuronal structure generally, including a lack of maturation on dendritic branching (Miller et al., 1990). Hannigan and Randall (1996) have reviewed the rat research which suggests that a subtype of dopamine receptors, D_1, of the mesolimbic dopamine system are the most affected compared to the tegmental or nigrostriatal dopamine systems. The authors suggest that a selective D_1 medication would be a preferred treatment choice for children with FAS and behavioral effects related to dopamine deficits.

Norepinephrine deficiency has also been documented by regional brain analyses in the hypothalmus, striatum, and septal areas in the offspring of alcohol-exposed rats (reviewed by Manteuffel, 1996). Beta-adrenergic receptors in the hippocampus have also been reported to be reduced, although muscarinic receptors are spared (Wigal et al., 1990). The only adrenergic agonist used in pharmacological studies of alcohol-exposed animals is clonidine, which has also been used to treat hyperactivity in children. Clonidine is an alpha$_2$-adrenergic agonist that actually lowers overall norepinephrine levels in children and adults. Clonidine decreases excessive locomotion in control mice, but it stimulates locomotion in alcohol-exposed mice (Weathersby et al., 1994).

Reductions in acetylcholine levels have also been found in the fetal and neonatal rat brain with in utero alcohol exposure. However, treatment with the acetylcholinesterase inhibitor physostigmine, which increases acetylcholine levels, reduced hyperactivity in alcohol-exposed rats but did not affect controls (Riley et al., 1986). Bond (1988) subsequently showed that neostigmine, a modified form of physostigmine that works peripherally, decreased hyperactivity in alcohol-exposed rats, whereas physostigmine increased hyperactivity. Although some of these preliminary results are conflicting, the improvement in hyperactivity with cholinergic agents suggests that cholinergic function mediates at least in part the hyperactivity problems in patients with FAS.

Prenatal alcohol exposure also significantly affects the serotonergic system by impairing the development of the cell bodies and their projections to target areas. Fetal serotonin levels have a trophic effect mediated by certain serotonin receptors (5-HT$_{1A}$) that modulate neuronal outgrowths to target areas and promote formation of collateral connections (Manteuffel, 1996). Treatment of pregnant alcohol-exposed rats with buspirone, a 5-HT$_{1A}$ agonist, prevented or reversed many of the serotonin abnormalities caused by alcohol exposure in the offspring (Kim and Druse, 1996). Buspirone treatment was not deleterious to the dopamine system and partially protected the norepinephrine system from the deleterious effects of alcohol. However, in controls a significant reduction in norepinephrine reuptake was seen in the dorsal raphe area with buspirone treatment (Gillespie et al., 1997).

Lastly, alcohol exposure inhibits the N-methyl-D-asparate (NMDA) receptor of the glutamatergic system, which is the main excitatory neurotransmitter system of the CNS. This system has important trophic effects in utero which are disrupted by alcohol exposure. In addition, NMDA receptors are essential for the synaptic plasticity in long term potentiation (LTP) which is important for cognition and memory. Fetuses chronically exposed to alcohol in utero have a significant reduction in NMDA receptors (Tsai and Coyle, 1998).

Medication studies in animals are helping to develop strategies for optimal psychopharmacological treatment of children with FAS. However, this work in both animals and humans is in its infancy. More work has been done with animals than with humans, and there is a great need for controlled research regarding the efficacy of psychopharmacological intervention in children with FAS.

Most important, the animal studies support the concept that deficits can occur in brain function secondary to alcohol exposure in utero without the presence of physical or dysmorphic features. This has been shown even in nonhuman primates, macaques, who were exposed to weekly doses of varying levels of alcohol similar to a binge drinking situation (Clarren et al., 1990). Many demonstrated dopamine abnormalities and ultrastructural changes in the caudate, even though they did not have gross structural abnormalities of their brains or bodies. The animal studies in the 1990s have shown that low-dose alcohol exposure prenatally causes changes in the brain, including neuronal changes or loss, neurochemical, or neurophysiological changes that are associated with neurobehavioral problems in the long term (reviewed by Streissguth, 1997). Human studies have also documented similar cognitive deficits in children with and without physical features who have been exposed to alcohol in utero (Mattson et al., 1997). The human longitudinal studies of even moderate to mild drinkers, for example, the seminal work of Striessguth and colleagues, have documented long-term neurodevelopmental problems well. Goodlett and West (1992) urge that abstinence during pregnancy is the only way to avoid these low-dose effects.

TREATMENT

Issues regarding treatment of children exposed to alcohol in utero are addressed according to the age of the child, beginning with the newborn period.

Infants

Very few reports are available regarding the neonatal withdrawal syndrome from alcohol. Robe et al. (1981) summarized 15 cases in the literature and compared them to 138 infants who had experienced withdrawal from narcotics. The paucity of reports suggests that severe withdrawal symptoms that are life-threatening are relatively rare in alcohol-exposed infants. However, in the 15 cases reviewed, seizures occurred in 33%, compared to only 1% in the narcotics group, and opisthotonus, apnea, cyanosis, and weight loss occurred only in the alcohol group (Robe et al., 1981). If a child is suspected of having alcohol or other drug exposure, it is worthwhile to collect a urine sample from the child after the child leaves the delivery room to detect alcohol or other drug exposures that occurred just prior to delivery (Bays, 1992). The blood alcohol level in the infant can also be drawn. The withdrawal symptoms may occur within the first 12 hours after birth, and the severe signs, including seizures, apnea, cyanosis, and even opisthotonus as prelude to seizures, are life-threatening and require treatment. Traditionally, phenobarbital at 5 mg/kg/d in divided doses can be used for treatment. Generally, medications are not necessary for treatment of withdrawal, but the following list of interventions should be helpful to mothers who are taking care of babies undergoing withdrawal (Bays, 1992):

1. Wrap the baby in a soft blanket (to help him or her feel secure).
2. Keep the lights dim (to decrease stimulation).
3. Drape the bed with a blanket or sheet (to decrease light and noise).
4. Keep the noise level low (to decrease stimulation).

5. Play soft, soothing music (to decrease stimulation).
6. Hold the baby frequently (to offer security).
7. Feed the infant frequently (to ease abdominal pain and provide extra calories).
8. Use a pacifier (to satisfy the need to suck).
9. Use unstarched, soft blankets or sheets to cover the bed (to prevent scrapes and rub marks).
10. Hold the baby firmly when he or she is held (to offer security).
11. Rock gently (to soothe).
12. Speak softly (to soothe/relax).
13. Gently massage the baby's back/arms/legs (to help relax).
14. Use a snuggly or front pack when carrying the baby to secure him or her and to offer comfort.

It is important for the mother to stay calm and to plan for resting and receiving appropriate child care, and many women need encouragement to do this. Infants withdrawing from alcohol are less irritable and hyperresponsive than infants withdrawing from narcotics (Robe et al., 1981). Unfortunately, many infants have combined exposures.

Coles and colleagues (1984) have studied infants exposed to drinking throughout pregnancy who do not show the dysmorphic features of FAS. They found that these infants had significant problems with tremors, sleeplessness, restlessness, hypertonia, hyperactive reflexes, excessive crying, and exaggerated mouthing movements compared with infants not exposed to alcohol and with infants whose mothers stopped drinking before the third trimester. They also found that these problems may not occur until the third day of life and may continue for a prolonged period, so the mothers need guidance regarding how to handle these problems at home.

Withdrawal problems in infants exposed to alcohol may include feeding difficulties and abdominal distention. Infants with FAS may have cleft lip or palate, which interferes with feeding, but more commonly they tire easily and are distractible during the feeding. Weight gain may be poor, and in severe cases a nasogastric tube is necessary (Van Dyke et al., 1982). Help from an oral feeding clinic or team that includes an occupational therapist will often be beneficial to stimulate oral motor coordination and to carry out a trial of various types of nipples. Swaddling, decreased environmental stimulation, and a consistent, frequent feeding schedule are necessary if the baby is irritable or hyperreactive (Bays, 1992).

An important issue in the newborn period is obtaining a drinking history from the biological mother. Questions need to be asked in a sensitive and nonjudgmental fashion regarding the amount, type, frequency, and timing of alcohol consumption during the pregnancy. The average daily and weekly alcohol consumption, in addition to information regarding bingeing, particularly the time and amount of binge drinking, is necessary. Documentation of other substance abuse, including smoking, is also necessary. When alcohol or drug exposure in utero is documented in the newborn period, the hospital social worker and subsequently the child protective services agencies must be notified. The infant should be observed for at least 3 days in the hospital, and a discharge conference should be held to arrange for appropriate follow-up and treatment for mother and child. Connecting the mother with an advocate or home visitation program such as the Birth to Three Program (Grant et al., 1996) will lead to the best outcome for the mother regarding her eventual rehabilitation and training for infant interactional skills. Such a program can enhance the development of the child and provide optimal follow-up for medical and developmental problems.

The examination of the baby must include a careful assessment for the dysmorphic features associated with FAS. If the clinician is inexperienced in such evaluations, referral to a geneticist, developmental pediatrician, or other physician with experience in the diagnosis of alcohol-related problems is important. Astley and Clarren (1997) have outlined the medical history questions and the physical examination in an easy-to-use format for clinicians. If cardiac abnormalities are detected on examination, such as a murmur or cyanosis, obtaining an EKG and a referral to a cardiologist are essential. Orthopedic problems should be evaluated by an X-ray initially and the baby referred to an orthopedist as necessary. Renal studies are not routinely recommended unless external abnormalities or infection are found. Hearing deficits are relatively common in patients with FAS, as described, so screening in the newborn period for deafness is essential. A auditory brainstem-evoked potential should be carried out if a screening study is positive. These children are also at high risk for conductive hearing loss from recurrent otitis media, so detailed clinical exams when illness or fever are present and follow-up tympanograms after treatment of otitis are recommended. For persistent otitis media, placement of polyethylene (PE) tubes in the tympanic membrane will normalize a conductive hearing loss. Visual problems are also common, so abnormalities on a visual exam require follow-up by an ophthalmologist.

The practical experience of parents linked in a parent support group can help address many issues that arise. A list of parent support groups around the country can be found in the resource list at the end of this chapter. In addition, a list of agencies which provide reading materials and video information regarding diagnosis and treatment of FAS and related conditions can be found in the resource section.

In evaluating a dysmorphic infant when the exposure to alcohol is uncertain or when the features are inconsistent with FAS, it is important to rule out other genetic disorders by means of a detailed clinical assessment, preferably with a dysmorphologist, and the use of high-resolution chromosomal testing and appropriate fluorescent in situ hybridization (FISH) studies when indicated (Battaglia et al., 1999). On rare occasions a child may have two disorders, such as FAS and XYY (Figure 1.5).

Toddlers and Preschool Children

It is essential for young alcohol-affected children to have consistent and predictable structure both at home and at school. Giving them activities which are develop-

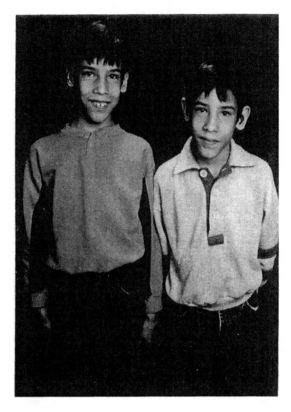

FIGURE 1.5:   Identical twin 9-year-old boys with FAS and XYY syndrome. The boy on the right is more severely affected with FAS, and he also has a sensory neural hearing loss.

mentally rather than chronologically appropriate helps to empower the child and allows hims or her develop a positive self-image. Because of deficits in one or more sensory systems, a multisensory teaching approach is generally useful, although each program must be individualized for a child's particular strengths and weaknesses (Kleinfeld and Westcott, 1993; Riley, 1997). Because language and motor deficits are common, most children qualify for early speech and language therapy and occupational therapy during the toddler and preschool period. Research has shown that language therapy based in a naturalistic setting with interactional strategies that support the child's language development is more effective in improving functional language for developmentally delayed children than traditional speech and language therapy (Kaiser et al., 1996). One model with demonstrated efficacy is enhanced milieu therapy (EMT). EMT trains the parent and teacher to enhance the child's language development through joint attention activities guided by the child's interests; through responsive interaction strategies, in which the parent models appropriate language responses; through use of social routines in which the child is relaxed and more talkative; and through contingent responsiveness, in which the parent's response is timely and appropriate to the child's communication attempt (Kaiser et al., 1996). Such a program can occur throughout the day and has shown significant improvements over traditional therapy in expanding the child's functional language abilities, even in children with developmental disabilities and mental retardation (Kaiser et al., 1996).

The approach to early intervention for the child with FAS should recognize the complexities of problems that these families face. Addressing the mother's issues even at this stage with advocacy that provides psychological support, help with obtaining services and entitlements, parent skills training, crisis intervention, guidance and feedback, and general encouragement has shown the best follow-up results in terms of maintaining environmental stability without alcohol use or abuse (Carmichael Olson and Burgess, 1997; Carmichael Olson et al., 1994; Grant et al., 1996).

Respite care, particularly for patients with significant behavioral problems, is an important issue for many families, especially if social supports are limited. The health care provider must often give guidance as to where respite care can be obtained. This is usually organized through social services, although the national organizations listed in the resource section may also have a national network for such services.

The optimal educational environment for children with FAS has not been studied using controlled methodology. Instead, only a handful of model treatment programs have been established for preschoolers exposed to alcohol or other drugs in utero. They include the Prenatally Exposed to Drugs (PED) Program in the Los Angeles Public Schools, Project DAISY from the District of Columbia, and the Ravenswood Parent and Child Intervention Program in California. Carmichael Olson and Burgess (1997) summarize these programs and provide useful anecdotal information. Other publications also provide information on educational approaches (Kleinfeld and Westcott, 1993; Riley, 1997; Soby, 1994; Tanner-Halverson, 1997). The general principles include a multidisciplinary staff, consistency in following daily routines, utilization of visual and auditory approaches or a multisensory approach, and attention to decreasing overstimulation and calming routines to decrease hyperactivity and improve attention. Many of these interventions have been advocated for children with significant ADHD who are disorganized or overreact to stimuli. Although Morse and colleagues (1995) have found an increase in sensory integration problems in children with FAS compared with controls, the efficacy of sensory integration therapy in this population has not been studied. General guidelines for teachers can be found in Table 1.2.

Preschoolers with FAS often show greater deficits in visual–spatial abilities than in language (Coles and Platzman, 1993), so it may appear at first glance that they do not need language therapy. However, on closer study, Abkarian (1992) found that although fluency and vocabulary levels may look appropriate in higher-functioning individuals, difficulties are usually present in comprehension, social discourse, and the pragmatics of speech. The social aspects of language, including

TABLE 1.2: Educational Strategies

Memory and Learning

Give simple directions using both verbal and nonverbal cues. Make sure the information is understood by having the child repeat the directions.

Model language by describing ongoing activities. Identify and label your feelings, the child's feelings, and those of others. Identify and model words to express the child's needs, wants, and fears.

Explain what a look, body gesture, or body language means.

Model appropriate problem solving.

Role-play cause and effect experiences.

Label objects in the classroom.

Practice new skills and review information for a prolonged period of time. Neural networks become better established the more they are used.

Use multisensory learning; for instance, writing things down helps the child to remember.

Generalize concepts whenever possible and tie in all sensory modalities in preschool. For instance, when studying red, paint with red paint, drink red juice, listen to a story with red pictures, and throw red balls at a red target.

Combine cues with questions to enhance recall.

Link new material to high-interest subjects to enhance learning and memory.

Use concrete objects and physical activities in learning presentations, for instance, when teaching money concepts, use coins and shopping experiences in play activities or in a field trip.

Read to the child!

Behavior Problems and ADHD

Structure the day with a schedule that is consistent. Children can create a visual reminder for themselves of what their schedule is with pictures of themselves doing each activity.

Avoid abrupt transitions by using verbal reminders for upcoming changes. A transition activity such as a sing song before a change is helpful, or provide them with a transitional object.

Have children use self-talk to stay on task.

Use positive reinforcement for good behavior, and do not reinforce undesirable behavior. Recognize a child's attempts, even when unsuccessful, with a smile or thank-you.

Use physical calming techniques such as a hug, holding the child's hand, or sitting beside the child.

Avoid overstimulation in the classroom and model strategies to deal with overstimulation or conflict, such as time-outs, walking away, talking, or negotiating. These strategies can be practiced in role-playing.

Never present a win–lose situation; always give choices.

Analyze noncompliant behavior for the deficits or miscomprehension that may be involved.

Motivate children by using high-interest areas and culture-specific or person-specific material when possible.

Use visual, physical, and tactile cues to redirect attention.

When attempting to change undesirable behavior, address one specific issue at a time.

Material presented here was derived from Kleinfeld and Westcott (1993), Riley (1997), Soby (1994), and Tanner-Halverson (1997).

reading verbal and nonverbal cues, labeling and understanding emotions, and controlling impulsive speech, are also problems. Becker et al. (1990) have documented frequent oral motor coordination deficits, articulation difficulties, and verbal dyspraxia in patients with FAS compared with controls. All of these difficulties in effective communication require early remediation because they have an impact on subsequent academic and social development and predispose to the secondary disabilities described previously in this chapter. Some of these problems can be addressed in the classroom, as described in Table 1.2, although most children with FAS benefit from specific language therapy either in or out of the classroom. An occasional patient may be severely retarded and nonverbal and require augmentative communication approaches in therapy.

Hyperactivity and distractibility often arise in the preschool period. Behavioral techniques may suffice in controlling hyperactivity in the home because significant concentration levels are not yet required at school. On occasion in the preschool period severe problems with hyperactivity, combined with tantrums or aggression, occur that do not respond to behavioral interventions at home or at school. Referral to a psychologist for more intensive therapy is usually helpful for both the child and the parents.

A trial of medication to decrease hyperactivity and impulsivity for the child who is 4 or older may be helpful in addition to the interventions described above. Clonidine, an alpha$_2$ presynaptic agonist which decreases norepinephrine levels both peripherally and centrally, may be helpful for the child who is easily overstimulated and severely hyperactive because it has an overall calming effect. The main side effect is sedation, so a low dose is recommended initially, such as 1/4 or 1/2 of a 0.1-mg tablet twice a day (Hagerman et al., 1998). An EKG is recommended at baseline if there is a history of cardiac problems such as fainting, dizziness, and murmur. Otherwise an EKG is recommended in follow-up, especially when clonidine is combined with stimulants because of a history of rare arrhythmias (Hagerman et al., 1998).

Clonidine often helps with sleeping problems, although if just sleep difficulties without hyperactivity occur, then a trial of melatonin should be considered. Melatonin is a sleep hormone that is normally produced by the brain when it is dark, but it is inhibited by the light (Brzezinski, 1997). It is not yet available by prescription, but it can be purchased at health food stores in the United States. Usually a dose of 1/2 to one tablet (3-mg tablets) by mouth at bedtime causes drowsiness and may help with sleeping difficulties. Studies regarding the efficacy of melatonin in children with FAS have not yet been carried out, although studies of developmentally disabled children with sleep difficulties show that melatonin is helpful for approximately 80% (Jan and O'Donnell, 1996). An alternative to medication is the *Baby Go to Sleep* tape (see Resources at the end of this chapter).

Stimulant medication can be used in the preschool period but is more likely to be helpful in the school-aged child for treatment of attention and concentration difficulties, so this will be discussed in the next section.

School-Aged Child

The school-aged child with FAS usually has significant language, motor, and cognitive deficits that continue to require language and motor therapy, in addition to special education support. Language therapy should build on the progress made in preschool, particularly in comprehension, social discourse, and the pragmatic aspects of speech (Abkarian, 1992). Group language therapy can be combined with a social skills building group so that social language and appropriate behavior can be modeled and incorporated. Similar models of social skill training have been developed for children with ADHD alone (Frankel et al., 1997) but may be useful for children with FAS. The parents should be involved in the social skill training so that consistency occurs both at school and at home regarding expectations and positive behavioral reinforcement (Frankel et al., 1997). In addition, work at home can also help to generalize the concepts taught at school. For instance, the child can count the utensils at the dinner table or write out the menu for the week with magnetic letters on the refrigerator. These learning activities at home should receive consistent positive reinforcement and can be naturally incorporated into everyday life.

The motor problems of children with FAS often also include sensory motor integration deficits. Children with FAS may easily overreact to stimuli, leading to disorganized, hyperactive, and tantrum behavior. Some of the sensory-motor calming techniques, such as a brushing program or use of a weighted vest to increase proprioceptive input, which are common interventions for children with fragile X syndrome (Scharfenaker et al., 1996), may also be helpful for children with FAS. Further research is needed in this area, but consultation with an OT therapist can be helpful for many children with FAS.

Computer Enhancement of Learning

Computers can enhance the learning process for children with FAS, because they provide structure, repetition of activities, consistent visual and auditory cues, and a way for children who have significant handwriting difficulties to produce written work. Specific computer programs can help improve areas of learning difficulty, including mathematics, problem solving, visual-perceptual skills, handwriting, and higher linguistic thinking. For instance, in the visual-spatial area, there are programs such as Kid Pixs (which enhances drawing and graphics), Blocks in Motion (which works on visual-spatial processing), and Trudy's Time and Place House (which focuses on early map and directional skills and develops visual-spatial skills through the manipulation of three-dimensional shapes; Tracy Kovach and Janet Blessinger, personal communication, 1998). More information about these programs can be found in the appendix 2 in this volume. These programs are quite helpful for enhancing visual-spatial processing through independent and exploratory learning experiences. Programs that require the child to improve problem-solving abilities through reading and listening to cues and planning adventures and trips also incorporate math and reading skills. These programs include Oregon Trails, Interactive Journeys, and Where in the World Is Carmen Sandiego. Mathematical concepts can be addressed ranging from the preschool period to higher math concepts such as geometry and algebra. Such programs include Millie's Math House, the Mighty Math series' Carnival Countdown, Zoo Zillions, and Cosmic Geometry, and the Math Blaster series.

Because visual-motor coordination problems are common in children with FAS, programs to enhance writing skills should be used, such as word prediction software that can guess what word the child is attempting to type from the first couple of letters typed. Auditory feedback can also be obtained through a talking word processor that can give information about the words they have written or read back what they have written. If the child has difficulty formulating words, an adapted expanded keyboard which is also programmable may be helpful in providing the child with whole word choices instead of simply individual letters (Tracy Kovach and Janet Blessinger, personal communication, 1998). The Co: Writer is a word prediction program, and its dictionary of words predicted can be limited or expanded depending on the needs of the child. Also helpful are Write: Outloud, a talking word processing program, and Intellikeys, a programmable expanded keyboard that can be adapted to send either letters, words, or whole sentences to the computer.

Telling stories or narratives can also be a problem for children with FAS. There are several computer programs available that can enhance the child's storytelling abilities. Living Books are animated stories in which words are high-lighted as the child reads and objects on each page can be manipulated. The McGee series includes simple stories in which the child chooses what will happen next for items on every page so the child can learn how to make decisions. Stanley's Sticker Stories and Storybook Weaver allow the child to illustrate and narrate his or her own story, which helps the child to focus because his or her interests are included in the story. The Imagination Express series and the Amazing Writing Machine allow the child to also write stories in addition to poems and letters in a fun and structured format. All of these programs will stimulate the child's imagination and improve attention by allowing the child to focus on his or her interest areas (Tracy Kovach and Janet Blessinger, personal communication, 1998).

Psychopharmacological Intervention

Considering the frequency of attention, concentration, and impulsivity problems in children with FAS and ARND, it is remarkable that at the time of this writing there is only one study published regarding the efficacy of stimulant medication use in FAS. Snyder and colleagues (1997) report 11 children aged 6 to 16 with FAS who were previously known responders to stimulants. In a controlled trial of stimulants, they found significant improvement in hyperactivity by parental questionnaire but no significant change in impulsivity or attention using a continuous performance task. The majority of the children were treated with methylphenidate at a dose of 5 to 20 mg twice a day, two of the children were treated with pemoline, and one with dextroamphetamine. Although the study did not evaluate the overall response rate to stimulants, one of the authors estimates that 70% of children with FAS are responsive to stimulant medication (Nanson, personal communication, 1997). In Denver, we surveyed 22 patients who had undergone 66 medication trials, and 63% responded well to stimulants, 88% responded well to mood stabilizers, and 82% responded well to selective serotonin reuptake inhibitors (Coe et al., 1999). Many patients have a combination of problems, such as mood swings, aggression, anxiety, obsessive–compulsive behavior, conduct disorder, or depression, in addition to impulsivity, poor attention, and poor social skills. Often a combination of medications, in addition to psychotherapy and special education support, is necessary (Coe et al., 1999).

CASE HISTORY: DAVID (1)

David is now an 8½-year-old young man who was diagnosed with fetal alcohol syndrome at 30 months of age. His biological mother was 17 years old at the time of his birth, and she drank alcohol and took other drugs throughout the pregnancy. David's birth weight, height, and head circumference were all at the 10th to 25th percentiles at the time of his birth. He was evaluated for failure to thrive in the first year of life, and his biological mother was known to be depressed and trying to seek treatment. At 16 months of age, he was placed in a temporary foster home because of severe malnutrition, and he subsequently was moved into two other foster homes where he thrived. At 30 months of age, he was noted to have several dysmorphic features, including microcephaly, prominent ears, small palpebral fissures, broad nasal bridge, long philtrum, thin upper lip, shortness of the fifth finger, and shortness of the second through fifth toes. Subsequent developmental testing on the Bayley scales demonstrated an MDI of 72 and a PDI of 61. A developmental preschool program with both language and motor therapy was recommended for him. Cytogenetic testing was negative at that time, and fragile X DNA testing was also negative. He was given a diagnosis of fetal alcohol syndrome at that time.

His medical history included recurrent ear infections beginning in the first year of life, and at 2 years of age PE tubes were placed. He has a history of milk allergy and chronic nasal congestion. At 1 year of age, he had a bilateral orchiopexy, and subsequently in the next year he had a revision of a failed circumcision, which had resulted in meatal stenosis.

At 3½ years of age, David was adopted by a family that has provided a very positive and loving home for him. At the time of his adoption, he was noted to have unsteady gait and difficulty with both fine and gross motor coordination. He learned to ride a tricycle at 4½ years of age, but he has always had difficulty in dressing himself. He has had occupational therapy and speech and language therapy through school on a weekly basis.

He was toilet trained at 3½ years of age and was dry for approximately 1 year, but at 5 years of age he developed nighttime enuresis (bed-wetting). A seizure disorder developed at approximately 3½ to 4 years of age, and he was noted to have staring spells on a daily basis, with some disorientation afterward. An EEG was carried out, and it demonstrated a right occipital spike focus with rare bicentral spiking during stage two sleep. He was treated with valproic acid for his seizures, and they have subsequently not reoccurred.

At 6 years of age, David was reevaluated for his language, learning, and attentional problems. His cognitive testing on the Kaufman Assessment Battery for Children demonstrated a mental processing composite of 80, with a sequential score of 89 and a simultaneous score of 77. He met criteria for ADHD and has significant impulsivity, which has caused problems in school. Imipramine was recommended at a dose of 10 mg twice a day to treat his ADHD symptoms and enuresis, and counseling was recommended for his behavioral problems. Kidney function studies and renal ultrasound were normal. Sensory integration occupational therapy was also recommended, in addition to his special education work.

The imipramine improved the enuresis, but there was not a significant improvement in his ADHD symptoms. His behavioral problems at school escalated, and he developed problems with stealing and lying, in addition to aggression toward other children. A behavior program was established at school, but the excessive negative reinforcement was not helpful for him. Consultation with a private psychologist was obtained with ongoing weekly therapy. A positive behavior reinforcement program was developed at school, which involved giving him a stamp or a sticker for positive feedback every 15 minutes when his behavior was appropriate. As David's behavior improved, the frequency of the positive reinforcer decreased from every 15 minutes to every hour. His private therapy outside of school has included discussions of appropriate social interactions both at home and at school, alternatives to aggression, and the regular playing of a board game which has been developed for children with ADHD. This game helps him to stop and think about possible alternatives for a variety of social situations before acting impulsively. He enjoys playing this game, so his focus and attention on this activity are quite good.

David's special education support in school has included the use of an aide to help him with mainstreaming in the regular classroom, in addition to pull-out help for his math and reading. When he was 8 years old and in second grade, a special education evaluation demonstrated significant problems with visual motor coordination and visual perception. On a test of visual-motor coordination he scored at the ninth percentile for his age. He was able to copy forms accurately at the 5-year age level, but he made major errors in visual spatial organization and directionality on more advanced forms. His visual perceptual skills ranged from the first percentile to the 84th percentile, with his lowest scores on memory subtest and tests of figure–ground perception. His math testing showed problems related to errors in counting, operational signs, and writing two-digit numerals, such as writing "41" for "14."

On the Wechsler Individual Achievement Test his basic reading standard score was 84, mathematics reasoning 88, spelling 82, reading comprehension 78, and numerical operations 78. These scores range from the seventh percentile to the 21st percentile for age. His overall reading composite scale was 78, with a math composite scale of 81. On the Peabody Individual Achievement Test his overall score on general information was 89, which is the 23rd percentile for age. On the developmental test of visual motor integration, his standard score was 80. Repeat cognitive testing using the WISC-III scale at age 8 demonstrated a Verbal IQ of 95, a Performance IQ of 75, and a Full-Scale IQ of 84.

David's therapist feels that his ADHD symptoms, with significant impulsivity combined with his significant motor coordination difficulties and handwriting problems in school, are his greatest difficulties at this time. To target his ADHD symptoms, he was given a trial of Adderall beginning at a dose of 5 mg each morning, and his imiprimine was discontinued before this trial. The Adderall, however, has not been helpful for his attentional problems, so it was discontinued, and methylphenidate was given a trial. It was recommended that he use a bell and pad apparatus to improve his intermittent bed-wetting problem (see appendix 4 to this volume).

His motor coordination problems included fine and gross motor incoordination, and problems with eating and swallowing. He tends to stuff his mouth, he does not chew his food, and then he frequently gags and may even vomit after eating. An oral feeding evaluation demonstrated normal oral motor structure and functional skills, but his eating difficulties were noted to be related to overall sensory integration problems. An occupational therapy sensory integration evaluation using a sensory integration and praxis test (SIPT) demonstrated significant sensory integration dysfunction. Many subtest scores were greater than 1 SD below the norm, including finger identification, graphesthesia, praxis on verbal command, design copying, postural praxis, oral praxis, sequencing praxis, and bilateral motor coordination. His lowest score was standing and walking balance, which was more than 2 SD below the norm. Overall, he demonstrated significant problems with visual motor skills, sensory processing abilities, and motor planning skills, in addition to difficulty with tactile perception. The lack of tactile feedback has interfered with his eating behavior, and this is the reason he overstuffs his mouth and has difficulty with swallowing and gagging. It was recommended that he receive occupational therapy with a sensory integration approach to help improve his processing of sensory information, fine and gross motor coordination, eating skills, and motor planning skills.

Because of the severity of his handwriting deficits, he was given a computer evaluation to assess the usefulness of computer technology to enhance his academic progress. He did remarkably well with the use of the Co:Writer software program (see appendix 2) to enhance his written language. The Co:Writer guesses what word he is trying to type after he types the first few letters. He was able to use this word prediction program to write a sentence much faster than using a typical word processing program. He was also independent in sounding out and spelling the desired words with the help of this program. In addition, it was recommended that he use computer software programs to enhance his sight word vocabulary, spelling, and reading skills. It was also recommended that he use books on tape to provide him with exposure to literature that is above his reading level but at his interest level (see appendix 3). Additional software that he enjoyed working with included the Living Books series, KidPix Studio, Amazing Writing Machine, and Story Book Weaver Deluxe (see appendix 2).

Because his school did not have some of this computer software available, a visiting computer team worked with the school as to how to obtain the appropriate computer technology and software for use by David and other students in need.

In summary, David's program consists of sensory integration occupational therapy and language therapy on a private basis which targets the development of abstract reasoning skills, in addition to the limited programming that is available at school. He also receives private counseling, and his therapist has worked with the school to develop and continue a positive behavior reinforcement program. His medication includes his anticonvulsant, Depakote and a stimulant medication, methylphenidate.

The main stimulants which are frequently used clinically are methylphenidate (Ritalin), dextroamphetamine (Dexedrine), a new preparation, Adderall, which is a mixture of four dextro and levo amphetamine salts, and pemoline (Cylert). Stimulants in general increase dopamine and norepinephrine levels in the CNS by blocking reuptake and enhancing release of these neurotransmitters at the synapse. The most significant effect is thought to be in the frontal regions, and previous PET scan studies have shown enhanced metabolism in some regions frontally, parietally, and in the striatum (Lou et al., 1984, 1989; Matochik et al., 1993; Vaidya et al., 1998). A recent PET scanning study by Volkow et al. (1997) has shown a consistent picture of enhanced metabolism in the cerebellum after methylphenidate in 15 normal males. Although dopamine is not present in the cerebellum, dopamine has a well-recognized role of modulating the activity of various brain regions. The effect in the cerebellum may be secondary to norepinephrine neurotransmission in the cerebellum or to action on the striatal-cerebellar tracts. Recently the cerebellum has been shown to have an important role in higher cognitive functions, including attention, memory, and learning (Andreasen et al., 1995; Leiner et al., 1989). Hopefully, the metabolic deficits in the cerebellum caused by prenatal alcohol exposure may be improved in some individuals with stimulant use.

In general, stimulants are relatively safe when used in low doses, with the main side effects being appetite suppression sometimes leading to weight loss and cardiovascular stimulation, which rarely can cause hypertension. Stimulants can also exacerbate tics in approximately 30% of individuals with tics or Tourette syndrome, so they should be used cautiously in these cases (see chapter 3, this volume). Other side effects include occasional headaches, stomachaches, sleeping difficulties, irritability, anxiety, and nail biting, all of which can worsen at high doses. Pemoline (Cylert) is unique among the stimulants because it can cause liver dysfunction, and follow-up of liver function studies is required (Shevell and Schreiber, 1997). In December 1996, Abbott Laboratories, the makers of Cylert, sent a letter to all physicians warning that 13 cases of acute hepatic failure had been reported to the FDA. They recommended not considering pemoline as a first-line treatment for ADHD because of the risk for liver toxicity. Although this risk is still relatively low, ranging from 1 : 70,000 to 1 : 300,000, it is recommended that liver function studies be carried out at least once every 6 months and after dose increases or after adding other medications (Johnston et al., 1996). Pemoline should never be given to someone with liver dysfunction and since alcoholism is common in patients with FAS, pemoline should be avoided if possible in this population.

There is some evidence for a better response rate to dextroamphetamine, compared to methylphenidate, in patients with alcohol spectrum disorders (O'Malley and Hagerman, 1998). In the longitudinal follow up of 23 patients with FAS/FAE, only 22% of those treated with methylphenidate had a positive response, whereas 79% of 19 patiens who were treated with dextroamphetamine had a positive response (Kieran O'Malley, personal communication, 1998). These preliminary data suggest that stimulants containing dextroamphetamine should be tried initially in patients with alcohol spectrum disorders and ADHD. Stimulants may need to be combined with other classes of medication, such as antidepressants, anticonvulsants, mood stabilizers, or even antipsychotics, because of the high rates of psychopathology in this disorder. These additional medications are described in the next section.

A thorough psychological evaluation must be carried out to identify comorbid psychopathology and to guide treatment, including counseling and medication. The report by Famy et al. (1998) found an unexpectedly high rate of psychotic thinking which should be assessed in a psychological evaluation. Usually long-term counseling and behavioral intervention (Watson and Gresham, 1998) are needed to treat significant psychopathology. However, the addition of social skills training which includes pragmatic aspects of language (Duke et al., 1996) is also important for the majority of children with alcohol spectrum disorders.

Adolescence and Adulthood

The high frequency of secondary disabilities in individuals with FAS, PFAS, or ARND is of great concern. One of the problems is the lack of recognition of the neurodevelopmental difficulties because many of these individuals are not retarded. Often young adults with FAS feel that programs for the developmentally disabled are not right for them because these programs usually have participants with mental retardation; the young adult with FAS may feel uncomfortable interacting with individuals who have lower cognitive abilities than they do. However, many young adults with FAS have failed job training for normal individuals. Intensive job training should start in high school and carry on after graduation with a long-term job trainer. In addition, the high rates of depression, anxiety, suicidal ideation, and impulsive behavior demonstrate the need for individual counseling or psychotherapy. Counseling should focus on concrete issues, such as temper control, social skills, drug or alcohol abuse if present, emancipation and independent living if possible, and depression or anxiety if present. An advocate can also help with job training, housing, money management, and daily living skills (Streissguth, 1997; Streissguth et al., 1995).

Psychopharmacological intervention may be helpful for the adolescent or adult with FAS. Stimulants may continue to be helpful for attention and concentration problems in adolescence, but they are usually not helpful in adulthood. For high rates of depression, the selective serotonin reuptake inhibitors (SSRIs) which enhance serotonin levels by blocking reuptake at the synapse can be helpful. Increasing serotonin levels can be helpful for aggression, mood lability, obsessive–compulsive behavior, and anxiety. Although no controlled studies have been carried out regarding the use of SSRIs in individuals with FAS specifically, clinical experience suggests that they are frequently helpful for the symptoms listed here. There is also a growing body of literature to support the uses of SSRI agents in individuals with developmental disabilities, particularly autism, fragile X syndrome, and disruptive behavior disorders (Zubieta and Alessi, 1993; see also chapters 2 and 3, this volume, for a more detailed discussion of SSRI agents). In the study by Coe et al. (1999) a high rate of mania was found with the use of sertraline (Zoloft) in children with FAS. This reflects significant mood instability in this population. A new SSRI agent, citalopram (Celexa) reports a lower rate of mania (0.2%) than with other SSRIs, and it is well tolerated in children (Thomsen, 1997). Controlled trials of the use of SSRI agents are warrented in individuals affected by alcohol-spectrum disorders.

Significant problems with mood instability or aggression occasionally occur in children or adolescents with FAS or ARND. Sometimes the use of SSRIs will improve aggressive behavior, particularly if this difficulty is related to anxiety or depression. In our experience, two patients with severe ADHD, FAS, and aggression did not improve on stimulants. Risperidone, a new atypical antipsychotic agent with a lower risk of extrapyramidal symptoms and tardive dyskinesia than other antipsychotics, was tried in a low dose, that is, 1 mg each day in these boys aged 11 and 12 years. Both boys made significant improvements in controlling aggressive behavior and hyperactivity on this medication. Such a response to risperidone has been seen in other clinical groups, including those with autism, pervasive developmental disorder, psychosis, and mental retardation of unknown causes (Fisman et al., 1996; Khan, 1997; McDougle et al., 1995; Quintana and Keshavan, 1995; Simeon et al., 1995; Vanden Borre et al., 1993). If psychotic symptoms are seen, then treatment with risperidone would also be indicated. Consultation with psychiatry is necessary if the treating physician is not experienced in psychopharmacology.

Mood instability may exacerbate behavior problems, including aggression. Anticonvulsants such as valproic acid and carbamazepine can be used to stabilize mood, and they are particularly helpful if the EEG is abnormal. Lithium, an older mood stabilizer, should be avoided if renal problems or hypoplastic kidneys are present (O'Malley and Hagerman, 1998). A new generation of anticonvulsants are presently on the market, and preliminary studies suggest that gabapentin (Neurontin) and tiagabine (Gabitril) are not only effective for seizure management but also may be helpful for mood stabilization (Shinnar, 1997; Ghaemi et al., 1998; Marcia Litzinger, personal communication, 1999). There are no controlled trials of these agents in individuals with FAS.

Many individuals with alcohol-related disabilities have been physically and/or sexually abused in the past, which is part of the reason that inappropriate sexual behavior is a common secondary disability. Much of this inappropriate behavior involves impulsive touching. Counseling is usually needed to address the past abuse and treat the inappropriate behavior. In adolescence or in some cases earlier, the family can address sex education issues. Often this issue is raised when the family reports masturbation within the family or public view. The principles of sex education for individuals with developmental disabilities includes teaching the difference between acceptable behavior in a private versus public setting and the right to refuse to be touched at any time (American Academy of Pediatrics Committee on Children with Disabilities, 1996). There are also several books that are helpful in this educational process (Edwards and Elkins, 1988; Kempton et al., 1985; McKee and Blacklidge, 1981).

CASE HISTORY: MARY

Mary is an 11-year-old young lady who was diagnosed with fetal alcohol syndrome when she presented to our child development unit at age 5½. She was the youngest of nine children, and her biological parents were both severe alcoholics. Her biological mother drank throughout her pregnancy on a daily basis, and her drinking included both beer and hard liquor. Mary was born full term with a birth weight of 5 lb 3oz, and she went immediately into foster care after delivery because of her mother's continuing alcoholism. She lived a year in foster care placement, subsequently lived with her older sister for 2 years, and then returned to her biological mother, who continued to drink. The biological mother abandoned her within that same year. She subsequently lived with her sister and then was adopted at age 6 by her present family.

Her original evaluation at age 5 years 5 months showed a history of delayed developmental milestones, including walking at 16 months, saying single words at 18 months, and toilet training at 3½ years of age. She had problems with severe hyperactivity throughout the day, in addition to destructive behavior, impulsivity, and distractibility. When left unsupervised, she smeared the walls and floor of her room with cosmetics. She was a picky eater, although occasionally she binged on food. On examination at age 5½, her weight was far below the fifth percentile, head circumference demonstrated microcephaly (less than the second percentile), and height was at the sixth percentile for age. She was in constant motion during the examination. She had epicanthal folds, in addition to hypertelorism and a flat nasal bridge. She had a thin upper lip with a flat and elongated philtrum. She had mild clinodactaly of the fifth fingers, and in general her extremities were long and thin. Chromosome testing at this time was normal, in addition to amino acids and organic acids.

Mary was diagnosed with fetal alcohol syndrome and ADHD at this time.

Stimulant medication was recommended, and she was started on methylphenidate (Ritalin) at a dose of 5 mg twice a day. She has continued on methylphenidate throughout her childhood, and her present dose is 15 mg three times a day. The methylphenidate has made a significant difference in improving her short attention span, distractibility, and hyperactivity. These are problems both at home and at school, and her ADHD is quite noticeable when she does not take her medication.

Cognitive testing was carried out at age 9 years 4 months, and Mary demonstrated a Verbal IQ of 85, a Performance IQ of 84, and a Full-Scale IQ of 84 on the WISC-III. Her verbal comprehension score was 91, but her Freedom from Distractibility score was 69, with a subtest score of 5 on Digit Span and 4 on Coding. A language and learning evaluation at age 5½ demonstrated visual motor integration scores at the early 4-year age level, expressive vocabulary within the average range, and receptive vocabulary within the low average range. A multidisciplinary approach was recommended for her educational setting, in addition to speech therapy with an emphasis on pragmatics and appropriate social interaction skills. Her attentional problems and hyperactivity interfered with all aspects of testing. At age 6½ an occupational therapy evaluation demonstrated poor praxis and motor planning abilities with poor fine and gross motor development, in addition to problems with hyperactivity and attention. An occupational therapy program with a sensory integrative basis was recommended twice per week, with an emphasis on improving vestibular, proprioceptive, and tactile processing; improving praxis; and improving motor coordination, including visual motor development.

Because of difficulties with settling down at bedtime, which has been a long-term problem for Mary, clonidine at a dose of 0.1 mg at bedtime was initiated at 11 years of age. A follow-up EKG was carried out because of the combination of clonidine and methylphenidate, and results were normal.

At age 11 Mary began to develop breast buds and pubic hair, and over the last 6 months her adoptive mother has seen an increase in mood fluctuations and temper outbursts. She becomes easily frustrated and angry, with yelling and stomping episodes at home on a daily basis. She did not appear to be depressed, but her moodiness and irritability led to a trial of a selective serotonin reuptake inhibitor, specifically sertraline (Zoloft), at a dose of ½ of a 50-mg tablet in the morning with an increase to 50 mg each morning after 2 months. Sertraline has been remarkably helpful, with an improvement in mood, a decrease in irritability and outburst behavior, and improvement in social skills.

Mary's most recent cognitive testing has included a Verbal IQ of 92, a Performance IQ of 90, and a Full-Scale IQ of 90 on the WISC-III. Her Verbal Comprehension score was 96, with a Freedom from Distractibility score of 81. Her lowest subtest scores continue to be Arithmetic at 6 and Digit Span at 7. In the academic area on the Wechsler Individual Achievement Test her basic reading score was 99, grammatics reasoning at 80, spelling at 82, numerical operations at 83, oral expression at 83, and written expression at 80.

On examination at age 11½, her weight continues to be significantly below the fifth percentile, her head circumference is at the second percentile, and her height is at the 25th percentile for age. She continues to have a broad and flat nasal bridge with slight evidence of epicanthal folds, long, thin extremities, thin torso, and a flat philtrum. Because of her normal intellectual testing, she was denied SSI services, with the statement from SSI that her disability "has ceased." She is receiving additional support in school for her attentional and learning problems, but she does not qualify for special education support in school. Her mother does not have the financial resources to provide appropriate counseling for Mary.

FUTURE DIRECTIONS

We are early in the process of developing effective psychopharmacological and educational interventions for children and adults affected by alcohol exposure in utero. For the last 2 decades, the focus of the FAS field has been on prevention. Although prevention efforts should continue, the focus of research should shift to treatment and amelioration of secondary disabilities. A more intensive effort must also be made to diagnose mildly affected individuals who may suffer from PFAS or ARND, because these individuals appear to have the most severe secondary disabilities in our society (Streissguth et al., 1996b).

Animal research has suggested that cholinergic agents may be beneficial for treatment of hyperactivity and cognitive deficits. Controlled studies should be carried out on acetylcholine precursors, acetylcholinesterase inhibitors, and muscarinic agonists, agents that affect the related activities of the cholinergic and glutamatergic systems to improve memory, cognition, and behavior. Piracetam and its derivatives, aniracetam and oxiracetam, enhance the cholinergic and the glutamatergic systems, but they are not licensed in the United States. They have been used in studies of Down syndrome, dyslexia, and Alzheimer's disease, with some mildly beneficial results (Compone, 1998).

Animal studies also suggest that enhancement of the serotonin system may have a protective effect in preventing some of the CNS dysfunction secondary to alcohol exposure. Controlled studies should be carried out with early intervention utilizing SSRIs including buspirone, which was utilized in animal studies, and other SSRIs which affect all of the serotonin receptors. Detailed neuropsychological testing should be included in these controlled studies so that improvements in executive function and working memory can be documented, in addition to behavioral improvements. The benefits of combined psychopharmacological approaches, such as the use of stimulants with SSRIs, must also be clarified.

Advances in educational interventions also require controlled studies in children with FAS. Innovative computer programs, such as the Fast Forward program, which utilizes a computerized slowing of speech to improve auditory processing deficits, have been shown to be helpful for children with language deficits and children with pervasive developmental delays but have not been studied in children with FAS (Merzenich et al., 1996; Tallal et al., 1996). There are numerous interventions presently available and many more that will become available in the future for children with FAS. As a society, we need to shift the monies that are presently spent on incarceration to early identification and intensive treatment of children who are affected by alcohol exposure in utero.

ACKNOWLEDGMENTS Thanks to Heather Carmichael Olson, Edward Riley, Sarah Mattson, Edward Goldson and Karen Riley for their thorough review of chapter 1 and cogent suggestions for improvement. This work was partially supported by the MCH training grant no. MCJ-089413 and the Denver Foundation. Thanks also to the Developmental Psychobiology Research group of the University of Colorado Health Sciences Center for intellectual support.

REFERENCES

Aase, J. M., Jones, K. L., Clarren, S. K. (1995) Do we need the term "FAE"? Pediatrics 95 (3): 428–30.

Abel, E. L. (1997) Was the fetal alcohol syndrome recognized in the ancient Near East? Alcohol and Alcoholism 32: 3–7.

Abel, E. L., and Sokol, R. J. (1991) A revised conservative estimate of the incidence of FAS and its economic impact. Alcoholism, Clinical and Experimental Research 15 (3): 514–24.

Abkarian, G. G. (1992) Communication effects of prenatal alcohol exposure. Journal of Communication Disorders 25: 221–40.

American Academy of Pediatrics Committee on Children with Disabilities (1996) Sexuality education of children and adolescents with developmental disabilities. Pediatrics 97 (2): 275–8.

Andreasen, N. C., O'Leary, D. S., Arndt, S., Cizadlo, T., Hurtig, R., Rezai, K., Watkins, G. L. (1995) Short term and long term verbal memory: A positron emission tomography study. Proceedings of the National Academy of Sciences, USA 92: 5111–5.

Aronson, M., and Olegard, R. (1987) Children of alcoholic mothers. Pediatrician 14: 57–61.

Astley, S. J., and Clarren, S. K. (1995) A fetal alcohol syndrome screening tool. Alcoholism, Clinical and Experimental Research 19 (6): 1565–71.

Astley, S. J., and Clarren, S. K. (1997) Diagnostic guide for FAS and related conditions. University of Washington, Seattle.

Battaglia, A., Bianchini, E., Carey, J. (1999) Diagnostic yield of the comprehensive assessment of developmental delay/mental retardation in an institute of child neuropsychiatry. American Journal of Medical Genetics 82: 60–66.

Bays, J. (1992) The care of alcohol- and drug-affected infants. Pediatric Annals 21 (8): 485–95.

Becker, M., Warr-Leeper, G. A., Leeper, H. A., Jr. (1990) Fetal alcohol syndrome: A description of oral motor, articulatory, short-term memory, grammatical, and semantic abilities. Journal of Communication Disorders 23 (2): 97–124.

Bihrle, A. M., Bellugi, U., Delis, D., Marks, S. (1989) Seeing either the forest or the trees: Dissociation in visuo-spatial processing. Brain and Cognition 11 (1): 37–49.

Bond, N. W. (1988) Prenatal alcohol exposure and offspring hyperactivity: Effects of physostigmine and neostigmine. Neurotoxicology and Teratology 10 (1): 59–63.

Brzezinski, A. (1997) Melatonin in humans. New England Journal of Medicine 336 (3): 186–95.

Carmichael Olson, H., and Burgess, D. M. (1997) Early intervention for children prenatally exposed to alcohol and other drugs. In: The effectiveness of early intervention. Guralnick, M. J. (ed.). Brookes, Baltimore, pp. 109–45.

Carmichael Olson, H., Streissguth, A. P., Bookstein, F. L., Barr, H., Sampson, P. D. (1994) Developmental research in behavioral teratology: Effects of prenatal alcohol exposure on child development. In: Developmental follow-up. Academic Press, San Diego.

Carmichael Olson, H., Streissguth, A. P., Sampson, P. D., Barr, H. M., Bookstein, F. L., Thiede, K. (1997) Association of prenatal alcohol exposure with behavioral and learning problems in early adolescence. Journal of the American Academy of Child and Adolescent Psychiatry 36 (9): 1187–94.

Church, M. W., and Gerkin, K. P. (1988) Hearing disorders in children with fetal alcohol syndrome: Findings from case reports. Pediatrics 82 (2): 147–54.

Church, M. W., Abel, E. L., Kaltenbach, J. A., Overbeck, G. W. (1996) Effects of prenatal alcohol exposure and aging on auditory function in the rat: Preliminary results. Alcoholism, Clinical and Experimental Research 20 (1): 172–9.

Church, M. W., Eldis, F., Blakley, B. W., Bawle, E. V. (1997) Hearing, language, speech, vestibular, and dentofacial disorders in fetal alcohol syndrome. Alcoholism, Clinical and Experimental Research 21 (2): 227–37.

Clarren, S. K., and Smith, D. W. (1978) The fetal alcohol syndrome. New England Journal of Medicine 298 (19): 1063–7.

Clarren, S. K., Astley, S. J., Bowden, D. M., Lai, H., Milam, A. H., Rudeen, P. K., Shoemaker, W. J. (1990) Neuroanatomic and neurochemical abnormalities in nonhuman primate infants exposed to weekly doses of ethanol during gestation. Alcoholism, Clinical and Experimental Research 14 (5): 674–83.

Coe, J. A., Sidders, J., Riley, K., Waltermire, J., Hagerman, R. J. (1999) A survey of medication responses in children and adolescents with fetal alcohol syndrome. Manuscript submitted for publication.

Coles, C. D. (1996) Early neurobehavioral assessment of children prenatally exposed to alcohol. In: Fetal alcohol syndrome: From mechanism to prevention. Abel, E. L. (ed.). CRC Press, New York, 145–70.

Coles, C. D., and Platzman, K. A. (1993) Behavioral development in children prenatally exposed to drugs and alcohol. International Journal of the Addictions 28 (13): 1393–433.

Coles, C. D., Platzman, K. A., Raskind-Hood, C. L., Brown, R. T., Falek, A., Smith, I. E. (1997) A comparison of children affected by prenatal alcohol exposure and attention deficit, hyperactivity disorder. Alcoholism, Clinical and Experimental Research 21 (1): 150–61.

Coles, C. D., Smith, I. E., Fernhoff, P. M., Falek, A. (1984) Neonatal ethanol withdrawal: Characteristics in clinically normal, nondysmorphic neonates. Journal of Pediatrics 105 (3): 445–51.

Compone, G. T. (1998) Drugs that increase intelligence: Application for childhood cognitive impairment. Mental Retardation and Developmental Disabilities Research Reviews 4: 36–49.

Duke, M. P., Nowicki, S., Martin, E. A. (1996). Teaching your child the language of social success. Peachtree, Atlanta, GA.

Edwards, J. P., and Elkins, T. E. (1988) Just between us: A social sexual training guide for parents and professionals who have concerns for people with retardation. Ednick Communications, Portland, Oregon.

Famy, C., Streissguth, A. P., Unis, A. S. (1998) Mental illness in adults with fetal alcohol syndrome or fetal alcohol effects. American Journal of Psychiatry 155: 552–54.

Fisman, S., Steele, M., Short, J., Byrne, T., Lavallee, C. (1996) Case study: Anorexia nervosa and autistic disorder in an adolescent girl. Journal of the American Academy of Child and Adolescent Psychiatry 35 (7): 937–40.

Frankel, F., Myatt, R., Cantwell, D. P., Feinberg, D. T. (1997) Parent-assisted transfer of children's social skills training: Effects on children with and without attention-deficit hyperactivity disorder. Journal of the American Academy of Child and Adolescent Psychiatry 36: 1056.

Frezza, M., Di Padov, C., Pozzato, G., Terpin, M., Baroana, E., Lieber, C. S. (1990) High blood alcohol levels in women: The role of decreased gastric alcohol dehydrogenase activity and first pass metabolism. New England Journal of Medicine 322: 95–9.

Ghaemi, S. N., Katzow, J. J., Desai, S. P., Goodwin, F. K. (1998) Gabapentin treatment of mood disorders: A preliminary study. Journal of Clinical Psychiatry 59 (8): 426–9.

Giedd, J. N., Castellanos, F. X., Casey, B. J., Kozuch, P., King, A. C., Hamburger, S. D., Rapoport, J. L. (1994) Quantitative morphology of the corpus callosum in attention deficit hyperactivity disorder. American Journal of Psychiatry 151: 665–8.

Gillespie, R. A., Eriksen, J., Hao, H. L., Druse, M. J. (1997) Effects of maternal ethanol consumption and buspirone treatment on dopamine and norepinephrine reuptake sites and D1 receptors in offspring. Alcoholism, Clinical and Experimental Research 21 (3): 452–9.

Goddard, H. H. (1912) The Kallikak family: A study in the heredity of feeble mindedness. Macmillan, New York.

Goodlett, C. R., and West, J. R. (1992) Fetal alcohol effects: Rat model of alcohol exposure during the brain growth spurt. In: Maternal substance abuse and the developing nervous system. Zagon, I. S., and Slotkin, T. A. (eds.). Academic Press, San Diego, pp. 45–75.

Goodlett, C. R., Peterson, S. D., Lundahl, K. R., Pearlman, A. D. (1997) Binge-like alcohol exposure of neonatal rats via intragastric intubation induces both Purkinje cell loss and cortical astrogliosis. Alcoholism: Clinical and Experimental Research 21 (6): 1010–17.

Grant, T. M., Ernst, C., Streissguth, A. P., Phipps, P., Gendler, B. (1996) When case management isn't enough: A model of paraprofessional advocacy for drug and alcohol abusing mothers. American Journal of Public Health 5: 3–11.

Habbick, B. F., Nanson, J. L., Snyder, R. E., Casey, R. E., Schulman, A. L. (1996) Foetal alcohol syndrome in Saskatchewan: Unchanged incidence in a 20-year period. Canadian Journal of Public Health. (Revue Canadienne de Sante Publique) 87 (3): 204–7.

Hagerman, R. J., Bregman, J. D., Tirosh, E. (1998) Clonidine. In: Psychotropic medication and developmental disabilities: The international consensus handbook. Reiss, S., and Aman, M. G. (eds.). Ohio State University Nisonger Center, Columbus, Ohio, pp. 259–69.

Hannigan, J. H., and Pilati, M. L. (1991) The effects of chronic postweaning amphetamine on rats exposed to alcohol in utero: Weight gain and behavior. Neurotoxicology Teratology 13: 649–56.

Hannigan, J. H., and Randall, S. I. E. (1996) Behavioral pharmacology in animals exposed prenatally to alcohol. In: Fetal alcohol syndrome: From mechanism to prevention. Abel, E. L. (ed.). CRC Press, New York, pp. 191–213.

Havers, W., Majewski, F., Olbing, H., Eickenberg, H. U. (1980) Anomalies of the kidneys and genitourinary tract in alcoholic embryopathy. Journal of Urology 124 (1): 108–10.

Jacobson, S. W., Fein, G. G., Jacobson, J. L., Schwartz, P. M., Dowler, J. L. (1984) Neonatal correlates of prenatal exposure to smoking, caffeine, and alcohol. Infant Behavioral Development 7: 253.

Jacobson, S. W., Jacobson, J. L., Sokol, R. J. (1994) Effects of fetal alcohol exposure on infant reaction time. Alcoholism: Clinical and Experimental Research 18 (5): 1125–32.

Jan, J. E., and O'Donnell, M. E. (1996) Use of melatonin in the treatment of paediatric sleep disorders. Journal of Pineal Research 21: 193–9.

Johnston, H. F., Witkovsky, M. T., Fruehling, M. L. S. (1996) Pemoline and liver function. Child Psychopharmacology Information Service 3: 1–2.

Jones, K. L., and Smith, D. W. (1973) Recognition of the fetal alcohol syndrome in early infancy. Lancet 2: 999–1001.

Jones, K. L., Smith, D., Ulleland, C. N., Streissguth, A. P. (1973) Pattern of malformation in offspring of chronic alcoholic mothers. Lancet 1: 1267–71.

Kaiser, A. P., Hemmeter, M. L., Hester, P. P. (1996) The facilitative effects of input on children's language development: Contributions from studies of enhanced milieu teaching. In: Research on communication and language disorders: Contributions to theories of language development. Adamson, L. B., and Romski, M. A. (eds.). Brookes, Baltimore, pp. 267–94.

Karp, R. J., Qazi, Q. H., Moller, K. A., Angelo, W. A., Davis, J. M. (1995) Fetal alcohol syndrome at the turn of the 20th century: An unexpected explanation of the Kallikak family. Archives of Pediatrics and Adolescent Medicine 149 (1): 45–8.

Kempton, W., Bass, M. S., Gordon, S. (1985) Sex and birth control for mentally handicapped people: A guide for parents. Planned Parenthood of Southeastern Pennsylvania, Philadelphia.

Khan, B. U. (1997) Brief report: Risperidone for severely disturbed behavior and tardive dyskinesia in developmentally disabled adults. Journal of Autism and Developmental Disorders 27 (4): 479–89.

Kim, J. A., and Druse, M. J. (1996) Protective effects of maternal buspirone treatment on serotonin reuptake sites in ethanol-exposed offspring. Developmental Brain Research 92 (2): 190–8.

Kleinfeld, J., and Westcott, S. (1993) Fantastic Antone succeeds: Experiences in educating children with fetal alcohol syndrome. Alaska University Press, Anchorage.

Klintsova, A. Y., Matthews, J. T., Goodlett, C. R., Napper, R. M. A., Greenough, W. T. (1997) Therapeutic motor training increases parallel fiber synapse number per Purkinje neuron in cerebellar cortex of rats given postnatal binge alcohol exposure: Preliminary report. Alcoholism: Clinical and Experimental Research 21 (7): 1257–63.

Ladrague, P. (1901) Alcoolisme et enfants. Universite de Paris, Paris.

Leiner, H. C., Leiner, A. L., Dow, R. S. (1989) Reappraising the cerebellum: What does the hindbrain contribute to the forebrain? Behavioral Neurosciences 103: 998–1008.

Lemoine, P., Harousseau, H., Borteyru, J.-P., Menuet, J. C. (1968) Les enfants de parents alcooliques: Anomalies obervees, a propos de 127 cas. Ouest Medical 21: 476–82.

Lemoine, P., and Lemoine, P. (1992) Outcome of children of alcoholic mothers (study of 105 cases followed to adult age) and various prophylactic findings. Annales de Pediatrie 39 (4): 226–35.

Lou, H. C., Henriksen, L., Bruhn, P. (1984) Focal cerebral hypoperfusion in children with dysphasia and/or attention deficit disorder. Archives of Neurology 41 (8): 825–9.

Lou, H. C., Henriksen, L., Bruhn, P., Borner, H., Nielsen, J. B. (1989) Striatal dysfunction in attention deficit and hyperkinetic disorder. Archives of Neurology 46 (1): 48–52.

Maier, S. E., Chen, W.-J., West, J. R. (1996) The effects of timing and duration of alcohol exposure on development of the fetal brain. In: Fetal alcohol syndrome: From mechanism to prevention. Abel, E. L. (ed.). CRC Press, New York, pp. 27–50.

Manteuffel, M. D. (1996) Neurotransmitter function: Changes associated with in utero alcohol exposure. In: Fetal alcohol syndrome: From mechanism to prevention. Abel, E. L. (ed.). CRC Press, New York, pp. 171–89.

Matochik, J. A., Nordahl, T. E., Gross, M., Semple, W. E., King, A. C., Cohen, R. M., Zametkin, A. J. (1993) Effects of acute stimulant medication on cerebral metabolism in adults with hyperactivity. Neuropsychopharmacology 8 (4): 377–86.

Mattson, S. N., and Riley, E. P. (1995) Prenatal Exposure to Alcohol: What the Images Reveal. Alcohol Health and Research World—Imaging in Alcohol Research 19 (4): 273–78.

Mattson, S. N., and Riley, E. (1996) Brain anomalies in fetal alcohol syndrome. In: Fetal alcohol syndrome: From mechanism to prevention. Abel, E. L. (ed.). CRC Press, New York, pp. 51–68.

Mattson, S. N., Gramling, L., Delis, D. C., Jones, K. L., Riley, E. P. (1996a) Global–local processing in children prenatally exposed to alcohol. Child Neuropsychology 2: 165–75.

Mattson, S. N., Riley, E. P., Delis, D. C., Stern, C., Jones, K. L. (1996b) Verbal learning and memory in children with fetal alcohol syndrome. Alcoholism, Clinical and Experimental Research 20 (5): 810–6.

Mattson, S. N., Riley, E. P., Gramling, L., Delis, D. C., Jones, K. I. (1997) Heavy prenatal alcohol exposure with or without physical features of the Fetal Alcohol Syndrome leads to IQ deficits. Journal of Pediatrics 131: 718–21.

Mattson, S. N., Riley, E. P., Sowell, E. R., Jernigan, T. L., Sobel, D. F., Jones, K. L. (1996c) A decrease in the size of the basal ganglia in children with fetal alcohol syndrome. Alcoholism, Clinical and Experimental Research 20 (6): 1088–93.

May, P. A. (1995) A multiple-level, comprehensive approach to the prevention of fetal alcohol syndrome (FAS) and other alcohol-related birth defects (ARBD). International Journal of the Addictions 30 (12): 1549–602.

McDougle, C. J., Brodkin, E. S., Yeung, P. P., Naylor, S. T., Cohen, D. J., Price, L. H. (1995) Risperidone in adults with autism or pervasive developmental disorder. Journal of Child and Adolescent Psychopharmacology 4: 273–82.

McKee, L., and Blacklidge, V. (1981) An easy guide for caring parents. Sexuality and Socialization: A book for parents of people with mental handicaps. Planned Parenthood of Contra Costa, Walnut Creek, California.

Merzenich, M. M., Jenkins, W. M., Johnston, P., Schreiner, C., Miller, S. L., Tallal, P. (1996) Temporal processing deficits of language-learning impaired children ameliorated by training. Science 271 (5245): 77–81.

Miller, M. W., Chiaia, N. L., Rhoades, R. W. (1990) Intracellular recording and injection study of corticospinal neurons in the rat somatosensory cortex: Effect of prenatal exposure to ethanol. Journal of Comparative Neurology 297: 91–105.

Moore, D. B., Ruygrok, A. C., Walker, D. W., Heaton, M. B. (1997) Effects of prenatal ethanol exposure on parvalbumin-expressing GABAergic neurons in the adult rat medial septum. Alcoholism: Clinical and Experimental Research 21 (5): 849–56.

Morse, B. A., Miller, A. L., Cermak, S. A. (1995) Sensory processing in children with fetal alcohol syndrome [Abstract]. Alcoholism: Clinical and Experimental Research 19: 101a.

Nanson, J. L., and Hiscock, M. (1990) Attention deficits in children exposed to alcohol prenatally. Alcoholism: Clinical and Experimental Research 14 (5): 656–61.

O'Malley, K. D., and Barr, H. (1998). Fetal alcohol syndrome and seizure disorder. Canadian Journal of Psychiatry 43 (10): 1051.

O'Malley, K., and Hagerman, R. J. (1998) Clinical practice guidelines for pharmacological interventions with alcohol-affected children. Presented September 11, 1998, at NIH conference "Intervening with children affected by prenatal alcohol exposure," Bethesda, MD.

Papara-Nicholson, D., and Telford, I. R. (1957) Effects of alcohol on reproduction and fetal development in the guinea pig. Anatomical Record 127: 438–9.

Quintana, H., and Keshavan, M. (1995) Case study: Risperidone in children and adolescents with schizophrenia. Journal of the American Academy of Child and Adolescent Psychiatry 34 (10): 1292–6.

Ramanathan, E., Wilkemeyer, M. F., Mittal, B., Perides, G., Charness, C. (1996) Alcohol inhibits cell–cell adhesion mediated by human L1. Journal of Cell Biology 133: 381–90.

Riley, E. P. (1990) The long-term behavioral effects of prenatal alcohol exposure in rats. Alcoholism: Clinical and Experimental Research 14 (5): 670–3.

Riley, E. P., Barron, S., Driscoll, C. D., Hamlin, R. T. (1986) The effects of physostigmine on open-field behavior in rats exposed to alcohol prenatally. Alcoholism: Clinical and Experimental Research 10 (1): 50–3.

Riley, E. P., Mattson, S. N., Sowell, E. R., Jernigan, T. L., Sobel, D. F., Jones, K. L. (1995) Abnormalities of the corpus callosum in children prenatally exposed to alcohol. Alcoholism: Clinical and Experimental Research 19 (5): 1198–202.

Riley, K. (1997) The child with prenatal alcohol exposure in the classroom. Prevention Works (Colorado Alcohol and Drug Abuse Division) 5: 1–3.

Robe, L. B., Gromisch, D. S., Iosub, S. (1981) Symptoms of neonatal ethanol withdrawal. Currents in Alcoholism 8: 485–93.

Roebuck, T. M., Simmons, R. W., Mattson, S. N., Riley, E. P. (1998) Prenatal exposure to alcohol affects the ability to maintain posture balance. Alcoholism: Clinical and Experimental Research, 22(1): 252–8.

Rosett, H. L. (1980) A clinical perspective of the Fetal Alcohol Syndrome. Alcoholism: Clinical and Experimental Research 4 (2): 119–22.

Rouquette, J. (1957) Influence de l'intoxication alcoolique parentale sur le developpement physique et psychique des jeunes enfants. Ph.D. dissertation, University of Paris.

Rueckert, L., and Levy, J. (1996) Further evidence that the callosum is involved in sustaining attention. Neuropsychologia 34 (9): 927–35.

Sampson, P. D., Kerr, B., Carmichael Olson, H., Streissguth, A. P., Hunt, E., Barr, H. M. (1997) The effects of prenatal alcohol exposure on adolescent cognitive processing: A speed-accuracy trade off. Intelligence 24 (2): 329–53.

Sampson, P. D., Streissguth, A., Bookstein, F. L., Little, R. E., Clarren, S. K., Dehaene, D., Hanson, J. W.,

Graham, J. M. (1997) Incidence of fetal alcohol syndrome and prevalence of alcohol-related neurodevelopmental disorder. Teratology 56: 317–26.

Sandor, S., and Elias, S. (1968) The influence of ethyl-alcohol on the development of the chick embryo. Revue Roumaine d'Embryologie Cytologie Serie d'Embryologie 5: 51–76.

Scharfenaker, S., O'Connor, R., Stackhouse, T., Braden, M., Hickman, L., Gray, K. (1996) An integrated approach to intervention. In: Fragile X syndrome: Diagnosis, treatment, and research. Hagerman, R. J., and Cronister, A. (eds.). 2nd ed. Johns Hopkins University Press, Baltimore, pp. 349–411.

Shevell, M., and Schreiber, R. (1997) Pemoline-associated hepatic failure: A critical analysis of the literature. Pediatric Neurology 16: 14–16.

Shinnar, S. (1997) Tiagabine. Seminars in Pediatric Neurology 4 (1): 24–33.

Simeon, J. G., Carrey, N. J., Wiggins, D. M., Milin, R. P., Hosenbocus, S. N. (1995) Risperidone effects in treatment-resistant adolescents: Preliminary case reports. Journal of Child and Adolescent Psychopharmacology 5 (1): 69–79.

Snyder, J., Nanson, J., Snyder, R. E., Block, G. W. (1997) Stimulant efficacy in children with FAS. In: The challenge of fetal alcohol syndrome: Overcoming secondary disabilities. Streissguth, A., and Kanter, J. (eds.). University of Washington Press, Seattle, pp. 64–77.

Soby, J. M. (1994) Prenatal exposure to drugs/alcohol: Characteristics and educational implications of fetal alcohol syndrome and cocain/polydrug effects. Thomas, Springfield, Illinois.

Sowell, E. R., Jernigan, T. L., Mattson, S. N., Riley, E. P., Sobel, D. F., Jones, K. L. (1996) Abnormal development of the cerebellar vermis in children prenatally exposed to alcohol: Size reduction in lobules I–V. Alcoholism: Clinical and Experimental Research 20 (1): 31–4.

Spohr, H. L. (1996) Fetal alcohol syndrome in adolescence: Long-term perspective of children diagnosed in infancy. In: Alcohol, pregnancy, and the developing child. Spohr, H.-L., and Steinhausen, H.-C. (eds.). Cambridge University Press, New York, pp. 207–26.

Spohr, H. L., and Steinhausen, H. C. (1987) Follow-up studies of children with fetal alcohol syndrome. Neuropediatrics 18 (1): 13–17.

Spohr, H. L., Willms, J., Steinhausen, H. C. (1993) Prenatal alcohol exposure and long-term developmental consequences. Lancet 341 (8850): 907–10.

Steinhausen, H. C., Willms, J., Spohr, H. L. (1993) Long-term psychopathological and cognitive outcome of children with fetal alcohol syndrome. Journal of the American Academy of Child and Adolescent Psychiatry 32 (5): 990–4.

Stockard, C. R. (1914) The artificial production of eye abnormalities in the chick embryo. Anatomical Records 8: 33–41.

Stoler, J. M., Huntington, K. S., Peterson, C. M., Peterson, K. P., Daniel, P., Aboagye, K. K., Lieberman, E., Ryan, L., Holmes, L. B. (1998) The prenatal detection of significant alcohol exposure with maternal blood markers. Journal of Pediatrics 133: 346–52.

Stratton, K. R., Howe, C. J., Battaglia, F. C. (1996) Fetal alcohol syndrome: Diagnosis, epidemiology, prevention, and treatment. National Academy Press, Washington, D.C.

Streissguth, A. P. (1983) Alcohol and pregnancy: An overview and an update. Substance and Alcohol Actions/Misuse 4 (2–3): 149–73.

Streissguth, A. P. (1994) A long-term perspective of FAS. Alcohol Health and Research World 18 (1): 74–81.

Streissguth, A. P. (1997) Fetal alcohol syndrome: A guide for families and communities. Brookes, Baltimore.

Streissguth, A. P., Herman, C. S., Smith, D. W. (1978) Intelligence, behavior, and dysmorphogenesis in the fetal alcohol syndrome: A report on 20 patients. Journal of Pediatrics 92: 363–7.

Streissguth, A. P., Herman, C. S., Smith, D. W. (1980) Teratogenic effects of alcohol in humans and laboratory animals. Science 209 (4454): 353–61.

Streissguth, A. P., Darby, B. L., Barr, H. M., Smith, J. R., Martin, D. C. (1983) Comparison of drinking and smoking patterns during pregnancy over a six-year interval. American Journal of Obstetrics and Gynecology 145 (6): 716–24.

Streissguth, A. P., Barr, H. M., Sampson, P. D., Darby, B., Martin, D. C. (1989) IQ at age 4 in relation to maternal alcohol use and smoking during pregnancy. Developmental Psychology 25 (1): 3–11.

Streissguth, A. P., Barr, H. M., Sampson, P. D. (1990) Moderate prenatal alcohol exposure: Effects on child IQ and learning problems at age 7½ years. Alcoholism: Clinical and Experimental Research 14 (5): 662–9.

Streissguth, A. P., Aase, J. M., Clarren, S. K., Randels, S. P., LaDue, R. A., Smith, D. F. (1991) Fetal alcohol syndrome in adolescents and adults. Journal of the American Medical Association 265 (15): 1961–7.

Streissguth, A. P., Barr, H. M., Sampson, P. D., Bookstein, F. L. (1994) Prenatal alcohol and offspring development: The first fourteen years. Drug and Alcohol Dependence 36 (2): 89–99.

Streissguth, A. P., Moon-Jordan, A., Clarren, S. K. (1995) Alcoholism in four patients with fetal alcohol syndrome: Recommendations for treatment. Alcoholism Treatment Quarterly 13 (2): 89–103.

Streissguth, A. P., Barr, H. M., Kogan, J., Bookstein, F. L. (1996a) Understanding the occurrence of secondary disabilities in clients with fetal alcohol syndrome (FAS) and fetal alcohol effects (FAE). University of Washington School of Medicine, Seattle.

Streissguth, A. P., Bookstein, F., Barr, H. M., Press, S., Sampson, P. (1998) A fetal alcohol behavior scale. Alcoholism: Clinical and Experimental Research 22 (2): 325–33.

Stromland, K. (1985) Ocular abnormalities in the fetal alcohol syndrome. Acta Ophthalmologica — Supplement 171: 1–50.

Stromland, K. (1987) Ocular involvement in the fetal alcohol syndrome. Survey of Ophthalmology 31 (4): 277–84.

Stromland, K., and Hellstrom, A. (1996) Fetal alcohol syndrome — an ophthalmological and socioeducational prospective study. Pediatrics 97 (6, Pt. 1): 845–50.

Sulik, K. K., Johnston, M. C., Webb, M. A. (1981) Fetal alcohol syndrome: Embryogenesis in a mouse model. Science 214 (4523): 936–8.

Sullivan, W. C. (1899) A note on the influence of maternal inebriety on the offspring. Journal of Mental Science 45: 489–504.

Swayze, V. W., II, Johnson, V. P., Hanson, J. W., Piven, J., Sato, Y., Giedd, J. N., Mosnik, D., Andreasen, N. C. (1997) Magnetic resonance imaging of brain anomalies in fetal alcohol syndrome. Pediatrics 99 (2): 232–40.

Tallal, P., Miller, S. L., Bedi, G., Byma, G., Wang, X., Nagarajan, S. S., Schreiner, C., Jenkins, W. M., Merzenich, M. M. (1996) Language comprehension in language-learning impaired children improved with acoustically modified speech. Science 271 (5245): 81–4.

Tanner-Halverson, P. (1997) A demonstration classroom for young children with FAS. In: The challenge of FAS: Overcoming secondary disabilities. Streissguth, A., and Kanter, J. (eds.). University of Washington Press, Seattle, pp. 73–83.

Taylor, C. L., Jones, K. L., Jones, M. C., Kaplan, G. W. (1994) Incidence of renal anomalies in children prenatally exposed to ethanol. Pediatrics 94 (2, Pt. 1): 209–12.

Thomsen, P. H. (1997) Child and adolescent obcessive-compulsive disorder treated with citalopram: Findings from an open trial of 23 cases. Journal of Child and Adolescent Psychopharmacology 7 (3): 157–66.

Tsai, G., and Coyle, J. T. (1998) The role of glutamatergic neurotrans—mission in the pathophysiology of alcoholism. Annual Reviews of Medicine 49: 173–84.

Uecker, A., and Nadel, L. (1996) Spatial locations gone awry: Object and spatial memory deficits in children with fetal alcohol syndrome. Neuropsychologia 34 (3): 209–23.

Ulleland, C. N. (1972) The offspring of alcoholic mothers. Annals of the New York Academy of Sciences 197: 167–9.

Ulleland, C. N., Wennberg, R. P., Igo, R. P., Smith, N. J. (1970) The offspring of alcoholic mothers. Pediatric Research 4: 474.

Vaidya, C. J., Austin, G., Kirkorian, G., Ridlehuber, H. W., Desmond, J. E., Glover, G. H., Gabrieli, J. D. E. (1998) Selective effects of methylphenidate in attention deficit hyperactivity disorder: A functional magnetic resonance study. Proceedings of the National Academy of Science. USA 95: 14494–9.

Vanden Borre, R., Vermote, R., Buttiens, M., Thiry, P., Dierick, G., Geutjens, J., Sieben, G., Heylen, S. (1993) Risperidone as add-on therapy in behavioural disturbances in mental retardation: A double-blind placebo-controlled cross-over study. Acta Psychiatrica Scandinavica 87 (3): 167–71.

Van Dyke, D. C., Mackay, L., Ziaylek, E. N. (1982) Management of severe feeding dysfunction in children with fetal alcohol syndrome. Clinical Pediatrics 21 (6): 336–9.

Volkow, N., Wang, G.-J., Fowler, J. S. L., Angrist, B., Hitzemann, R., Lieberman, J., Pappas, N. (1997) Effects of methylphenidate on regional brain glucose metabolism in humans: Relationship to dopamine D2 receptors. American Journal of Psychiatry 154: 50–55.

Walpole, I., Zubrick, S., Pontre, J., Lawrence, C. (1991) Low to moderate maternal alcohol use before and during pregnancy, and neurobehavioural outcome in the newborn infant. Developmental Medicine and Child Neurology 33 (10): 875–83.

Wang, P. P., and Bellugi, U. (1993) Williams syndrome, Down syndrome, and cognitive neuroscience. American Journal of Diseases of Children 147 (11): 1246–51.

Watson, S., and Gresham, F. M. (eds.) (1998) Handbook of child behavior therapy. Plenum Press, New York.

Weathersby, R. T., Becker, H. C., Hale, R. L. (1994) Reduced sensitivity to the effects of clonidine on ethanol-stimulated locomotor activity in adult mouse offspring prenatally exposed to ethanol. Alcohol 11 (6): 517–22.

West, J. R. (1986) Long-term effects of developmental exposure to alcohol. Neurotoxicology 7 (2): 245–56.

Wigal, S. B., Amsel, A., Wilcox, R. E. (1990) Fetal ethanol exposure diminishes hippocampal beta-adrenergic receptor density while sparing muscarinic receptors during development. Developmental Brain Research 55 (2): 161–9.

Zubieta, J. K., and Alessi, N. E. (1993) Is there a role of serotonin in the disruptive behavior disorders? A literature review. Journal of Child and Adolescent Psychopharmacology 3: 11–35.

RESOURCES

Organizations/Resource Centers

National Organization of Fetal Alcohol Syndrome (NOFAS)
1819 H Street, NW, Suite 750
Washington, DC 20006
telephone: (202) 785-4585
fax: (202) 466-6456
e-mail: NOFAS@erols.com
http://www.nofas.org/material.htm

Family Empowerment Network: Supporting Families Affected by Fetal Alcohol Syndrome and Effects
University of Wisconsin
519 Lowell Hall
610 Langdon Street
Madison, WI 53703
telephone: (800) 462-5254
fax: (608) 262-6590
e-mail fen@mail.dsc.wisc.edu

This organization publishes the *Fen Den* newsletter and provides support, conferences, and training for families.

Fetal Alcohol Information Service
P.O. Box 95597
Seattle, WA 98145-2597

This organization publishes the *Iceberg* newsletter, which includes information regarding education and new developments about FAS and related conditions.

National Association for Perinatal Addiction Research and Education (NAPARE)
11 E. Hubbard Street 200
Chicago, IL 60611
Ira J. Chasnoff, President

Alcohol and Drug 24-Hour Help Line
telephone: (800) 562-1240

This is sponsored by the Washington State Substance Abuse Coalition.

Fetal Alcohol Education Program
Boston University School of Medicine
1975 Maine Street
Concord, MA 01742
telephone: (978) 369-7713

This program carries out training and education and also provides materials, including articles and books regarding fetal alcohol syndrome and related disorders.

FAS/FAE Information Service Canadian Center on Substance Abuse
75 Albert Street, Suite 300
Ottawa, Ontario, Canada K1P5E7
telephone: (800) 559-4514 (within Canada); (613) 235-4048 (outside Canada)

This service provides English and French information regarding fetal alcohol syndrome and related conditions and links support groups, projects, and resource centers.

FAS Family Resource Institute (FAS*FRI)
P.O. Box 2525
Lynnwood, WA 98036
telephone: (800) 999-3429
fax: (253) 531-2668
e-mail: vicfas@hotmail.com

Fetal Alcohol and Drug Unit
University of Washington
180 Nickerson Street, Suite 309
Seattle, WA 98109
telephone: (206) 543-7155

This center carries out clinical evaluations, conducts research, and disseminates information on fetal alcohol syndrome and related disorders.

Child Development Unit
University of Colorado Health Sciences
Center—Child Development Unit, B-140

The Children's Hospital
1056 East 19th Avenue
Denver, CO 80218
telephone: (303) 861-6630
fax: (303) 764-8086

This center offers clinical evaluations and treatment programs and also conducts research regarding fetal alcohol syndrome and related disorders.

National Clearing House for Alcohol and Drug Information (NCAID)
P.O. Box 2345
Rockville, MD 20852
telephone: (800) 729-6686

National Council on Alcoholism and Drug Dependence (NCADD)
12 West 21 Street
New York, NY 10010

National Perinatal Information Center
One State Street, Suite 102
Providence, RI 02908

General Resources

Association for Retarded Citizens of the United States (ARC)
National Headquarters
2501 Avenue J
Arlington, TX 76006
telephone: (817) 261-6003

This is an association in support of individuals with mental retardation.

March of Dimes Birth Defects Foundation
National Headquarters
1275 Mamaroneck Avenue
White Plains, NY 10605
telephone: (888) MO-DIMES; (206) 624-1373

This national organization funds research and also disseminates educational materials.

General Reading

Dorris, M. (1989) The broken cord. New York: HarperCollins.
Kleinfeld, J. K., and Wescott, S. (eds.). (1993) Fantastic Antone Succeeds! Experiences in educating children with fetal alcohol syndrome. Fairbanks: University of Alaska Press.
Melner, J., Shackelford, J., Hargrove, E., Daulton, D. (1997) Resources related to children and their families affected by alcohol and other drugs. 3rd ed. NECTAS. Chapel Hill, North Carolina. (919) 962-2001.
Steinmetz, G. (1992) The preventable tragedy: Fetal alcohol syndrome. National Geographic 181 (2): 36–9.
Streissguth, A. P., and Kanter, J. (eds.). (1997) The challenge of fetal alcohol syndrome: Overcoming secondary disabilities. Seattle: University of Washington Press.
Streissguth, A. (1997) Fetal alcohol syndrome: A guide for families and communities. Baltimore, MD: Brookes.

Video Information

Clinical Diagnosis of Fetal Alcohol Syndrome by John Aase (1994), available from Flora and Company Multimedia, P.O. Box 8263, Albuquerque, NM 87198. Telephone: (505) 255-9988.

The Fabulous FAS Quiz Show, published by the March of Dimes Foundation, Washington State Department of Health and State Superintendent of Public Instruction (1994) Available by calling (206) 624-1373. This video is a teacher's guide that also targets middle school students regarding prevention of babies born with FAS.

David with FAS (1996), available from Films for the Humanities and Sciences,

P.O. Box 2053, Princeton, NJ 08543-2053, or call (800) 257-5126. This video is about the life of David Vandenbrink, a 21-year-old man with FAS and multiple problems.

Honor of All (1986). Available from North American Public Broadcasting Consortium, P.O. Box 8311, Lincoln, NE 68501. It documents the Canadian Indian Reserve as it establishes sobriety.

What's Wrong with My Child? (1992). This was produced for television for 20/20 in New York with the American Broadcasting Company and includes interviews of families and children with FAS. It also includes an interview with writer Michael Dorris and his adopted son, who has FAS. It can be obtained by calling (800) CALL-ABC.

Slides

Alcohol, Pregnancy and the Fetal Alcohol Syndrome (1994), developed by A. P. Streissguth and R. E. Little. This is a package of 79 slides and accompanying text giving a comprehensive overview of fetal alcohol syndrome, including dysmorphology, current research, and public health issues. Telephone: (800) 432-8433.

FAS/FAE Web sites

The National Organization on Fetal Alcohol Syndrome
http://www.nofas.org/material.htm

The ARC's Q&A on FAS
http://TheArc.org/faqs/fas.html

FAS/FAE Information Service
http://www.ccsa.ca/fasgen.htm

FAS Information
http://www.geocities.com/HotSprings/Spa/2131/fas.html

Clean Water International, an organization for FAS
http://www.shadeslanding.com/clean-water/about.html

A case history of an FAS child and information on FAS
http://www.pclink.com/jwebb

National resources for FAS/FAE
http://mirconnect.com/specificnational/fas.html

FAS links
http://www.irsc.org/fas.htm

"Educating Children with FAS/FAE"—Guides for educators
http://www.taconic.net/seminars

"Resource appendix of Fetal Alcohol Syndrome"—Organizations, support groups, videos, and slides
http://www.pbrookes.com/catalog/extras/streiapp.htm

National Crime Prevention Council—Studies of the behavior patterns of FAS/FAE children
http://www.acbr.com/fas/offpro_e.htm

"FAS/E Symptoms," FAS Family Resource Institute—Behavioral symptoms of adolescents with FAS/E through the eyes of parents
http://www.accessone.com/~delindam

"Awareness of Chronic Health Conditions: What the Teacher Should Know," British Columbia Ministry of Education, Skills and Training.
http://www.educ.gov.bc.ca/.specialed/www/awareness/contents.html

Parents and Professional Discussion Group

FASlink

An e-mail discussion group dedicated to exchanging information and offering support relating to fetal alcohol syndrome issues. To join or subscribe to this discussion, send an e-mail message to <list@ccsa.ca> with the message: join faslink. Put this command in the body of the message, not in the subject field. Do not attach a signature, because the listserv will try to interpret your signature as a command.

You will then receive a welcome message notifying you that you have been added to the discussion group ("list"). A copy of each message sent to the list will then be forwarded to the e-mail address given. If you want messages sent to a different address, use the command: JOIN faslink <e-mail-address>.

To send a message to the list after you have joined, send your e-mail message to: faslink@ccsa.ca.

2

Fragile X Syndrome

Although fragile X syndrome (FXS) is the most common inherited cause of mental retardation that is known, it also causes a broad spectrum of involvement, ranging from mild emotional problems or learning disabilities through all levels of mental retardation (Hagerman, 1996b). It affects both males and females, but females are less affected because they have two X chromosomes; the second X chromosome compensates for the mutated X. The mutation that causes FXS is located on the bottom end of the X chromosome at Xq27.3.

The history of FXS began in 1943, when Martin and Bell first reported a large pedigree with 11 retarded males and a few mildly involved females. They reported that this pedigree represented a sex-linked or X-linked cause of mental retardation that affected males more severely than females (Martin and Bell, 1943). It was not until 1982 that cytogenetic studies showed that this family had FXS (Richards and Webb, 1982). It has been known since the last century, however, that there are approximately 24% more retarded males than females (Johnson, 1897), but it was not until the 1900s that the X-chromosomal causes of mental retardation became apparent. Although Penrose (1938) noted that more retarded males than retarded females were institutionalized, he thought that this was related to aggression in males, which more frequently precipitated institutionalization. It was Lehrke (1974) who argued that the preponderance of mentally retarded males was due to X-linked genes. Today we know that over 100 genes on the X chromosome cause mental retardation and that approximately 30% of cases of X-linked mental retardation are secondary to FXS (Lubs et al., 1996; Sherman, 1996).

Neurodevelopmental Disorders: Diagnosis and Treatment, by Randi Jenssen Hagerman. New York: Oxford University Press, 1999. © Oxford University Press, Inc.

The history of the development of the fragile X field is an exciting story that has been recounted by Turner (1983) and Sherman (1996). Lubs (1969) reported a family with four retarded males who demonstrated a cytogenetic marker or break on the bottom end of the X chromosome. This report, however, was forgotten, although others in the 1970s also began to report families with X-linked mental retardation and a cytogenetic marker (Escalante and Frota-Pessona, 1973; Giraud et al., 1976; Harvey et al., 1977). Grant Sutherland in Australia demonstrated the marker in a family with mental retardation but subsequently found that the marker disappeared when a different tissue culture media was used to grow the cells before cytogenetic examination. After further studies, Sutherland reported in 1977 that the cell culture media had to be deficient in folic acid to stimulate expression of the fragile site on the bottom end of the X chromosome (Sutherland, 1977). This and subsequent reports (Sutherland, 1979; Sutherland et al., 1985) stimulated others throughout the world to look for the fragile site using appropriate tissue culture media. Subsequently, numerous reports of this disorder appeared in the 1980s. It was named FXS because of the fragile site or marker on the bottom end of the X chromosome. In 1978, Turner and colleagues showed that macroorchidism (large testicles) was also associated with the mental retardation that demonstrated the fragile site on the X chromosome.

The original Martin and Bell pedigree of 1943 was reevaluated in 1982 and found to demonstrate typical physical features of FXS, including prominent ears, macroorchidism, and the fragile site on the X chromosome (Richards and Webb, 1982). In the 1980s, the typical physical and behavioral characteristics associated with FXS were described, but in 1991 the field advanced significantly with the discovery of the Fragile X Mental Retardation 1 gene (FMR1) (Verkerk et al., 1991).

FMR1 MUTATION

In the spring of 1991, laboratories in France, England, and Australia identified a trinucleotide repeat expansion, CGG, that was present in individuals who were carriers and also affected by FXS (Bell et al., 1991; Vincent et al., 1991; Yu et al., 1991). Individuals who were affected were found to be hypermethylated in this region. Subsequently, an international collaboration among the laboratories of Ben Oostra in the Netherlands, David Nelson in Texas, and Steve Warren in Atlanta cloned the fragile X gene and named it FMR1 (Verkerk et al., 1991). At the 5' end of the gene is a CGG expansion that was subsequently found to be transcribed but not translated into protein. The length of the CGG region was found to be highly variable in normal individuals, with a range of between 6 and 54 CGG repeats (Fu et al., 1991). The average number of repeats in the normal population is 29 to 30 (Brown, 1996b; Snow et al., 1993). Individuals who are carriers for fragile X and do not have cognitive involvement have 55 to approximately 200 CGG repeats (premutation) that are usually unmethylated, and the protein produced from the FMR1 gene is normal (Devys et al., 1993). Individuals with more than 230 CGG repeats (full mutation) usually have methylation of the gene, which prevents transcription and translation of the gene into the FMR1 protein (FMRP).

The CGG repeat expansion is usually punctuated by an AGG repeat at every 9 to 10 CGG repeats (Zhang et al., 1995). These AGG anchors appear to provide stability of the CGG repeat during replication. Carriers with the premutation are usually missing one or more AGG anchor. Approximately two-thirds of males with the premutation have no AGG anchors, and one-third have only one AGG anchor at the 5' end of the repeat (Zhang et al., 1995). Individuals who have 40 to approximately 55 repeats are considered to be in the gray zone (Eichler et al., 1994) because instability may be present, particularly if AGG anchors are missing. The smallest premutation size in a mother that has expanded to the full mutation within one generation is 59 CGG repeats (Nolin et al., 1996). Expansion to a full mutation only occurs when a female with the premutation passes the mutation on to her offspring. Expansion to a full mutation does not occur when a male with the premutation passes it on. Carrier males will pass on the premutation to all of their daughters but to none of their sons. The daughters of males with less than 80 CGG repeats usually demonstrate a small expansion over their father's CGG repeat number, although it always remains within the premutation range (Nolin et al., 1996). The daughters of males with 80 to 99 repeats have a similar likelihood to expand (44%) or contract (34%); however, daughters of males with 100 repeats tend to contract in size (67%) (Nolin et al., 1996).

The offspring of mothers with the premutation almost always have an expansion of the repeat number. The higher the number of CGG repeats in the mother, the greater the risk of expansion to the full mutation range in the offspring (see Table 2.1). Essentially, women with 90 or more CGG repeats expand to a full mutation in almost 100% of cases. There is a low risk of contraction, and in three of 393 cases there was contraction of the CGG repeat allele to the normal range (Nolin et al., 1996). Individuals with a gray zone allele between 40 and 49 CGG repeats are unstable in 7.7% of cases; that is, they may experience expansion of the repeat number, although the expansion is usually minimal, and it has never been reported to expand to the full mutation size (Nolin et al., 1996). Individuals with a gray zone allele between 50 and 60 repeats are unstable in 25% of cases (Nolin et al., 1996).

Individuals who are diagnosed with FXS through cytogenetic testing should have testing with molecular methodology, including polymerase chain reaction (PCR) and Southern blot testing to document the presence of the mutation at FMR1 and the methylation status of the mutation (Brown, 1996b; Gringras and Barnicoat, 1998). Approximately 5% of individuals who were cytogenetically positive and identified during the 1980s were found to be negative on DNA testing and did not demonstrate the mutation at FMR1 (Hagerman, 1992). Some of the individuals who are negative for the FMR1 mutation but cytogenetically positive may have the FRAXE or the FRAXF mutation (Jacky, 1996). The FRAXE mutation also has a CGG repeat and is slightly distal to the FMR1 mutation (Nelson, 1998). It is associated with a mild degree of mental retardation in most cases,

TABLE 2.1:   Risk of Expansion to the Full Mutation in the Offspring of Mothers with the Premutation

Maternal repeats	Expansion to full/Total (No.)	Offspring with full mutation (%)
56–59	3/22	13.4
60–69	7/34	20.6
70–79	59/102	57.8
80–89	78/107	72.9
90–99	83/88	94.3
100–109	81/81	100
110–119	46/47	97.8
120–129	24/24	100
130–199	26/27	96.3

Data were derived from Nolin et al. (1996) and represent the combined figures of Nolin et al. (1996), Fu et al. (1991), and Snow et al. (1993).

although the physical phenotype is quite variable (Brown, 1996a; Mulley et al., 1995; Russo et al., 1998). The *FRAXF* locus is approximately 600 kb distal to the *FRAXE* locus, and it also is a CGG trinucleotide repeat; however, the presence of the full mutation at this location is not consistently associated with mental retardation (Parrish et al., 1994).

The prevalence of the *FMR1* premutation has been documented to be 1 in 259 women in the general population (Rousseau et al., 1995). Rousseau's study included more than 10,000 women in Quebec who donated blood to a blood bank. Spence et al. (1996) found a similar prevalence in a smaller study of 474 women who had no family history of mental retardation and who were screened at the time of pregnancy. Three of 474 were positive for the premutation, with 60 or greater repeats. In a screening of males in the general population, approximately 1 in 700 carried the premutation (Rousseau et al., 1996).

The prevalence of the full mutation in the general population is uncertain because of limited screening studies. In previous cytogenetic reports, approximately 1 in 1,250 males and 1 in 2,500 females in the general population have mental retardation and FXS (Webb et al., 1986). Subsequent molecular studies, however, decreased this prevalence figure to 1 in 4,000 since several cytogenetically positive individuals did not demonstrate the full mutation (Turner et al., 1996). A similar prevalence rate of 1 in 4,000 was found in Australia when males with significant mental retardation and typical physical features of FXS were screened (Slaney et al., 1995; Turner et al., 1996). These studies did not evaluate, however, the full spectrum of involvement in FXS, including those who present with higher cognitive abilities or simply learning disabilities, because only those with significant mental retardation were screened. A recent study in the Netherlands demonstrated the prevalence of FXS at approximately 1 in 6,000 for males (de Vries et al., 1997). This study screened five institutions and 16 special schools for individuals with mental retardation. It was estimated that at present in the Netherlands more than 50% of individuals with FXS are undiagnosed (de Vries et al., 1997).

DELETIONS AND POINT MUTATIONS

It is possible to have the fragile X phenotype without a CGG expansion in the full mutation range. A deletion of the *FMR1* gene would lead to no FMRP, and it is the absence of FMRP that causes the phenotype of FXS. In fact, it is theoretically possible for a deletion patient to have a more severe phenotype since individuals with a full mutation would have a period early on in fetal development when methylation has not yet occurred and the presence of FMRP would exist for a short period of time in utero until methylation takes place. Individuals with a deletion, however, would never have the presence of FMRP in utero (Hirst et al., 1995). Deletions can also cause a more severe phenotype when more genetic material than the *FMR1* gene is deleted. An example is the case reported by Quan et al. (1995b) in which a patient had typical features of FXS in addition to anal atresia and the deletion involved the *FMR1* gene and a region more proximal to this gene.

The presence of repetitive CGG sequences within the premutation range or the full mutation range causes a hot spot for deletions (de Graaff et al., 1995). Although many patients with a typical fragile X phenotype have been reported with a large deletion that removes the *FMR1* gene (Birot et al., 1996; Gedeon et al., 1992; Tarleton et al., 1993), there are also cases of patients who have a deletion of only part of the *FMR1* gene and still have typical phenotypic features (Gu et al., 1994; Hart et al., 1995; Hirst et al., 1995; Meijer et al., 1994; Quan et al., 1995a; Trottier et al., 1994; Wohrle et al., 1992). Deletions have also been reported in females who have typical features of FXS, including mental retardation (Clarke et al., 1992; Schmidt, 1992). Grønskov et al. (1997) reported a female who had deletion of the CGG repeat plus minimal flanking markers; she produced normal levels of FMRP, even though her other X chromosome had a large terminal deletion without the *FMR1* gene. Therefore, the absence of the CGG repeats in this case did not block protein production from the *FMR1* gene. However, deletion of a 1.6-Kb area proximal to the CGG repeat of the *FMR1* gene, thought to contain a promoter region, caused absence of FMRP in four retarded males in a family, in addition to other typical features of FXS (Meijer et al., 1994).

It is also possible to have the FXS phenotype with a point mutation within *FMR1*. This was reported in an individual who had severe mental retardation and remarkable macroorchidism when a T-to-A point mutation caused an isoleucine to aspartate amino acid change in the second KH domain within the FMRP (de Boulle et al., 1993). Subsequently, two additional patients who have a typical

FXS phenotype were described without a CGG expansion. One patient had a single de novo nucleotide deletion leading to a frameshift and premature translational stop, which led to an absence of the normal FMRP (Lugenbeel et al., 1995). The second patient had a two-base-pair change, which led to the loss of exon 2 and premature termination of the protein, also leading to an absence of FMRP and the FXS phenotype (Lugenbeel et al., 1995). Wang and colleagues (1997) have reported three patients who have a point mutation leading to deletion of exon 10 and premature termination of translation leading to the typical phenotype of FXS.

FMRP, FXR1, AND FXR2

Fragile X syndrome is caused by the absence or reduction of the FMR1 protein (FMRP). There are 17 exons within the FMR1 gene, but the start codon for translation of the FMR1 message into protein is actually 69 base pairs after the CGG repetitive sequence (Oostra, 1996). Therefore, the CGG repeats are not included in the FMRP structure. A variety of alternative splicing of the FMR1 mRNA message exists, such that there are approximately 12 isoforms of FMRP (Ashley et al., 1993). There do not appear to be significant tissue differences in the presence of isoforms of FMRP (Verkerk et al., 1993). The structure of FMRP includes two KH domains, which are regions of protein structure that are typical of RNA binding proteins (Imbert et al., 1998). In addition, an RGG box is present, which is also typical for nuclear RNA binding proteins. Without the presence of the RGG box, FMRP cannot bind RNA (Siomi et al., 1993). FMRP binds to approximately 4% of human fetal brain messages, including its own message (Ashley et al., 1993).

Within the structure of FMRP there is a nuclear transport signal and also a nuclear export signal (Warren, 1997). Therefore, FMRP travels from the cytoplasm into the nucleus, and it has been shown to pick up RNA messages and then move into the cytoplasm and bind to ribosomes (Khandjian et al., 1995; Warren, 1996; Imbert et al., 1998). FMRP appears to regulate translation of multiple messages in conjunction with two other fragile X–related proteins, FXR1 and FXR2 (Imbert et al., 1998; Liu et al., 1996). The amino acid sequences of FMR1, FXR1, and FXR2 are very similar, including the presence of KH domains and an RGG box. FXR1 and FXR2 are encoded by autosomal genes located at 3q28 and 17p13.1, respectively (Coy et al., 1995; Siomi et al., 1995; Zhang et al., 1995). Although the expression of FXR1 and FXR2 proteins is normal in patients with FXS, it appears that FMRP requires the presence of FXR1 and FXR2 to regulate translation at the ribosome (Liu et al., 1996). It is postulated that a mutation at FXR1 and FXR2 may cause an FXS-like phenotype, but this has not been documented. An important future goal is to identify the mRNA messages that appear to be regulated by FMRP, FXR1, and FXR2. The lack of FMRP probably leads to dysfunction in the translation of these messages to which it binds, and the lack of these additional proteins may cause the pleiomorphic phenotype which is typical of FXS and described later.

Recent studies of the severely affected patient reported by de Boulle et al. (1993) who has a point mutation in the KH domain region have shown that the mutated FMRP binds to mRNAs but does not associate with translating ribosomes (Feng et al., 1997a). It appears, therefore, that the severe phenotype is caused by the sequestration of the FMRP-bound mRNAs from their normal pathway of translation. A more typical patient with FXS who is lacking FMRP may have these same mRNAs partially translated by an alternative system instead of completely sequestered (Feng et al., 1997a).

Animal and human fetal studies have demonstrated that FMR1 RNA expression is widespread in multiple tissues, with the highest transcription rates in brain, placenta, testes, cartilage, lungs, and kidneys (Abitbol et al., 1993; Hinds et al., 1993). Lower expression was found in liver, skeletal muscle, and pancreas, with an unusual mRNA transcript in the heart. In human fetuses of 9 weeks, FMR1 RNA expression was generally seen in proliferating and migrating tissues within the CNS, but in the 25-week human fetus, expression was most dense in the cholinergic neurons of the nucleus basalis magnocellularis, in the pyramidal neurons of the hippocampus, and in the cerebellum (Abitbol et al., 1993). These findings in the normal human fetus are important because the cholinergic neurons innervate the limbic system and some of the phenotypic expression in FXS involves emotional difficulties that are related to the function of the limbic system. The cerebellum is important for sensory processing, attention, motor coordination, and even complex learning, all of which are problematic in patients with FXS. As described later in this chapter, the hippocampus is a very important brain structure for both memory and emotional regulation; in individuals with FXS, this structure, among others, is larger than in normal patients (Reiss et al., 1994).

Detailed neuroanatomic studies in humans and rats show FMRP associated with the polysomes in dendrites and dendritic spines, suggesting that FMRP plays a role in the translation of proteins related to dendritic function (Feng et al., 1997b). FMRP was present in large and small caliber dendrites, dendritic branch points, at the origin of spine necks and in the spine heads (Feng et al., 1997b). Very little staining for FMRP was seen in axons because axon terminals do not have ribosomes; therefore, the function of FMRP is mainly postsynaptic. Weiler et al. (1997) have shown that synaptic stimulation of metabotropic neurons leads to rapid synthesis of FMRP. They hypothesize that FMRP production then regulates structural changes of the synapse and dendrite that are important for normal maturation of synaptic connections. Feng et al. (1997b) speculate that altered protein synthesis in the dendrites and spines of patients with FXS causes their mental retardation.

In studies of fetuses with the *FMR1* mutation, chorionic villi sampling (CVS) at 11 weeks demonstrated lack of methylation of the *FMR1* full mutation with documentation of gene transcription; however, with fetal tissues obtained at 13 weeks, complete methylation of *FMR1* was seen with no mRNA expression (Sutcliffe et al., 1992). Delayed methylation past 13 weeks in a fetus with the full mutation could conceivably lead to milder clinical involvement because of the prolonged presence of FMRP in early gestation.

PHYSICAL PHENOTYPE

Facial Features

The broad spectrum of involvement in FXS is related to the level of FMRP that is present in patients. In addition, background gene effects can cause variability in the presentation of both physical and behavioral features. Some clinicians depend on the typical facial features in FXS to suggest the diagnosis, although these features may not be present in 25 to 30% of children. The classic facial features associated with FXS include a long face, prominent ears, and a prominent chin, or prognanthism. The long face and prognanthism are more common after puberty (Figures 2.1 and 2.2). Prominent ears are seen in approximately 70%, and they show cupping of the upper part of the pinnae (Hagerman, 1996b; Simko

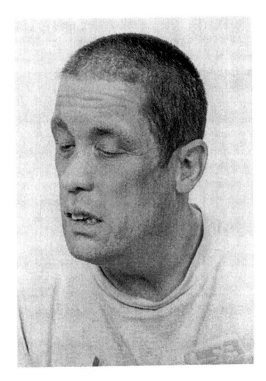

FIGURE 2.1:   Note long face and mildly prominent chin in this adult male with FXS.

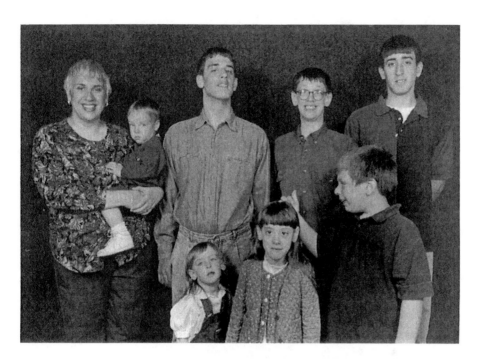

FIGURE 2.2: A family with five children who have FXS. The baby held by the mother and the young man on the far right are the only children who do not have FXS. Note the prominent ears in the children affected by FXS.

et al., 1989; Figure 2.3). Individuals who have a significant lack of methylation of their full mutation are less likely to have prominent ears (see Table 2.2) (Merenstein et al., 1996). On occasion, patients may have surgical pinning of prominent ears, particularly if the ear prominence is dramatic or psychologically stressful to the child. A broad ear width is also typical in FXS (Butler et al., 1991).

The facial changes, particularly the ear prominence in FXS, appear to be related to the connective tissue dysplasia associated with FXS (Hagerman et al., 1984; Opitz et al., 1984). Preliminary elastin studies have demonstrated abnormal elastin fibers that are short and more sparsely distributed in the dermis (Waldstein et al., 1987). This study also demonstrated an absence of the normal elastin arborization that occurs between the dermis and epidermis in patients with FXS. Additional facial features that are common in patients with FXS include puffiness around the eyes, narrow palpebral fissures, a large head relative to the body, prominent forehead, epicanthal folds, strabismus, and hypotonia (Hagerman, 1996b; Hockey and Crowhurst, 1988; Simko et al., 1989).

A high arched palate is seen in the majority of cases, and this is commonly associated with dental crowding or malocclusion. A cleft palate has been reported in 8% of males with FXS (Partington, 1984). The Pierre-Robin malformation sequence, including a cleft palate and large tongue, has been reported in FXS

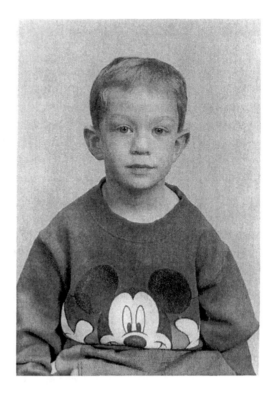

FIGURE 2.3:   Young boy with FXS and prominent ears because of cupping of the upper part of
the ear pinnae. Also note broad forehead and epicanthal folds.

(Lachiewicz et al., 1991). Loesch et al. (1992) and Piussan et al. (1996) have
reported patients with cleft lip and palate, in addition to limb anomalies consistent
with FG syndrome in patients with FXS.

Females with FXS also demonstrate typical facial stigmata (Figure 2.2). Fryns
et al. (1986) found that 14% of females with normal intelligence and FXS demonstrated a long face, prominent forehead, and mandibular prognanthism, whereas
these features were seen in 55% of females with mental retardation. Loesch and
Hay (1988) found typical facial features, including prominent ears, in 37% of
adult females with FXS and 14% of girls with FXS. Typical physical features were
found to be more common in females with the full mutation than in females
with the premutation and in controls (Hull and Hagerman, 1993; Riddle et al.,
1998). Table 2.2 identifies the frequency of physical features in females with both
the premutation and the full mutation, in addition to males with FXS. The degree
to which a female with the full mutation demonstrates physical features of FXS
is dependent on the activation ratio—that is, the percentage of cells that have

TABLE 2.2:   Percentage of Males and Females with Typical Physical Features of FXS

	Fully methylated postpubertal males $n = 64$	Fully methylated prepubertal males $n = 97$	<50% methylation prepubertal males $n = 5$	Mosaic prepubertal males $n = 29$	Premutation females $n = 114$	Full mutation females $n = 41$
Long face	80	64	40	63	30	66
Prominent ears	66	78	20	86	20	43
High arched palate	63	51	100	36	43	59
Hyperextensible finger joints	49	81	80	86	14	24
Double-jointed thumbs	48	58	80	62	18	42
Hand calluses	52	18	20	13	0	10
Flat feet	60	82	80	82	16	24

Adapted from Merenstein et al. (1996) and Riddle et al. (1998).

the normal X as the active X. The activation ratio directly correlates with the amount of FMRP production (Riddle et al., 1998; Tassone et al., 1998). Some females with the premutation have mild physical involvement, particularly prominent ears, which are significantly different from controls (Hull and Hagerman, 1993; Riddle et al., 1998).

Recurrent otitis media infections and recurrent sinusitis are common problems in children with FXS. In a study of 30 boys with FXS, 63% had recurrent otitis infections, compared with 15% of their normal siblings and 38% of developmentally delayed children without FXS (Hagerman et al., 1987). The majority of children with FXS who have recurrent otitis media require the insertion of one or more sets of PE tubes in the tympanic membranes (Hagerman, 1996b). In addition, 23% of individuals with FXS have sinusitis infections. Both the otitis media infections and the sinusitis infections may be related to the facial structural changes in FXS. Perhaps the connective tissue dysplasia and hypotonia may also lead to collapsible eustachian tubes, which inhibit drainage of the middle ear. A rare patient with FXS has also been documented to have transient hypogammaglobulinemia with IgG subclass deficiencies, although this may be a secondary phenomenon to recurrent infection (Hagerman, 1996a).

Ophthalmologic Findings

Preliminary studies in patients with FXS demonstrated a high incidence of ophthalmologic problems, including strabismus (lazy eye) in 30 to 56% (King et al., 1995; Maino et al., 1991; Schinzel and Largo, 1985; Storm et al., 1987). The types of strabismus include esotropia, exotropia, and hyperdeviation, but refractive errors, including myopia and hyperopia, are also common. Nystagmus (lateral jerking of the eye) is only occasionally seen in FXS (King et al., 1995). The high frequency of eye problems reported initially may be related to a selection bias in those who were studied; that is, children with eye problems are more commonly referred to the ophthalmologist or optometrist. In a recent prospective study regarding eye abnormalities in 44 children diagnosed with FXS, 25% demonstrated significant eye findings, including strabismus, which was present in 9%, and refractive errors, primarily hyperopia and astigmatism, in 18% (Hatton et al., 1997).

Skin/Joint Problems

The skin of patients with FXS has often been described as soft and velvet-like (Turner et al., 1980). This is most likely related to the elastin abnormalities that have been documented in case studies (Waldstein et al., 1987). The connective tissue problems also lead to joint laxity, and 73% of children younger than 11 years with FXS had joint laxity with hyperextensible metacarpal phalangeal (MP) joints (MP extension ≥90°), whereas 56% of those 11 to 19 years of age and only 30% of those older than 20 years had this finding (Davids et al., 1990). Hyperextensible finger joints are thought to be related to the connective tissue abnormality, but it also appears as if the ligaments tighten with age; these findings are less common in adult patients (Table 2.2). Flat feet, or pes planus, also appears to be related to joint laxity, and approximately 80% of younger patients and 60% of older patients with FXS have this finding (Table 2.2). Flat feet are usually not associated with pain or disability, although they can cause uneven shoe wear. Flat feet can be treated with foot orthoses or orthopedic shoes that can improve the gait and shoe wear, although this is not a necessity. On rare occasions, foot surgery may be required (Davids et al., 1990).

Joint dislocations are also related to hyperextensibility and connective tissue problems. They are uncommon and occur in only 3% of patients (Hagerman, 1996b). Joint dislocations have included recurrent dislocations of the patella, hip dislocations noted at birth, and shoulder dislocations. The connective tissue dysplasia also predisposes patients to hernias, and 15% have had this problem (Table 2.3). Most hernias are inguinal, although umbilical hernias are also seen.

Macroorchidism

Macroorchidism, or large testicles, occurs in 80–95% of adolescent and adult males with FXS (Butler et al., 1992; Hagerman, 1996b; Lachiewicz and Dawson, 1994b). Macroorchidism is defined in late adolescence and adulthood by a testicular volume of greater than 30 ml. Longitudinal studies have demonstrated that enlargement of the testicles beyond the normal range usually begins at approximately 8 to 9 years of age, although an occasional prepubertal patient will have a testicular volume greater than or equal to 4 ml (Lachiewicz and Dawson, 1994b). Macroorchidism begins to occur prior to the onset of pubic hair, and the testicles increase in size until approximately 15 to 16 years of age (Butler et

TABLE 2.3: Medical Problems of Males with Fragile X Syndrome

Problem	No. of patients evaluated	Percentage of patients with problem
Emesis	147	31
Failure to thrive in infancy	138	15
Strabismus	161	36
Glasses	148	22
Hernia	230	15
Joint dislocation	150	3
Orthopedic intervention	171	21
Otitis media	291	85
History of sinusitis	43	23
Seizures	288	22
History of apnea	139	10
Diagnosis of autism	211	20
Diagnosis of ADHD	224	80
Motor tics	188	19
Psychotic ideation	146	12

From Hagerman (1996a); reprinted with permission of the Johns Hopkins University Press.

al., 1992). The average adult testicular volume is 45 ml, with the 95th percentile at 70 ml, in a study of 185 males with FXS (Butler et al., 1992).

The cause of macroorchidism is not known, although endocrine dysfunction, presumably the increase of gonadotropin stimulation, is thought to account for this problem (Hagerman, 1996b). Mild elevations in gonadotropin levels (FSH and LH) have been reported by Turner et al. (1975), Ruvalcaba et al. (1977), and McDermott et al. (1983).

Males with FXS are fertile and have produced offspring; however, the majority of males with FXS are mentally retarded and are usually not sexually active because of their cognitive and social deficits (Hagerman, 1996b). The sperm of males with the full mutation have a premutation (Reyniers et al., 1993). Although this finding first suggested that the gametes were protected against a CGG expansion early on in embryonic development, subsequent studies by Malter et al. (1997) suggest that this is not the case. In this study, the oocytes of a female fetus with the full mutation at 16 weeks gestation carried the full FMR1 mutation on one of her two X chromosomes; her mother was a premutation carrier. The same study also evaluated the testes of a 13-week male fetus who had the full mutation. There was no evidence of a premutation, even though the mother carried a premutation. Immunohistochemistry studies on testicular tissue sections of the 13-week fetus demonstrated an absence of FMRP staining. In the testes of a 17-week male fetus with the full mutation, there was a faint band on DNA testing of 135 repeats. Immunocytochemistry studies demonstrated some evidence of

FMRP expression in this 17-week fetus. The authors hypothesize that contraction of a full mutation occurs in the male germ cells sometime after week 13 of development, and that this process is combined with selection for FMRP-expressing germ cells, leading to the production of mature spermatozoa that have the premutation (Malter et al., 1997). All female offspring of males with the full mutation and FXS will be carriers of the premutation.

Growth and Endocrine Studies

There is a tendency for increased growth in males and females during childhood, including increased height and weight and increased head circumference (Butler et al., 1992; Loesch et al., 1995; Sutherland and Hecht, 1985). Although the timing of puberty is usually normal in patients with FXS, there is a decrease in the pubertal growth spurt such that adult growth parameters demonstrate a tendency for short stature (Loesch et al., 1995).

Hypothalamic dysfunction has been postulated in the FXS (Fryns, 1984). Some patients with FXS have a Sotos syndrome-like phenotype, including cerebral gigantism, developmental delays, and generalized overgrowth (de Vries et al., 1995). Endocrine studies in two males with FXS and the Sotos syndrome–like phenotype demonstrated an elevation of insulin-like growth factor one (IGF1) and insulin-like growth factor binding protein 3, although thyroid function, growth hormone, and gonadotropin levels, in addition to plasma testosterone levels, were normal (de Vries et al., 1995). A Prader-Willi-like phenotype has also been documented in FXS, including hypogonadism in childhood, short fingers and toes, and excessive eating with lack of satiation (de Vries et al., 1993; Schrander-Stumple et al., 1994). Hypothalamic dysfunction also occurs in Prader-Willi syndrome, and there appears to be phenotypic overlap perhaps related to protein dysfunction overlap that may occur with the lack of FMRP translation regulation in FXS.

An occasional case of precocious puberty in females with FXS is further evidence of hypothalamic dysfunction (reviewed by Hagerman, 1996b; Kowalczyk et al., 1996). A blunted thyroid-stimulating hormone response to thyrotropin-releasing hormone stimulation has also been reported in FXS (Wilson et al., 1988). A normal testosterone response to human chorionic gonadotropin stimulation has been documented in males with FXS, although mild elevations of androstenedione, 17-hydroxyprogesterone, and progesterone were noted (Berkovitz et al., 1986).

Cardiac and Kidney Involvement

Mitral valve prolapse, or a floppy mitral valve, was reported in 22 to 55% of adults with FXS (Loehr et al., 1986; Sreeram et al., 1989). In addition, tricuspid leaflet prolapse was seen in 15% of 13 males and females with FXS (Puzzo et al., 1990). However, when young children with FXS were studied (16 boys and 1 girl), only one patient demonstrated auscultation findings consistent with mitral valve prolapse, and none showed echographic findings of mitral valve prolapse (Crabbe et al., 1993). These problems, therefore, appear to develop in adolescence or adulthood. In addition, mild dilation of the aortic root has been documented in 18 to 52% of adults with FXS (Loehr et al., 1986; Sreeram et al., 1989). On longitudinal follow-up, however, this mild dilation does not appear to be progressive. Sudden death, secondary to an arrhythmia perhaps precipitated by mitral valve prolapse, is a very rare occurrence and has been seen only twice by this author and rarely by others (Hagerman, 1996b; Waldstein and Hagerman, 1988; Loesch, 1998, personal communication). Our two patients were not taking medication but both had evidence of mitral valve prolapse. The role of FMRP in the heart has not been clarified in normal individuals, much less the effect of the absence of FMRP on cardiac function.

Hypertension is relatively commonly seen in adult males with FXS during a clinic evaluation, although anxiety in these circumstances is common and may be causal to the elevated blood pressure (Hagerman, 1996b). Perhaps connective tissue problems, specifically abnormal elastin fibers in vessels, affect the resiliency of the vessel wall and predispose males with FXS to hypertension, although this has never been studied. The enhanced sympathetic response to stimuli and lower vagal tone described subsequently in males with FXS may also lead to hypertension.

Abnormal elastin fibers may also impact the ureters. I have had three patients who have required a nephrectomy because of renal scarring secondary to severe reflux. I also know of two patients with hypospadius, but this frequency is typical for the general population and appears not to have a higher frequency in FXS.

Neurologic and Neuroanatomical Findings

Young children with FXS often present with hypotonia and motor incoordination. The hypotonia appears to be a general effect of CNS dysfunction in FXS and may also relate to other physical features such as joint laxity and a long face (Hagerman, 1996b). Finelli et al. (1985) described hyperreflexia in FXS, but this is not a consistent finding in young children and is more common in adults (Hagerman, 1996b). Sudden infant death syndrome (SIDS) occurred in 8% of 209 male offspring with FXS and in 4% of 169 female offspring of obligate carrier women (Fryns et al., 1988). Sleep apnea has been reported by Tirosh and Borochowitz (1992) in four patients with FXS who underwent extensive sleep apnea studies, although it was not seen in seven patients with FXS studied by Musumeci et al. (1996). Snoring is common in young children with FXS, and apnea during sleep by history has occurred in 10% (Table 2.3). Children with significant snoring or a history of sleep apnea often improve with a tonsillectomy and adenoidectomy. The apnea is often of the obstructive type and may be exacerbated by hypotonia and connective tissue problems. Questions regarding apnea and snoring should always be asked when taking the medical history.

The most common neurological abnormality in FXS is seizures, which occur in approximately 20% of patients with FXS (Table 2.3). Spike wave discharges are common in EEGs, and their similarity to the central and temporal spikes in benign rolandic childhood epilepsy has been reported (Musumeci et al., 1988a; Musumeci et al., 1988b). Most of the time seizures are well controlled with anticonvulsants in FXS, and often seizures are outgrown before adulthood (Musumeci et al., 1999; Wisniewski et al., 1991). Seizures may also be present in females with FXS, and they have been reported in 7.8% of adult women and 5% of girls (Loesch and Hay, 1988). The seizures in males and females include partial complex seizures, generalized tonic clonic, and absence seizures.

Sleep problems are common in FXS and may be related to melatonin deficiency (O'Hare et al., 1986). In sleep studies comparing children with FXS and their normal siblings or controls, a significant decrease in total sleep time and more frequent wakefulness throughout the night was documented (Holloway et al., 1999). An EEG study of sleep demonstrated a decrease in total sleep time and a decrease in rapid eye movement (REM) sleep in patients with FXS (Musumeci et al., 1996).

Detailed volumetric MRI studies have been carried out over the last several years by Reiss and colleagues, and these studies have demonstrated a smaller cerebellar vermis in both males and females affected with FXS, in addition to a larger caudate, thalamus, and hippocampus (Mostofsky et al., 1998; Reiss et al., 1991a, 1991b, 1994, 1995a). The cerebellum is activated in tasks that involve the discrimination and processing of sensory information and in tasks that involve attention and learning (Gao et al., 1996; Raymond et al., 1996), so these problems in the phenotype of FXS may be related to the smaller cerebellar vermis. In a study of 37 females with FXS, the size of the posterior cerebellar vermis predicted the scores on both Verbal and Performance IQ of the WISC III, in addition to the outcomes of both visual spatial tasks (block design and Rey Figure) and executive function tasks (Wisconson Card Sorting categories) (Mostofsky et al., 1998). In addition, in another study of females with FXS, the degree of stereotypic behavior correlated inversely with the size of the posterior cerebellar vermis (Mazzocco et al., 1997a).

A mouse model for FXS has been developed in which the *FMR1* gene is eliminated or knocked out (Bakker et al., 1994; Oostra and Willems, 1998). Recent studies of the neuroanatomy of the knockout mouse have demonstrated immature neuronal connections and an increase in dendritic branches (Comery et al., 1997). These mice are deficient in FMRP because they are missing the *FMR1* gene. Comery and colleagues have hypothesized that there is a lack of the normal pruning process and maturation of neuronal connections in patients and mice that are deficient in FMRP. Such a lack of pruning in development would lead to a larger brain size, as reported in patients with FXS by Schapiro et al. (1995) and Reiss (1994, 1995b) in certain areas of the brain. The lack of the normal pruning process would lead also to neuronal overconnectedness, which may relate to the hyperarousal in the behavioral phenotype in FXS described in the next section.

BEHAVIORAL PHENOTYPE

Boys with FXS present with a characteristic behavioral phenotype beginning in early childhood. Although language delays and hyperactivity are usually seen within the first 2 to 3 years, patients are also noted to be unusually sensitive to stimuli, causing tantrums with transitions, tantrums in crowded situations, or tantrums when overwhelmed by too much stimulation or activity. A number of autistic-like features have been associated with this syndrome, including poor eye contact, tactile defensiveness or sensitivity to touch, hand biting, hand flapping, other hand stereotypies, and perseveration or repetition in speech and behavior. These features are described as autistic-like because they are often seen in children who have autism or pervasive developmental disorder (Bailey et al., 1998; Hagerman, 1996b). Patients with FXS are easily hyperaroused or hypersensitive to certain stimuli, and this problem may be the cause of the autistic-like features. Often children with FXS are shy and socially anxious, but they are usually interested in social interactions and so this core feature of autism is usually not present with FXS. Eye contact provides a significant degree of stimulation, which can be overwhelming for the child, so they will often avoid eye contact or look fleetingly at people. Children with FXS can also be sensitive to noises, which can sometimes be overwhelming or irritating, causing the child to cover his ears. Some children have been noted to have an acute sensitivity in hearing and can hear sirens or other noises in the distance before normal individuals can hear them. Children with FXS can also be very sensitive to touch, so that tags in clothing or certain textures of clothing can irritate them. They may even be sensitive to the texture of some food in early childhood, which may lead to eating difficulties or even failure to thrive. The hypersensitivity to stimuli is thought to be related to the neurological organization of the brain, including the overconnectedness or excessive dendritic branching between neurons (Comery et al., 1997).

Recent studies of electrodermal activity—that is, the measure of sweat response to stimuli—have shed light on the issue of hypersensitivity to stimuli. The eccrine sweat glands are innervated by the cholinergic fibers of the sympathetic system. A preliminary study demonstrated enhanced electrodermal responses to sensory stimuli in two individuals with FXS (Belser and Sudhalter, 1995). A subsequent controlled study of 25 patients with the *FMR1* mutation demonstrated that males with FXS had an enhanced electrodermal response and poor habituation to visual, auditory, tactile, olfactory, and vestibular stimulation compared with age-matched controls (Miller et al., 1999). Males with FXS had a dramatic increase in amplitude and number of peaks in their electrodermal response to stimuli, characterizing an enhanced reactivity. In addition, their ability to calm this enhanced reactivity to repetitive stimuli was deficient because they could not habituate or phase out the electrodermal response with repetitive stimuli. The electrodermal studies appear to represent the neurological underpinnings of the phenomena of hyperarousal with stimuli, since the enhanced sweat response is an enhanced sympathetic response to stimuli. Recent studies of cardiac activity have shown a generally faster heart rate and lower vagal tone or parasympathetic activity in boys with FXS than in normal controls (Roberts, 1998). These preliminary electrophysiological studies are demonstrating autonomic dysfunction in FXS, which appears to be related to the behavioral phenotype.

Although most children with FXS are interested in social interaction, approximately 15% will have an overall diagnosis of autism (Baumgardner et al., 1995; Hagerman, 1996b). Children who are more cognitively impaired and who have severe sensory integration problems are more likely to be autistic (Bailey et al., 1998; Hagerman, 1996b; Turk et al., 1997). Often children with FXS who are autistic are nonverbal, with early developmental testing on the Bayley Scales of less than 50. Children with FXS and autism or severe autistic-like features usually improve over time with speech, language, and occupational therapy, such that by mid-childhood they may no longer meet criteria for autism (Baumgardner et al., 1995). Children with FXS typically show appropriate emotional perception and face recognition, unlike children with autism (Turk and Cornish, 1998; Simon and Finucane, 1996).

Hyperactivity, in addition to a short attention span, is seen in approximately 80% of boys with FXS and in approximately 35% of girls with FXS (Hagerman, 1996b). Even when hyperactivity is not a problem for boys, a short attention span with distractibility, such that they are only able to focus on a task for moments or minutes, is seen in almost all males with a deficiency of FMRP. For the school-aged child, the main focus of intervention is to improve the attention span, so that their ability to focus and concentrate on a task can be enhanced to improve learning. The use of stimulant medications and other interventions to improve ADHD symptoms is discussed in detail in the section on treatment.

COMMENTS FROM JOSHUA'S MOTHER

Joshua was born with both eyes crossed. From day 6 he screamed constantly with colic and was a very difficult baby to raise. I can remember when he was a week old, lifting him up, staring into his crossed eyes, "Where are you, Josh? I can't connect with you." He constantly vomited and gagged. His nickname was "Chunky." As he couldn't see properly for the first 8 and one-half months of his life he became very anxious and fearful of his surroundings and the noises around him. We could never put him down to play or to explore. After his eye operation at 8 and one-half months old, we expected to see a great improvement. His operation was a great success. He saw for the first time people's faces and places. He was awake and alive to the world around him. We knew that he would be slightly delayed in his development, but we thought a lot of his anxiousness would be relieved, but Joshua was as intense as ever.

He was walking independently by 14 months but would constantly fall over. The greatest difference to other children seemed to be his anxiousness to new surroundings and people—he would just scream—and his lack of exploring and getting into mischief. He loved music, and it was our greatest calming technique. It still is today.

I remember feeling depressed many times. He needed constant care, he was always putting objects in his mouth, losing balance, walking off edges, and gagging on food. He never wanted to sleep at night. He tested my patience and perseverance beyond belief. I doubted my ability as a mother. He challenged my very being. I felt useless, we always have to keep coping, staying abreast of Josh, sheltering him from the storm of anxiousness and hyperactivity—calming him when he is incapable of stopping, having to know where he is at every moment of the day—finding the path of least resistance, siphoning out irrelevant stimuli, and knowing the environmental situations to steer clear of.

By Rachel Calvert; reprinted with permission from *HEAR: I AM*, the Queensland fragile X support group newsletter, November 1997.

In females with FXS, shyness and social anxiety are common (Lachiewicz, 1995; Mazzocco et al., 1998; Sobesky et al., 1995). In a controlled study of girls with FXS compared with age- and IQ-matched controls, a psychiatric diagnosis of avoidant personality disorder or avoidant disorder in childhood was present in the majority of females with the full mutation (Freund et al., 1993). In behavioral ratings, 40% of girls with FXS who were older than 9 had an anxiety rating in the clinical range (Lachiewicz and Dawson, 1994a). On occasion, severe shyness and social anxiety may lead to selective mutism in girls with FXS, particularly in those who do not suffer from ADHD. Selective mutism is the inability to speak in certain social situations, particularly in school. We have seen this problem in seven females with the full mutation (Hagerman et al., 1999). Females who have ADHD are usually more impulsively outgoing and appear to be less likely to have selective mutism. Treatment for selective mutism includes counseling or psychotherapy, in addition to medication, specifically selective serotonin reuptake inhibitors (SSRIs) as described later in this chapter.

Hyperactivity and a short attention span may be present in approximately 30% of girls with FXS (Freund et al., 1993; Hagerman et al., 1992). Usually the degree of hyperactivity in girls with FXS is less severe than in boys with FXS, and the girls also respond well to stimulant medication. ADHD symptoms in girls with FXS are linked to the executive function deficits described in the next section. Although boys with FXS also experience shyness and social anxiety, it is usually masked by the more significant degree of hyperactivity and tantrum behavior. Shyness and social anxiety are such significant core features in FXS that they also occasionally occur in individuals who only carry the premutation (Franke et al., 1996). These problems will be described in more detail in the section on premutation carriers.

COGNITIVE PHENOTYPE

The degree of cognitive involvement in FXS also relates to the variations in the FMR1 mutation and the amount of FMRP produced in each individual (Tassone et al., 1998). Males with a full mutation that is fully methylated have a mean IQ of 41, whereas males who are mosaic (some cells with the premutation and some cells with the full mutation) have a mean IQ of 60, and males with a full mutation with only partial methylation (less than 50% methylation) have a mean IQ of 88 in adulthood (Merenstein et al., 1996). More recent studies of FMRP expression as measured in peripheral blood using immunocytochemical techniques developed by Willemsen and colleagues (1995, 1997) have demonstrated that the level of FMRP production explains 38% of the variance in overall IQ in males with a mosaic pattern and 68% of the variance in IQ in males with a partially methylated full mutation (Tassone et al., 1999). The FMRP in lymphocytes was produced by the cells that had the premutation pattern in mosaic males and by the cells that had a lack of methylation in males with a partially methylated full mutation. Because of the variations at the molecular level, there is a broad spectrum of involvement in males related to production of FMRP. Approximately 13% of males with FXS will present with an IQ that is not in the retarded range (Hagerman et al., 1994). These high-functioning individuals may also have fewer of the physical and behavioral features of FXS than do males typically affected by FXS (Figure 2.3).

The cognitive profile of individuals with FXS includes weaknesses in processing and remembering auditory sequences and abstract or complex information but strengths in object memory (Freund and Reiss, 1991; Kaufmann et al., 1990). They usually do best in utilizing simultaneous processing to solve tasks in which they view the overall gestalt visually (Kemper et al., 1986; Kemper et al., 1988). On the Kaufman Assessment Battery for Children (K-ABC), the Simultaneous Processing Composite score is almost always higher than the Sequential Processing Composite score, and the Achievement score; reflecting that what is learned from the environment, is always higher than the overall IQ, which is based on novel problem-solving tasks (Hodapp et al., 1992; Kemper et al., 1986, 1988). The Arithmetic score on the K-ABC is usually the lowest achievement score in both boys and girls affected by FXS. In girls with FXS, remediation services are usually necessary for math, even when reading and spelling are at grade level (Hagerman et al., 1992). Because of early strengths in language and long-term memory, young boys with FXS may appear to be less affected in the preschool years (Bennetto and Pennington, 1996; Freund et al., 1995).

IQ Decline

Approximately 30% of males and females with FXS will experience significant IQ decline over time (Wright Talamante et al., 1996). This finding was first reported by Lachiewicz et al. (1987), and it has been subsequently studied by several authors (Dykens et al., 1989; Fisch et al., 1992; Hagerman et al., 1989; Hodapp et al., 1990). Many patients will demonstrate a steady growth in IQ until mid- to late childhood, when mental age tends to plateau (Dykens et al., 1989). Typically, children with FXS do not lose skills; instead, they fail to develop abstract reasoning compared with normal children and, since more demands are made in reasoning on IQ testing as the child ages, a decline in IQ scores can be seen over time (Hagerman et al., 1989). It has recently been shown that individuals with less than 50% methylation of the full mutation do not demonstrate a significant IQ decline (Wright Talamante et al., 1996).

The first prospective longitudinal study of cognitive development in young boys with fragile X was carried out by Bailey and colleagues (1998). For the first 72 months of life overall development was significantly delayed and progressed on average at half the rate expected for typically developing children. On the Battelle Developmental Inventory, motor and adaptive domains were consistently the highest scores, but overall there was great variability between individuals related to background gene effects and variation in the *FMR1* mutation.

Females

The spectrum of involvement in females with the full mutation is related to the X activation ratio—that is, the percentage of cells that have the normal X as the active X. A significant correlation between cognitive measures and the activation ratio has been documented (Abrams et al., 1994; Riddle et al., 1998). In a careful study of the effects of the *FMR1* mutation compared with background genetic effects in which the parental IQs were studied in females with the full mutation, it was found that the parental IQ predicted 26% of the variance in the IQ of the daughters with FXS, whereas the activation ratio predicted 33% of the IQ variance (Reiss et al., 1995b). Recently it was found that FMRP levels in peripheral blood correlated with the IQ in females with the full mutation, but FMRP levels predicted only 24% of the variance in IQ in these females (Tassone et al., 1999). There are differences in the activation ratio between tissues in females, and neither the activation ratio nor the FMRP production in peripheral blood may represent these variables in brain tissue.

In females with the full mutation, approximately 71% demonstrate a significant cognitive deficit—that is, an IQ in the borderline or mentally retarded range (de Vries et al., 1996b). This study documents a higher percentage of females with cognitive involvement than do reports that show 50% (Hagerman et al., 1992; Rousseau et al., 1994a) because they evaluated females in their homes, so individuals were included who were too anxious to come into the clinic. The activation ratio correlated with the Wechsler Scales Performance IQ and the Full-Scale IQ but not the Verbal IQ (de Vries et al., 1996b). Similar findings were reported by Riddle et al. (1998), so it appears that the *FMR1* mutation has a more significant effect on overall Performance IQ than on Verbal IQ.

In a study that evaluated executive function abilities, which include attentional abilities, planning and organizational abilities, working memory, inhibition, and ability to shift set in problem solving, the executive function abilities correlated more strongly with the activation ratio then with the overall IQ (Sobesky et al., 1996). In the past, approximately one-half to two-thirds of women with the full mutation but with normal intellectual abilities have been shown to demonstrate executive function deficits (Mazzocco et al., 1993; Sobesky et al., 1996; Thompson et al., 1994). Therefore, subtle learning problems that include attention and organization difficulties, in addition to impulsivity, commonly occur in women with the full mutation who have a normal IQ because of these executive function deficits (Bennetto et al., 1996). The degree of executive function problems also correlates with other emotional difficulties, including shyness, social interactional difficulties, impulsivity, and moodiness (Sobesky et al., 1995; Sobesky et al., 1996).

Language

The language of boys and girls with FXS is characterized by perseveration on words, phrases and topics. Mumbling is common and the speech is often cluttered—that is, fast, bunched together, and difficult to understand (Hanson et al., 1986). Oral motor coordination problems consistent with an oral motor dyspraxia are common in males with FXS (Abbeduto and Hagerman, 1997; Scharfenaker et al., 1996). Approximately 11% of males are essentially nonverbal at age 5, and this severe involvement correlates with severe cognitive and motor deficits (Taylor et al., 1998).

The majority of males with FXS are verbal with a characteristically deviant pattern to their speech that includes perseveration, pragmatic (social and interpersonal language) deficits, high associate word responses, poor topic maintenance, and impulsive automatic phrases (Abbeduto and Hagerman, 1997; Sudhalter et al., 1990, 1991). The presence of ADHD and executive function deficits leads to the poor topic maintenance and impulsive or disinhibited aspects of speech. The perseveration is likely related to frontal lobe deficits, and the high associate word responses may be related to the enhanced interconnectedness between neurons. It is also difficult to inhibit a prepotent response when the inhibitory system, which is part of executive functions, is suboptimal.

High-Functioning Males

There have been several reports of high-functioning or nonretarded males with FXS (de Vries et al., 1996a; Lachiewicz et al., 1996; Loesch et al., 1993; McConkie-Rosell et al., 1993; Merenstein et al., 1994; Míla et al., 1994; Rousseau et al., 1994b; Smeets et al., 1995; Steyaert et al., 1996; Taylor et al., 1994; Wang et al., 1996; Wohrle et al., 1998) (Figure 2.4). Most of these individuals have a variant DNA pattern usually lacking methylation or a high level of mosaicism. In our experience, approximately 13% of males with FXS present in this high-functioning category, and it is essential to carry out DNA testing, which documents the percentage of methylation present or the percentage of cells that demonstrate the premutation (Hagerman et al., 1994). Wöhrle and colleagues (1998) found an unmethylated full mutation in 22 of 119 (18%) samples with a CGG expansion. High-functioning or nonretarded males with FXS usually demonstrate executive function deficits, in addition to significant emotional and behavioral problems. Strengths in reading and spelling are often seen, but math is usually deficient (Hagerman, 1996b; Merenstein et al., 1994). Their behavioral problems may

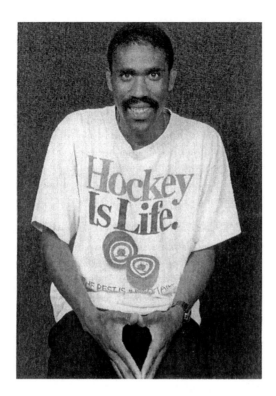

FIGURE 2.4: A young adult male who has a mild form of FXS because he is producing approximately 37% of normal FMRP levels from his full mutation, which is almost completely unmethylated. Note the lack of prominent ears, although his face is mildly long.

include schizotypal features that really represent autistic-like features, including poor eye contact, odd mannerisms, difficulty in modulating speech, poor pragmatic language, and difficulties with social interaction or extreme shyness. Some of these individuals have been previously diagnosed with Asperger syndrome, which is characterized by high-functioning individuals with autistic features or social deficits (Hagerman, 1996b). Problems with obsessive-compulsive behavior and sometimes attentional problems, in addition to their shyness and social anxiety, frequently occur. Sometimes problems with aggression can be a major difficulty for these individuals.

CASE HISTORY: ERIC

Eric is a 13-year-old male with fragile X syndrome; DNA testing demonstrates a premutation with 66 repeats in 84% of his cells and a full mutation that is methylated with 230 repeats in 16% of his cells. Seventy percent of his lymphocytes are positive on immunocytochemical studies for the presence of FMRP (Tassone et al., 1999). His history includes occasional hand flapping in childhood, hyperactivity, and a short attention span. He had recurrent ear and sinus infections, which required a tonsillectomy and adenoidectomy when he was 7 years old. Tantrums and angry outbursts have been a problem for him throughout his childhood, and they occur approximately once per week. Because of his ADHD, he was started on dextroamphetamine (Dexedrine) at 8 years of age, and this improved his ADHD symptoms at school and at home. His dose has been gradually increased through childhood to a 15-mg spansule in the morning at the present time.

At age 12 the WISC-III demonstrated a Verbal IQ of 99, a Performance IQ of 107, and a Full-Scale IQ of 103. Although his Verbal Comprehension Index is 103 and his Perceptual Organization Index is 114, his Freedom from Distractibility index is 84, which is reflective of his ADHD symptoms. Eric tends to oversimplify in processing incoming information, and his impulsivity amplifies his hasty processing. He has an angry and oppositional defiant style in relating to his environment, and he has demonstrated significant aggression to some of the individuals in his environment. Counseling on an intensive basis was recommended for him, and this has been quite helpful.

Clonidine at a dose of one-half of a 0.1-mg tablet was added to Eric's medication regimen on a three-times-a-day schedule to help with aggression both at home and at school. Although this was helpful, his aggression continued, and fluvoxamine (Luvox) was added. However, his behavior became more hyperactive on this medication, so it was discontinued. Because of ongoing problems with aggression, risperidone (Risperdal) was added to his regimen, with one-half of a 1-mg tablet given twice a day. Risperidone has helped his mood fluctuations and aggression, although intermittent problems continue at school. It is recommended that he be placed in a day treatment program for a more intensive psychotherapeutic environment.

Sometimes a carrier grandfather will be found on DNA testing to carry an unmethylated full mutation with very few features of FXS (Wöhrle et al., 1998). A detailed DNA analysis was carried out in multiple tissues at autopsy in a grandfather who was relatively unaffected except for an articulation deficit, math difficulties, attentional problems, and mood lability (Taylor et al., 1999). In blood he had a CGG expansion that ranged from 80 to more than 500 repeats and was unmethylated. In almost all organ tissues he had a methylated full mutation at 480 CGG repeats. In the brain he had an unmethylated smear (similar to the blood) in almost all areas, except for one sample taken from the saggital sulcus, including the motor strip and the parietal lobe. Perhaps his articulation difficulties are related to the full mutation in this region of his brain. Mosaicism of somatic tissues, particularly in the brain, can lead to a milder or unusual cognitive or behavioral phenotype, although autopsy studies are rare to further document the frequency of this finding.

PREMUTATION CARRIERS

Women who are carriers of the premutation have been shown to be unaffected intellectually (Mazzocco et al., 1993; Reiss et al., 1993). Executive function deficits are also not a significant problem in women with the premutation (Sobesky et al., 1996). However, a recent study of 17 women with the premutation demonstrated a lowered Performance IQ compared with the Verbal IQ, and the Performance IQ correlated with the activation ratio in fibroblasts (Allingham-Hawkins et al., 1996).

Women with the premutation may demonstrate some involvement in the physical and emotional aspects of the phenotype. More prominent ears and chin and an overall higher score on an index of physical characteristics typical of FXS has been documented in women with the premutation than in controls (Hull and Hagerman, 1993; Riddle et al., 1998). Premature ovarian failure or premature menopause occurs in approximately 20% of women with the premutation, which is significantly higher than controls (Partington et al., 1996; Schwartz et al., 1994). In addition, a high twinning rate three times the incidence in normals has been found in women who carry the premutation (Turner et al., 1994).

In our experience, the most significant problems for women with the premutation are emotional. Although some women with the premutation do not have these difficulties, approximately 50% suffer from significant anxiety, obsessive worrying, depression or mood lability (Sobesky, 1996; Sobesky et al., 1994a, 1994b; Thompson et al., 1996). A controlled study of 29 women with the premutation compared with the mothers of children with autism who do not have FXS and mothers of normal children demonstrated that 45% of women with the premutation experienced an affective disorder, 17% an anxiety disorder, and 10% social phobia (Franke et al., 1996). The high rate of affective disorder was significantly different from normal controls, and the prevalence of an anxiety disorder was threefold higher than in mothers of normal controls and mothers of autistic children. The age of onset of these problems usually predated the diagnosis of FXS or mental retardation and often began in adolescence (Franke et al., 1996). It is therefore unlikely that the cause of these emotional problems is only related to the stress of raising a child with FXS.

A subsequent study by Franke and colleagues (1998) found that social phobia was significantly more common in mothers with a full mutation (31%) than in mothers of autistic children (5%) or controls (0%). Social phobia was also seen in mothers with the premutation (18%) and in siblings with the premutation who were not mothers (6%). Major depression was most frequent in mothers with the premutation (20%) compared to mothers with the full mutation (15%), mothers of autistic children (10%), and premutation sibling controls (0%). However, there was a trend for bipolar affective disorder to be associated with the *FMR1* mutation in any form, including full-mutation mothers (15%), premutation mothers (12%), and premutation siblings (12%) compared to sibling controls without the *FMR1* mutation (0%) and mothers of autistic children (5%). Personality studies were also carried out; schizotypal and avoidant disorders were most common in full-mutation mothers each with 23%, but they were seen in fewer than 10% of premutation mothers and in fewer than 3% of controls. When the prevalence of social phobia is combined with avoidant and schizotypal personality disorders, 77% of full-mutation mothers had these problems, compared to 31% of premutation mothers, 12% of premutation siblings, and 7% of mothers with autistic children (Franke et al., 1998). There appears to be a continum of emotional involvement correlating with the severity of the mutation at FMR1. Why some individuals with the premutation have no problems and others are impacted with emotional difficulties or on rare occasion with cognitive deficits may relate to several different mechanisms. There may be occult expansion in other tissues compared to the premutation in blood (Hagerman, 1996b); there may be a mild FMRP deficit in a limited number of premutation carriers, as previously reported in three males with the premutation (Hagerman et al., 1996); there may be a different molecular mechanism of involvement in some individuals with the premutation such as translational dysfunction, as suggested by Tassone et al. (1999) in her report of retarded males with the premutation who demonstrated an elevation of mRNA levels for FMR1 and a significant deficit of FMRP; or there may be the co-occurrence of other genes that cause cognitive deficits or emotional problems which have an additive influence to the FMR1 premutation, such as a mutation in the serotonin transporter leading to autism (Cook et al., 1997). Landau et al. (1999) hypothesized an additive effect in a premutation carrier male who also is a carrier for spinal muscular atrophy and has experienced cognitive deficits combined with cerebral and cerebellar atrophy in later life.

COMMENTS FROM A MOTHER: RACHEL

Although I only have a premutation of fragile X of 133 CGG repeats, I suffer extreme anxiousness and depression. I have always felt different to other people and have never coped well socially. At high school I averaged two to three days attendance every week. Academically I was above average and entered University.

I struggle with fragile X inside me every moment of every day. I know how my children feel inside, the frustrations of being trapped in a fragile X mind, the wanting to partake in everything, the not being able to speak out and say—I want to have a go. The wanting so desperately to have a go.

I look through my fragile X eyes to see my fragile X children, to understand my children and this gives greater patience, greater perseverance, and keeps me trying.

By Rachel Calvert; reprinted with permission from HEAR: I AM, the Queensland fragile X support group newsletter, November 1997.

WHO TO TEST

Children and adults who present with mental retardation or autism without a specific known etiology should be tested for FXS (Brown et al., 1996). The use of both DNA and cytogenetic testing is recommended, because when the DNA is negative the cytogenetic testing may often reveal the presence of other cytogenetic disorders in approximately 5% of individuals, particularly if significant dysmorphic features are present (Jacky, 1996). The use of *FMR1* DNA testing is essential because some individuals who are negative cytogenetically for the fragile X site may be positive for a mutation at *FMR1*. Individuals who have significant learning disabilities, in addition to physical or behavioral features that are typical for FXS, should also be tested. This is particularly important in girls, because they usually do not present primarily with mental retardation but instead with learning disabilities. Not all individuals who evidence hyperactivity, ADHD, or learning disabilities need to be tested for FXS. In a screening of 1,014 school children who had academic difficulties but no mental retardation, only one premutation was detected (Mazzocco et al., 1997b). However, if typical physical or behavioral features are present, particularly autistic-like features, then DNA testing should be carried out (Hagerman, 1996b).

A variety of checklists has been developed to help clinicians in identifying individuals who are at high risk for FXS (de Vries et al., 1997; Giangreco et al., 1996; Hagerman et al., 1991; Nolin et al., 1991). It is particularly important to consider the diagnosis of FXS in individuals who have Sotos syndrome, Asperger syndrome, Prader-Willi syndrome, FG syndrome, or Pierre Robin sequence, because these disorders have been reported to be associated with FXS. In addition, sex chromosomal abnormalities, such as Kleinfelter syndrome (XXY), 45,X, XYY, and 47,XXX have all been reported in association with FXS (reviewed by Hagerman 1996b; Figure 2.5). There may be an increased rate of nondisjunction events in heterozygotes, and this may also lead to children with Down syndrome and FXS. It is important to clarify whether FXS occurs in combination with these other disorders for genetic counseling reasons and also because the treatment program should include interventions for FXS, as described in the next section.

Widespread population screening for fragile X is presently possible because of the relatively low cost of *FMR1* DNA testing. Newborn screening will allow early intervention for affected individuals and subsequent genetic counseling for all family members. Prenatal screening, however, will allow the family to make a decision about whether or not to continue an affected pregnancy. A recent cost analysis of screening efforts in the general population has found that prenatal screening would be the most cost effective (Wildhagen et al., 1998). Preconceptual screening had the second best cost saving balance, and it would also allow the couple to consider all reproductive options, including egg donation, in vitro fertilization, and adoption (Cronister, 1996).

TREATMENT

Although at the present time there is no cure for FXS, there are a variety of treatments and interventions that can be helpful for both children and adults who are affected by this disorder. This section reviews psychopharmacological interventions, individual therapy interventions, and educational and computer

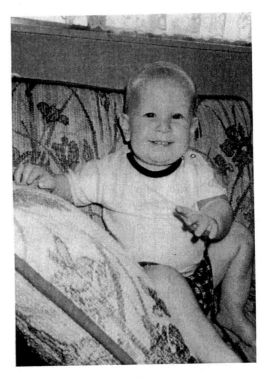

FIGURE 2.5:   An 18-month-old baby with FXS
and Kleinfelter syndrome. His development has
been normal so far.

techniques, and presents case studies. It is important for professionals to work
together to obtain an optimal treatment program that can work synergistically.
For instance, if an appropriate medication is found to improve attention and
concentration and decrease hyperactivity, the child can make more progress in
an appropriate educational setting, in addition to significant gains in language
and motor therapy. Often stimulants for attention and concentration will also
help with motor coordination.

It is necessary to have a key person to coordinate a treatment program; this
is often the physician who is overseeing the case, such as the developmental
pediatrician or the psychiatrist who is also prescribing the medications. Although
the American Academy of Pediatrics has produced guidelines for health supervision for children with FXS (1996), these guidelines do not include adequate
information regarding medications, which is clarified here (Hagerman, 1997).
This section is divided into age groupings, reviewing a variety of treatment approaches at each time interval. One of the most important interventions will be
addressed first: genetic counseling, which is necessary at whatever age the child
is diagnosed.

Genetic Counseling

It is essential for a genetic counselor or a professional who is experienced in working with fragile X to describe in detail to the family how the mutation can change through the generations. The counselor should draw the family tree and sort out who is at risk for being a carrier and who may be affected by FXS. A detailed family history must include questions regarding the physical and cognitive features of fragile X—for instance, asking whether other individuals in the family have learning disabilities, school problems, math deficits, or known mental retardation, in addition to such physical characteristics as a long face, prominent ears, hyperextensible finger joints, and so forth. The history of other family members should also include questions about the emotional phenotype, such as depression, anxiety, mood lability, outburst behavior, obsessive-compulsive symptoms, hyperactivity, and panic attacks (Staley Gane et al., 1996).

An example of a family tree can be seen in Figure 2.6, and this can be used as a model to demonstrate how the CGG repeat number changes through the generations. It is important to point out that male carriers will have daughters who are obligate carriers of the premutation. None of the sons of male carriers will carry the *FMR1* mutation because they receive the Y chromosome from their father. It is also important to point out to families that the expansion to a full

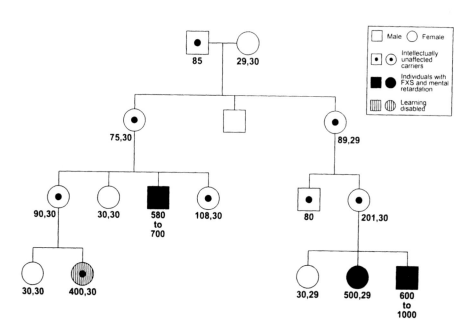

FIGURE 2.6: A typical family tree with a great-grandfather who is a premutation carrier. The numbers below the squares and circles represent the CGG repeat number for each X chromosome.

mutation will occur only when it is passed on by a woman. The risk for expansion to the full mutation at various sizes of the CGG repeat in the mother is outlined in Table 2.1. Women who have greater than 90 CGG repeats are basically at almost 100% risk for passing on the full mutation to their offspring who inherit the X chromosome with the *FMR1* mutation. The variability of phenotypic involvement in individuals with the full mutation, whether they are males or females, should also be explained in detail to the family. If an individual has been diagnosed through cytogenetic testing, it is important to carry out DNA testing to clarify the molecular parameters, including the CGG repeat number, the presence of methylation, or whether a mosaic status occurs. Some individuals who have typical physical and behavioral features of FXS may be negative on cytogenetic testing, but the mutation can be documented with DNA testing (Gringras and Barnicoat, 1998). This result is often seen in individuals who are high functioning and have a lack of methylation, which will suppress the expression of the fragile site in cytogenetic studies.

Some families find it difficult to disseminate information to other family members because of fear of rejection or anger or lack of acceptance of the diagnosis. The genetic counselor can help with these difficulties by sending a general letter explaining the fragile X diagnosis (McConkie-Rosell et al., 1995). The family should be encouraged to inform relatives directly, and individuals who are at risk for being carriers or affected by FXS should undergo DNA testing. Siblings in the family who have developmental problems, school difficulties or, emotional problems should also be tested as soon as possible with DNA testing to clarify whether their problems are related to FXS. Siblings who have had normal development and are without emotional problems may also benefit from DNA testing to clarify whether they are carriers. In a survey of carrier women, 60% felt having information about the carrier status would have been helpful to their children by ages 12 to 15 years and over 90% feel having this information is helpful by high-school age (McConkie-Rosell et al., 1997). Therefore, most mothers prefer testing of normal siblings in childhood rather than having them learn this information when they are adults. Normal siblings can be fearful about testing because of concern that they may be positive or that they may eventually demonstrate problems like those their siblings have. It is important to reassure normal or mildly affected siblings that they will never have the problems that their more affected brother or sister suffers from.

One of the most important reasons for genetic counseling is to offer prenatal diagnosis for future pregnancies (Cronister, 1996). With the advent of molecular testing in the 1990s, the ability of carrier females to make informed choices has resulted in a tenfold decrease in the prevalence of affected males in Australia (Robinson et al., 1996). DNA testing can be done with chorionic villis sampling (CVS), which is performed at 10 to 11 weeks' gestation. Amniocentesis can be done at 15 to 16 weeks' gestation, and it carries a relatively low risk of pregnancy loss (<0.5%) (Cronister, 1996). Both of these procedures can be done on an outpatient basis, but FMR1 DNA testing is not routinely carried out and must be specifically requested by the OB-GYN physician (Hagerman et al., 1998c). A third option is fetal blood sampling, which can take place at 18 weeks of gestation; when performed by an experienced team, the pregnancy loss rates are approximately 1% (Ryan and Rodeck, 1993). This procedure is carried out less commonly than CVS and amniocentesis in the United States. In all of the prenatal diagnostic procedures, the premutation can be differentiated from the full mutation. However, methylation has often not taken place by 11 weeks of gestation and sometimes not even by 15 weeks, so that methylation levels cannot be used to predict the degree of involvement in prenatal studies. Families should be informed regarding the risks of cognitive and emotional involvement from FXS in male or female individuals with the full mutation. Families will make their own decision regarding whether to terminate the fetus, and whatever decision they make is the right decision for them and should be supported by the genetic counselor and the medical team (Staley Gane et al., 1996).

New reproductive technologies, such as in vitro fertilization and egg donation, should be discussed with families, along with adoption, as alternative strategies that can be utilized to have a normal child. Genetic counselors can be supportive to families in a variety of ways besides counseling for prenatal diagnosis and reproductive options. Counselors can help families adjust to and cope with the stresses of having a child with FXS. Genetic counselors are frequently asked about issues regarding treatment, and they should be knowledgeable about professionals to whom to refer a family for optimal intervention for their child. The genetic counselor should have a long-term relationship with families who have a child with FXS, because the parents and also extended family members may intermittently require prenatal diagnosis, information regarding newer reproductive technologies, and general support (Cronister, 1996; Staley Gane et al., 1996).

Infancy

Fragile X syndrome can be diagnosed in infancy or even in utero, particularly when there is a known family history. The infant should be examined carefully for evidence of connective tissue problems or malformations, including cleft palate, club foot, congenital hip dislocation, and hernias. There is a risk of sudden infant death, so episodes of apnea or obstructed breathing should be looked for in the medical history. Infants should always be put to sleep on their backs instead of prone because of the increased risk for SIDS in prone position.

Most babies with FXS do relatively well in the newborn period, although occasionally problems with gastroesophageal reflux or difficulties with coordinating a suck occur. Vomiting associated with gastroesophageal reflux requires positioning upright after meals and thickening of feedings (Sondheimer, 1994). On occasion, severe gastroesophageal reflux may require medication such as metoclopromide (Reglan), which will improve the gastric emptying time and enhance lower esophageal sphincter pressure, or bethanacol, which will also improve the lower esophageal sphincter pressure. Cisapride (Propulsid), a prokinetic agent which stimulates smooth muscle cell contraction, will also improve gastric emptying time and the lower esophageal sphincter pressure. However, cisapride must be used cautiously in infants and use with medication such as erythromycin, which interfere with the cytochrome P_{450} system should be avoided because toxic levels of cisapride can cause cardiac arrhythmias (Ward et al., 1999).

Most infants are hypotonic and require early infant intervention, which usually includes infant stimulation and a motor program. Frequent otitis media infections usually begin in the first year of life. They require vigorous therapy, including the use of antibiotics and placement of PE tubes to avoid a conductive hearing loss which can interfere with language development (Hagerman et al., 1987).

Psychotropic medications are not used in the first year of life; however, folic acid is an exception to this. In approximately 50% of families, parents have noted an improvement in behavior, particularly attention and concentration, with folic acid, although controlled studies have not demonstrated consistent support for this (Hagerman, 1996a; Turk, 1992). Folic acid can be tried at a dose of 1 mg/kg up to 10 mg/day. It comes in a 1-mg tablet form and can also be used in a liquid preparation (5 mg/ml) that can be mixed by pharmacies on special request (Hagerman, 1996a). Side effects of folic acid include loose stools, and a rare patient may become more irritable or hyperactive on folic acid. Vitamin B_6 and zinc deficiency have been documented to occur with high-dose folic acid use. Blood testing to document vitamin B_6 and zinc levels should be done at least once a year. Patients can be easily supplemented with a multiple vitamin that has B_6, and, if zinc deficiency occurs, zinc supplementation can be given.

Toddlers and Preschoolers

Hypotonia and motor delays are frequently noted in the toddler and require occupational therapy that utilizes a sensory integration approach with a focus on improving both fine and gross motor coordination, motor planning, joint stability, hyperarousal to stimuli, and tantrums (Scharfenaker et al., 1996; Schopmeyer and Lowe, 1992). The physical therapist can also be helpful to the child who is having severe problems with motor coordination. Toddlers may still be involved in an infant stimulation program, but sometime between the ages of 2 and 3, enrollment into a special education preschool program is recommended. Perhaps the most remarkable developmental delay occurs in the language area; most children with FXS are not developing phrases or sentences by 2 years of age. Developmental testing can be carried out in infants and toddlers with the Bayley Scales of Infant Development to help the physician and therapist monitor progress in all developmental areas.

Early speech and language intervention is recommended, and this can be instituted even before 2 years of age. The speech and language therapist should focus on oral motor coordination, oral hypersensitivity to stimuli, and development of both receptive and expressive language skills, including boosting vocabulary, but also working with concept formation such as sorting, matching, and early cause-and-effect concepts. Some children have a significant oral motor dyspraxia or incoordination of the muscles of articulation that interfere with expressive language. Oral motor exercises and other interventions, such as pulling on taffy, blowing bubbles, using whistle toys, or blowing the harmonica or the kazoo, can help to develop the muscles of articulation (Scharfenaker et al., 1996).

Approximately 10% of the children seen in our fragile X clinic have no language or have severe delays in language which require intensive intervention, including the use of augmentative communication, to stimulate language development (Reinhartsen et al., 1997; Scharfenaker et al., 1996; Taylor et al., 1998). Combining speech, language, and occupational therapy so that rhythm and movement and singing and dancing can be utilized to further stimulate oral language development is often helpful. The following case illustrates examples of interventions for a child with severe language delays.

CASE HISTORY: JOHN (1)

John is a 6-year-old boy with FXS who was diagnosed at 2 years of age when cytogenetic testing demonstrated that 35% of his lymphocytes had the fragile X chromosome. Subsequent DNA testing demonstrated a full mutation that was fully methylated. The mother's pregnancy was normal, and John's birth weight was 8 lbs. 2 oz. after a full-term delivery. John sat at 6 months and walked at 15 months, but he has had severe language delays and he does not use words, even at 6 years of age. He has a history of hand flapping and hand biting, beginning in the first year of life, in addition to obsessive chewing on objects. Eye contact has always been poor, and he has had significant tactile defensiveness. He is described as hyperactive with a short attention span, and he perseverates in his behavior.

His medical history includes recurrent otitis media infections, and three sets of PE tubes were placed between 6 months and 2 years of age. He has never had problems with sinus infections, seizures, apnea, or strabismus.

At 3 years 9 months, John scored at the 16-month age level on the Bayley Scales, and his Vineland Adaptive Behavior Assessment demonstrated an overall Adaptive Behavior Composite of 52, Communication Domain of 53, Daily Living Skills of 60, Socialization of 59, and Motor Skills of 55. He was placed in a preschool environment that included occupational therapy and language therapy, in addition to special education support. A trial of folic acid did not help his behavior. Clonidine was tried, but it made him irritable, so this was discontinued. At age 5 years, he was started on one-half of a 5-mg methylphenidate (Ritalin) tablet in the morning, and this improved his attention and concentration, but twice-a-day dosing seemed to decrease his energy.

At age 6 years, he does not speak; instead he makes a moaning sound which may change somewhat in its inflection. On physical exam at age 6 years 3 months, his height is above the 95th percentile for age, weight is at the 93rd percentile for age, and OFC is at the 80th percentile for age. He has a very short attention span and extremely poor eye contact. He has a long face with ears that are not prominent. His eyes demonstrate epicanthal folds, his palate is high and narrow, and oral motor coordination problems were noted. Extremities show finger hyper-extension to 90 degrees, he is double-jointed in his left thumb, and his feet are flat bilaterally. He will toe walk when he is not wearing his shoes.

John's treatment program involves many professionals with a focus on improving his most significant area of deficit, language. To enhance his communication, he needs access to picture communication displays at home and in school. They should be incorporated into his daily routine, and their use should be modeled by adults who are interacting with him. The Mayer Johnson Picture Symbols (see Appendix 3) should be available at home and in school with the recommended computer software. He can also utilize a small communication book attached to a key chain to wear on a belt loop or carry in a fanny pack. Each page should contain three to four symbols to relate to a favorite topic or activity and frequently used vocabulary messages that he needs in all environments such as, "I need a bathroom" and "I am hungry." A remnant communication book can be used that is personalized for him and communicates relevant information, including drawings of people, places, and activities that are meaningful to him, and magazine pictures and photographs of people who are important in his family and environment. Objects, such as souvenirs from activities or events, can be incorporated into this communication book. This book, including the symbols, pictures and objects, can facilitate talking about past events and conversations about activities that he is currently doing. A Velcro book can be made to which symbols can be attached with a Velcro patch on the back (Coreen Jacks, personal communication, 1997). The events or schedule of the day can be organized on the Velcro strips, and positive or negative feedback can be given by attaching a smiling or frowning face to the end of an activity sequence.

A small portable voice output communication aid (VOCA), such as the BIGMac (see Resources at the end of this chapter) can be used for single messages such as requesting an item during classroom activity or at home. A Cheap Talk voice output aid (see Resources) can be used for up to four programmed messages, and more sophisticated VOCAs can eventually be used in structured settings (see chapter 6.

In John's individual therapy, his speech and language pathologist needs to work on oral motor coordination because of the severity of his oral motor dyspraxia. The use of rhythm and movement and singing should be intensified in his programs. He clearly responds best to intervention that includes music and rhythms. His strengths in imitation and modeling can also be utilized, as his speech and language therapist model oral motor movements. Mirror work may also be helpful for this; a talk-back mirror which records up to 20 seconds of verbalizations that can immediately be played back can be obtained (see Resources at the end of this chapter). He should continue in physical therapy and in occupational therapy with a sensory integration approach. Utilizing sensory integration techniques, such as calming techniques, deep pressure back rubs, and perhaps even a hot bath, may help improve his attention and subsequent vocalizations.

To improve his attention and concentration, we are also increasing his methylphenidate to a 5-mg dose; this can be tried two to three times a day. The physician must be mindful of a quieting effect of higher doses of methylphenidate and make sure that this dose not suppress any emerging vocalization.

Treatment of Seizures

In the preschool period, it is also important to take a careful history for possible seizures, since these occur in approximately 20% of children with FXS. If a history of seizure activity occurs, an EEG should be carried out, and medication for treatment of seizures can be utilized, particularly if spike wave discharges occur on the EEG. The most commonly used seizure medication treatment in FXS is carbamazepine (Tegretol). Carbamazepine is an iminostilbine with a tricyclic structure which is the drug of choice for partial motor, partial complex, and secondary generalized tonic clonic seizures. It is usually well tolerated, although approximately 30% of individuals may experience sedation. The starting dose is 10 mg/kg/day, and the maintenance dose is usually 20 to 40 mg/kg/day, although serum levels must be checked in the morning before a dose is given to document whether the patient is in the therapeutic range (7–12 micrograms/ml).

Carbamazepine can have a number of side effects, including liver toxicity, rash, hyponatremia, decrease in the white blood cell count, and a very rare possibility of agranulocytosis (Pellock, 1987). Several medications can interfere with the metabolism of carabamazepine, including erythromycin, fluoxetine, and other SSRIs. When other medications are taken in addition to carbamazepine, the serum levels must be followed more closely to avoid toxicity from carbamazepine. At high levels of carbamazepine, individuals can experience lethargy, ataxia, vomiting, nausea, and double vision (Pippenger, 1987). Most important, in approximately 3% of patients, an allergic or hypersensitivity reaction may develop, usually within 2 to 4 weeks of initiating the medication. This reaction can include a skin rash, in addition to edema in the face, sore throat, hepatitis, and leukopenia. Patients who are started on carbamazepine must be told to discontinue the medication if a rash develops.

Carbamazepine can be very helpful for mood disorders because it tends to stabilize mood and decrease aggressive outbursts or episodic dyscontrol (Keck et al., 1998). This beneficial response can be seen even when a patient does not suffer from seizures or has a normal EEG. Controlled studies of carbamazepine's efficacy in FXS has not been carried out, but anecdotal reports have demonstrated that this medication is helpful for behavioral problems, particularly mood instability, in eight of nine patients with FXS (Gualtieri, 1992).

Individuals who have absence seizures or major motor seizures may respond more effectively to valproate or divalproex sodium (Depakene or Depakote) (Friis, 1998). This medication is probably also effective for partial motor seizures and also has the beneficial effect of stabilizing mood in a manner similar to carbamazepine.

Valproate acid has been shown to be as effective as lithium in the treatment of mania in adults with bipolar disorder (Bowden et al., 1994; Freeman and Stoll, 1998). The side effects of valproate include appetite changes, weight gain, hair thinning, low platelet count, and, most important, hepatic toxicity and pancreatitis. Hepatic failure can occur with the greatest risk in young patients treated with multiple drugs (Dreifuss and Langer, 1987). A newly reported side effect of valproate is the onset of polycystic ovarian disease in adolescence and adulthood in some women who have been treated with valproate long term (Isojarvi et al., 1993).

Over the last few years there has been a plethora of new anticonvulsants released for adjunctive treatment of seizures. These new anticonvulsants include lamotrigine (Lamictal) which reduces the excitatory neurotransmitter glutamate, but it may interfere with the metabolism of valproate and may cause a rash which on rare occasion leads to Steven-Johnson syndrome (Besag, 1999); vigabatrin (Sabril), which increases the inhibitory neurotransmitter GABA and is recommended for infantile spasms and as an add-on therapy for partial onset drug resistent epilepsy (Ylinen, 1998); gabapentin (Neurontin), which increases GABA in the brain, inhibits voltage-activated sodium channels, and increases serotonin levels in the brain, has demonstrated efficacy as add-on treatment for refractory partial epilepsy (Mikati et al., 1998); tiagabine (Gabitril), which inhibits the re-uptake of GABA and is an effective adjunctive therapy for all partial seizure types in adolescents and adults (Kälviäinen, 1998); and topiramate (Topamax), which has multiple mechanisms of action, including sodium channel blocking, enhanced GABA at GABA-a receptors, blocking of glutamate receptors, and weak inhibition of carbonic anhydrase, has demonstrated efficacy in adjunctive treatment of partial epilepsy, generalized epilepsy and Lennox-Gastaut syndrome (Kerr, 1998). For review of drug interactions and side effects, see Alvarez et al. (1998). Usually the seizures in FXS are well controlled with carbamazepine or valproate, so experience is limited with these newer agents. However, some of these agents have been utilized for mood stabilization, as described later in this chapter.

Toilet training problems are common in children with FXS, and many children may be delayed in toilet training. It is likely that some children may not experience the sensory signals of having a full bladder or a full bowel, and this adds to an inability to go to the toilet at appropriate times. Often placing the child on the toilet before the typical time when a bowel movement occurs will result in stooling in the toilet, which should be followed by ample positive reinforcement. A videotape has been developed for teaching children with pervasive developmental disorders how to use the toilet (see the Resources at the end of this chapter). The use of music and jingles can help the child become enthusiastic about toilet training, and positive reinforcement can be helpful for maintaining the behavior. For more information regarding toilet training techniques to be used with children with FXS, see Crepeau-Hobson and O'Connor (1996) and the appendix 4 of this book. Also, for an excellent review about behavioral approaches to toilet training, see Luxem and Christopherson (1994).

Ophthalmologic problems are common in children with FXS, including strabismus in up to 30 to 40% and refraction errors. An ophthalmologic evaluation is recommended by 4 years of age or earlier if strabismus or other difficulties, including ptosis, nystagmus, or visual difficulties, are noted.

Sometimes significant tantrums can be a great difficulty in the preschool period. Often the use of positive behavior reinforcement can alleviate some of these problems, but when they are severe, the use of counseling to give the family additional guidance regarding behavioral interventions is quite helpful. For discussions regarding counseling techniques in children with FXS, see Brown et al. (1991) and Sobesky (1996).

Psychopharmacology

Psychopharmacological intervention can be utilized for the child in the preschool period, particularly if tantrums are excessive with hyperarousal or ADHD. Often stimulants can cause irritability or an increase in tantrums when they are used before 5 years of age; therefore, behavioral interventions, counseling, and sensory integration occupational therapy should be utilized before a medication trial. The most commonly used medication in the preschool period with a child 3 years of age or older is clonidine (Catapres). This medication is an antihypertensive agent which acts as an α_2-adrenergic presynaptic agonist. The overall effect is to decrease norepinephrine activity at the synapse, both centrally and peripherally (Hagerman et al., 1998a). Clonidine has an overall calming affect for hyperarousal and hyperactivity, and it often decreases aggression. It can be used to treat ADHD, but it does not help attention and concentration as much as the stimulant medications that are described later in this chapter. Clonidine may also be helpful in reducing anxiety in children (Salee et al., 1998).

The side effects of clonidine include sleepiness, which is dose-dependent and usually improves after the first 2 to 3 weeks of medication. The dosing of clonidine is started low—that is, just one-quarter or one-eighth of a tablet twice a day in the preschool period. Each tablet is 0.1 mg, and the dose can be gradually increased to approximately 4 to 5 micrograms/kg/day for school-aged children. The side effect of sleepiness usually helps bedtime wakefulness or sleep disturbances in children with FXS or children with ADHD (Hagerman et al., 1995; Wilens et al., 1994). Clonidine also comes in a patch (Catapres TTS one, two, or three patches). With a young child, the patch can be cut to decrease the overall strength. It is usually effective for approximately 5 days, and it is placed in the mid-back area, preferably where the child cannot reach. It can be dangerous to use the patch in the preschool period, however, because a young child may tear off the patch and eat it, which will lead to a toxic overdose of clonidine and coma. The patch can also be irritating to the skin in approximately 30 to 40% of the patients. To decrease skin irritation, a steroid spray, such as Vancenase AQ double strength or Beconase AQ nasal spray, can be sprayed on the back and allowed to dry before placing the patch (Hagerman et al., 1998a).

The follow-up of patients on clonidine involves monitoring the blood pressure and heart rate. EKG changes can occur, including prolongation of conduction or an occasional dysrhythmia (Chandran, 1994; Dawson et al., 1989). There have been reports of four cases of sudden death in children treated with clonidine and methylphenidate together (Cantwell et al., 1997; Swanson et al., 1995). In review of these cases, the cause of death does not appear to be related to the clonidine (see more detailed discussion in chapter3). However, EKG studies both before and after administration of clonidine, particularly when this medication is prescribed with other medications, are warranted (Delahunty et al., 1999; Hagerman et al., 1998a). The blood pressure should be measured periodically in patients taking clonidine, and a history should be taken for any problems related to dizziness, fainting, or chest pain. When clonidine is discontinued, it must be slowly tapered over a few days to avoid an abrupt rebound in blood pressure which can lead to headaches. The patch can be discontinued abruptly, since there will be a gradual taper of the medication from skin stores once the patch is removed.

If clonidine causes excessive sedation, guanfacine (Tenex) can be used. Guanfacine is a more specific α_{2A}-adrenergic presynaptic agonist which has a longer half-life and causes less sedation. Guanfacine comes in a 1-mg tablet, which is 10 times the milligram strength of the clonidine tablet. For a young child, one-half or even one-quarter of a tablet at bedtime, with a gradual increase to twice a day usage, is usually adequate. There is little experience with guanfacine in children, although it has been reported to improve hyperactivity and attention in children with ADHD (Hunt et al., 1995). There are no controlled studies regarding guanfacine's use in FXS, but anecdotal reports suggest that it causes less sedation than clonidine.

Sleep disturbances are common in the preschool and school-aged child with FXS (Holloway et al., 1999). One small study demonstrated a melatonin deficiency in adult males with FXS (O'Hare et al., 1986), but melatonin levels have not been studied in children with FXS. However, our anecdotal experience suggests that a bedtime 3-mg dose of melatonin is helpful in the majority of patients with FXS who suffer from sleep difficulties, including wakefulness in the middle of the night. Studies of melatonin's efficacy in over 100 children with developmental disabilities and sleep disturbances demonstrates that it is helpful for over 82% (Jan and O'Donnell, 1996). No significant side effects were encountered even with long term use for greater than four years (Jan and O'Donnell, 1996).

School-Aged Children

It is important for the coordinator of a treatment program of a school-aged child with FXS to ensure that special education support, speech and language therapy, and OT therapy are included in the educational program. When inadequate therapy is available through the school system, the clinician can guide the family to arrange private therapy, which can often be covered by medical insurance. We recommend, whenever possible, inclusion in the regular classroom, or mainstreaming, since children with FXS have a great ability to model the behavior of the children with whom they interact. Children can be pulled out of class during the day for one-to-one therapy, or group intervention can be included in the regular classroom. Many children with FXS require an educational aide or special education teacher who can modify assignments for them to optimize inclusion in the regular classroom (Braden, 1997; Spiridigliozzi et al., 1994; Wilson et al., 1994). Girls with FXS are usually easily integrated into a regular classroom, although individual remediation is usually needed for math. Approaches are reviewed by Miezejeski and Hinton (1992).

Treatment of ADHD

Attentional problems and hyperactivity can interfere significantly with an educational program. Helpful intervention techniques in the classroom include enhancing structure, having the child sit in the front of the classroom, using a study carrel, allowing the child to go on errands when he becomes restless, or giving the child other special privileges, such as erasing the chalkboard and so forth. Further intervention ideas and treatment suggestions in a therapy situation can be found in Keogh (1992), Dykens et al. (1994), Wilson et al. (1994), and Braden (1997). Behavior checklists such as the Conners' or the Child Behavior Checklist (Achenbach) can be utilized; they are reviewed in Barkley (1990). A clinical assessment of the child is required to evaluate the degree of ADHD symptoms. The assessment includes a physical and neurological examination, along with monitoring attention and concentration during play and tasks that require attention (Hagerman, 1984).

Psychopharmacological intervention is often required for treatment of ADHD. Stimulant medications are the treatment of choice and are most effective in children who are 5 years of age or older, although occasionally they can also be helpful for the child under 5. In general, children with FXS appear to be sensitive to higher levels of stimulant medication, and at higher doses problems related to irritability or tantrum behavior may increase. It is therefore helpful to start at a low dose of stimulant medication to avoid these problems (Hagerman, 1996a). The most commonly used stimulants include methylphenidate (Ritalin), dextroamphetamine (Dexedrine), Adderall (a mixture of four dextro- and levo-amphetamine salts), and pemoline (Cylert). Both methylphenidate and amphetamine salts have been documented to be helpful in patients with normal IQ and in patients with mental retardation (Aman et al., 1993; Gillberg et al., 1997; Handen et al., 1994; Mayes et al., 1994). These studies demonstrate the efficacy of stimulants for treatment of ADHD symptoms in children with mild to moderate mental retardation, although efficacy in children with profound mental retardation is not established. Although the response to stimulants in children with ADHD but without mental retardation is approximately 80 to 95% (Barkley et al., 1991), the response rate to stimulants in children with mental retardation and/or FXS is approximately 60% (Hagerman et al., 1988). In a double-blind crossover trial of methylphenidate and dextroamphetamine compared with placebo in 15 prepubertal children with FXS, 10 patients were clinical responders (Hagerman et al., 1988). For children up to 5 years of age, a starting dose would be 2.5 mg of methylphenidate or dextroamphetamine or Adderall once or twice a day. The dosing can be gradually increased to two or three times a day with short-acting methylphenidate or dextroamphetamine. Adderall is a longer-acting medication, and often dosing just once a day is sufficient. Adderall is a mixture of four dextro- and levo-amphetamine salts that are metabolized at different rates so that there is a gradual lessening of effect in the afternoon. Some families have reported less irritability in the afternoon than with methylphenidate. In a controlled study, Adderall has been shown to be significantly helpful for attention, concentration, deportment, and academic performance in children with ADHD (Swanson et al., 1998a, 1998b).

In some individuals who become irritable on methylphenidate, dextroamphetamine, or Adderall, pemoline may be helpful, particularly in a low dose such as 18.75 mg or 37.5 mg given once a day. However, a recent FDA report of liver failure in 13 patients who had been treated with pemoline over the last 20 years of pemoline's use stimulates caution among practitioners and the need to document liver function studies on a regular basis in children taking pemoline (Adcock et al., 1998; Rosh et al., 1998). Pemoline is not the first choice of medication because of this side effect, but it may be helpful in individuals who do not tolerate the other stimulant medications.

In general, stimulant medication enhances both dopamine and norepinephrine neurotransmission, and this is the mechanism for improving attention and concentration. These neurotransmitter systems are particularly important for frontal or executive function, and they also help with organization and improving motor coordination and handwriting skills. Side effects of stimulant medication include appetite suppression and cardiovascular stimulation. Height and weight growth percentiles need to be followed closely by the clinician, and children should be seen at least twice a year to monitor growth and cardiovascular function. EKGs do not need to be done when stimulant medications are used alone, but when they are combined with clonidine, an EKG in follow-up is essential (Delahunty et al., 1999; Hagerman et al., 1998a).

Alternative medications can be used to treat ADHD. These medications include amantadine (Symmetrel), which is an antiviral agent but which also stimulates the dopaminergic system to improve attention and concentration and decrease hyperactivity. Response rate to amantadine in individuals with hyperactivity and mental retardation is approximately 40% (Gualtieri, 1990). Anecdotal reports suggest that it is helpful for treatment of ADHD in children with FXS (Gualtieri, 1992). Tricyclic medication can also improve ADHD symptoms and was beneficial in one patient with FXS (Hilton et al., 1991), but the cardiac side effects, including prolongation of cardiac conduction and the need for following EKGs, along with the risk of death with overdose, relegates this group of medication to a second-line approach for treatment of ADHD. We have seen the occasional occurrence of increased outburst behavior when tricyclics are used in the treatment of children with FXS (Hagerman, 1996a). Lastly, buspirone

(Buspar), an anxiolytic agent which is a partial agonist at some serotonin receptors, in addition to modest stimulation of dopamine and α-adrenergic systems, has been shown to be helpful in the treatment of ADHD in an open trial (Malhotra and Santosh, 1998). Although trials have not been carried out in FXS, anecdotal experience has shown that buspirone is often helpful for anxiety in FXS, but the effect on ADHD has not been dramatic.

Selective Serotonin Reuptake Inhibitors (SSRIs) and Mood Stabilizers

School-age and adolescent children with FXS may also experience difficulties with anxiety, social phobia, obsessive-compulsive behavior, mood lability, and aggression. The shyness and social anxiety is a more severe problem in girls with FXS than in boys. Aggression, however, is typically a more severe problem for boys with FXS than for girls. Both of these problems can also be treated with a selective serotonin reuptake inhibitor (SSRI) (Alderman et al., 1998). This group of medications blocks the reuptake of serotonin, which is a neurotransmitter that is important in the limbic system, the emotional center of the brain. Low levels of serotonin are associated with depression, anxiety, obsessive-compulsive behavior, aggression, and suicidal ideation. The SSRIs are generally considered antidepressant medications, but they also help anxiety, obsessive-compulsive behavior, moodiness, and aggression. Depression is not common among children affected by FXS, although it is relatively common in carriers of the premutation (Sobesky, 1996; Sobesky et al., 1996). The SSRIs can be given to children, adolescents, and adults with FXS to target one or more of these behaviors. In FXS, SSRIs are most commonly used for anxiety, and the improvement that is seen in aggression is probably secondary to the effects of decreasing anxiety (Hagerman, 1996a). For instance, outbursts may occur when a child or adolescent is put in a new situation or after a transition that is anxiety-provoking. Mood may abruptly change, and anger or aggression can lead to outburst behavior with either verbal or physical aggression.

In a study regarding the use of fluoxetine (Prozac) in FXS, 18 females (including 6 with the premutation only) and 17 males with FXS were surveyed after being placed on fluoxetine for treatment of anxiety or aggression (Hagerman et al., 1994). Fluoxetine overall was helpful in 83% of females, particularly for treatment of depression, mood lability, anxiety, panic attacks, outburst behavior, and obsessive-compulsive symptoms. In males, fluoxetine was helpful in 71%; it was usually prescribed for treatment of physical or verbal outbursts. Twenty-nine percent of the males either did not improve or became worse on fluoxetine. Some of these individuals experienced significant activation from fluoxetine, which presented as an increase in hyperactivity or an increase in aggression. Other side effects included nausea in 12%, insomnia in 6%, weight gain in 6%, and weight loss in 6% of the males. One female experienced suicidal ideation on fluoxetine, but this was also a problem before starting fluoxetine. Individuals with significant behavior or emotional problems should be in counseling before initiating the use of an SSRI.

In females with the premutation, SSRIs are particularly helpful in decreasing obsessive worries which sometimes interfere with sleep at night.

COMMENTS FROM THE MOTHER OF MAX

Even before Max was born I was anxious, intense, and high-strung. Max's arrival only compounded my difficulties; his care and maintenance put me over the edge. My determination to give my child what nature did not became all-encompassing. Therapies, doctors, operations, medications, home-schooling, individual educational plans (IEPs), research, reading; all these tools, despite their yields, were wearing me down. I was on overload and didn't have a clue. My usual low-grade depression deepened. I was crying a lot, snapping at my family constantly, and nervous/anxious all the time. I could not stop moving, moving, moving, or relax. I could not maintain any emotional equilibrium or anticipate my outbursts. It was dreadful. There was no peace for me. After beginning medication (Prozac) (Dr. Hagerman suggested to me that I was depressed and could be helped), I found, to my relief, that I was the same. However, I could pace myself better and was crying much less, had more mood equilibrium, and was less edgy. I could control my tongue when frustrated and better control my temper. With my developing self-control I also felt better about myself.

The knowledge that I am a carrier and awareness of the resulting genetic liability has been a great relief to me. With medication I can compensate and be proactive. My "heavy" temperament is lighter, and so is my heart.

Amy Gleicher—mother of Max; Livingston, New Jersey

Controlled studies regarding the use of fluoxetine and other serotonin agents are necessary to understand the overall efficacy in individuals with FXS and in carriers of the premutation. In general, these medications are relatively safe and well tolerated; they do not irritate the liver or the heart, and they do not require follow-up blood testing.

A recently approved SSRI, fluvoxamine (Luvox), has been shown to be effective for children with obsessive-compulsive behavior (Riddle et al., 1996). Anecdotally, this medication has been quite helpful in treatment of children and adults with FXS who experience significant anxiety, mood lability, or aggression.

At times, the activation effect of a SSRI may be quite helpful for social withdrawal or even treatment of selective mutism in girls with FXS (Hagerman et al., 1998b). This medication can facilitate verbalizations in individuals with selective mutism, and it also improves social interaction. Such an effect has also been reported in autism (Cook et al., 1992). It appears that the beneficial effects in the language area are related to decreasing anxiety, but it is unclear if a direct effect on language could be present. Kramer (1993) reported a case of improved language skills in an intellectually normal female who was treated for depression with fluoxetine.

If the activation effect is severe or if mania developes with an SSRI agent, then the dose should be lowered or the medication should be discontinued. Such effects suggest that mood stabilzation is required. Medication such as lithium and/or anticonvulsant mood stabilizers described previously are usually helpful for severe mood instability problems (Freeman and Stoll, 1998). Some of the newer anticonvulsants, such as gabapentin (Neurontin) can be added to valproate or carbamazepine or lithium as an adjunctive mood stabilizer. Most of the experience in bipolar disorder or with individuals who have intellectual disability is anecdotal, and there are no reports of combined therapy in individuals with FXS. For a review of combined therapy for treatment of mood instability, see Keck et al. (1998) and Freeman and Stoll (1998).

An easy-to-read, user-friendly booklet regarding the use of a variety of psychotropic medications in patients with FXS has been developed by the FRAXA Research Foundation and can be obtained by contacting them directly (Tranfaglia, 1996; see Resources at the end of this chapter).

Psychosis

A severe disturbance in thinking with psychotic features can be seen in fewer than 10% of children, adolescents, and adults with FXS (Hagerman, 1996a; Khin et al., 1998). These individuals should be evaluated by a psychiatrist for consideration of neuroleptic or antipsychotic medication. Perhaps one of the safest neuroleptics on the market at this time is risperidone (Risperdal), a new atypical antipsychotic, because of the decreased risk for extrapyramidal symptoms (EPS). This is because risperidone blocks both serotonin receptors and dopamine receptors, leading to a low risk for EPS when doses are kept under 8 mg/day (Kapur and Remington, 1996; Livingston, 1994). Risperidone has not only been used to treat schizophrenia and psychosis but has also been helpful in treating severe behavior problems including mood instability in individuals with mental retardation or pervasive developmental disorder (Fishman and Steele, 1996; Khan, 1997; Purdon et al., 1994). Risperidone has also been used to augment SSRI treatment in individuals with severe obsessive-compulsive disorder (McDougle et al., 1995; Saxena et al., 1996). It is described in more detail in chapter 3.

An even newer atypical antipsychotic agent, olanzapine (Zyprexa), has been developed. It is related to clozapine but does not cause the side effect of neutropenia (drop in white blood cell count) or seizures (Reus, 1997). Although olanzapine is not as effective as clozapine for treatment of schizophrenia, it is safer than clozapine, and it has a low risk of EPS compared with other antipsychotics (Kumra et al., 1998). We have occasionally used olanzapine in patients with FXS when risperidone was not effective for controlling aggression or psychotic symptoms, and it has been helpful in more than 50% of trials. However, this is a new medication with limited experience in children and adults, and further studies are warranted (Krishnamoorthy and King, 1998).

Educational Interventions

In addition to the educational strategies outlined here for treatment of ADHD behaviors, several general principles should be remembered in educating children with FXS (Braden, 1997; Scharfenaker et al., 1996; Spiridigliozzi et al., 1994; Wilson et al., 1994).

1. They usually respond best to a multimodality approach that combines both visual and auditory input with frequent repetition.
2. They are very sensitive to environmental stimuli, so avoid loud noises, crowded situations, flickering lights, alarms, or other distracting stimuli.
3. They often require support and preparation for transitions.
4. Signs of escalating behavior, such as red ears, sweating, loud voice, increase in cluttering, or agitation require calming interventions, such as a calm voice or moving to a quieter environment, or OTSI techniques such as brushing, joint compression, deep pressure massage, calming music, or a favorite video.
5. Utilize high-interest areas in academic lessons.
6. Allow frequent breaks involving physical activity, such as lifting, pushing, and carrying.
7. Allow oral activities, such as gum chewing or eating taffy or beef jerky.
8. Use modeling and imitation strengths.
9. Assign a buddy to facilitate peer acceptance and peer modeling.
10. Use visual cueing, that is, hand signs or pictures, to prompt appropriate behavior.
11. Follow a similar routine on a daily basis, which is reinforced with a set of pictures depicting the routine.
12. Utilize computers to enhance academic and language development.

School-aged children with FXS continue to benefit from occupational and speech and language therapy during elementary education. Therapy can occur both individually and in a group (Scharfenaker et al., 1996). Some goals are best addressed in a group setting, such as pramatic language skills that use role-playing (see Appendix 3). Many children with FXS will require an aide when they are included in the regular classroom. The aide can modify the assignments so that the child with FXS can participate as much as possible and understand the lesson. Often a computer modification can be used, such as designing a word-picture match on Kid Pix instead of taking a spelling test (see Appendix 2).

Some children with FXS and moderate to severe cognitive deficits require an intensive behavioral and educational training program similar to what Lovaas and colleagues have developed for children with autism (Smith et al., 1997).

Computers and Assistive Technology

Computers should be used as often as possible in the academic setting and at home. Most children with FXS enjoy working with computer programs, and it is an area in which they usually excel. Computers and assistive technology can be utilized to enhance literacy, language development, all academic areas, leisure activity, augmentative communication, and even inclusion (Erickson and Koppen-haver, 1995; Patzer and Pettegrew, 1996; Wershing and Symington, 1995). The programs that work best for children with FXS have bold, clear graphics and include active participation with auditory and visual feedback, so that the child's attention and focus is drawn to the program. The Edmark software series and the Living Books meet these qualifications and are favorites for many children we follow (Kristen Gray, personal communication, 1998). Usually children with FXS do not do well if time pressure is included in the program because it escalates anxiety (Kristen Gray, personal communication, 1998). Computers can be utilized even in the preschool period to develop concepts, such as colors, shapes, body parts, sound-symbol associations, sorting, and categorizing. Younger children can use a Touch Window system, but even preschoolers can learn to use a mouse or track ball. With IntelliKeys (see Appendix 2) the keyboard can be modified and programmed so that it is age-appropriate (Figure 2.7). Don Johnston produces zoom caps or stickers on keys, in addition to a programmable keyboard called Discover Board. A particularly versatile program is Kid Pix, which allows the child to draw and create learning tasks, including word problems (see Appendix 2 to this volume).

Auditory feedback in word processing is available from Don Johnston and IntelliTools; Co:Writer can predict possible word choices when the first letter or more is typed. These programs and more can enhance literacy skills (see Appendix 2 to this book). Favorite programs for different ages are outlined in Table 2.4.

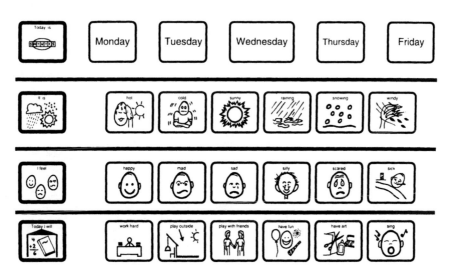

FIGURE 2.7: An example of a modified keyboard using IntelliKeys, which can facilitate age-appropriate written language.

TABLE 2.4: Computer Technology for Individuals with FXS

Ages	Uses	Companies	Favorite software	Adaptations
Preschool	Enhance language	Edmark	Millie's & Bailey's preschool	IntelliKeys
	Early childhood concepts	Brøderbund	IntelliPics	Motivating stickers on mouse or keyboard
	Enhance attention	IntelliTools		Assisted Access
School-aged	Language development	Edmark	IntelliPics	Track ball
	Inclusion	Brøderbund	Kid Pix	IntelliKeys
	Literacy	Don Johnston	IntelliTalk	Assisted Access
	Academic concepts	IntelliTools	Mighty Math Series	Zoom Caps
			Living Books Series	
Adolescents	Vocational transition to community	Attainment	Co:Writer	IntelliKeys
	Independent skills	Edmark	IntelliTalk	Assisted Access
	Academics	Don Johnston	Spending Money	Zoom Caps
	Literacy	IntelliTools	Community Words	
Adults	Vocational	Attainment	Spending Money	IntelliKeys
	Literacy		Community Words	Assisted Access
	Recreation			

Adapted from information presented by Kristen Gray (personal communication, 1998). For more information about software, see Appendix 2 to this volume.

Many programs are targeted for adolescents and adults, because they focus on community living, independence, and vocational skills. The company Attainment has developed specific programming in these areas.

Adolescents and Adults

The problem of mitral valve prolapse (MVP) is more common in adolescents and adults with FXS than in children with FXS. It can be detected by hearing a click or short murmur on auscultation, but the diagnosis of MVP should be confirmed by echocardiogram (Hagerman, 1996a). MVP is usually not associated with arrythymias, but the use of prophylactic antibiotics for dental procedures or surgery associated with bacteremia to avoid infective endocarditis is recommended when the MVP is associated with regurgitation (Durack, 1995).

The onset of puberty is associated with hormonal changes which also affect behavior. Mood lability and anxiety may become more problematic for both males and females with FXS. Aggression is more likely to occur in males at this time, and it is a problem for approximately 50% (Hagerman, 1996b). Mood swings, crying spells, and irritability around the menstrual period are manifestations of premenstrual syndrome (PMS) which may be more exaggerated in females with FXS than in those without FXS. Usually these behaviors respond well to an SSRI, and fluoxetine (Prozac) has been shown to have efficacy in treatment of PMS (Steiner et al., 1995). SSRIs can also be used to treat aggression, as described previously.

On occasion, the anxiety may be severe and unresponsive to SSRIs, buspirone, clonidine, guanfacine, or beta blockers. In such cases, benzodiazepines can be considered, including alprazolam (Xanax), lorazepam (Ativan), or clonazepam (Klonopin). Occasionally with benzodiazepines, a paradoxical reaction can occur with an increase in agitation or outburst behavior.

Vocational training is an important issue for the adolescent, and a plan for development of vocational skills should be incorporated into the individual education plan (IEP) by age 14. Although hyperactivity usually improves in adolescence, significant attentional problems often persist and may interfere with vocational activities. Sensory integration problems are also an issue in vocational settings, and crowds, excessive stimuli, disturbing noises, smells, or flickering lighting should be avoided. Adults with FXS may need frequent breaks from their work routine to promote sensory regulation (Jennifer Hills, personal communication, 1998). On-the-job training with a job coach demonstrating hands-on modeling is usually necessary. Use of a videotape of the patient or a trainer demonstrating appropriate behavior on the job can also be helpful. Utilizing a consistent routine with appropriate visual cueing leads to fewer behavioral problems. Koegel and colleagues (1992) have developed a training program to teach self-management of behavior with a positive approach that is useful in patients with FXS. Patients can be taught to recognize positive and negative behaviors and reward themselves for positive behaviors (Wilson, 1992).

Counseling is often helpful for the adolescent or adult with FXS who is having behavior problems or emancipation difficulties. The counselor can facilitate the transition from family living to living independently or semi-independently and can promote self-esteem, anger management, and self-monitoring (Bregman, 1991; Brown et al., 1991; Nezu and Nezu, 1994). Counseling is also helpful for individuals with the premutation who are experiencing problems with anxiety, phobias, or depression (Sobesky, 1996). Sex education and sexuality issues can also be addressed in counseling. There are several guides available regarding how to approach sex education in individuals with developmental disabilities (Craft, 1994; Fegan et al., 1993; Rowe and Savage, 1987; Turnbull et al., 1989).

Social skills training is essential for many individuals affected by FXS, both males and females. It is particularly important in adolescence when the demands for appropriate social interactions escalate. Girls with FXS usually have significant problems with shyness and social anxiety, although many also have impulsivity, distractibility, and moodiness, which may also interfere with social interactions. Group therapy that addresses social skills and utilizes modeling of appropriate behavior can be useful for many adolescents (Marcia Braden, personal communication 1998). Programs which a therapist can follow to build social skills include *Let's Talk* (Mundy, 1991) and *Social Skills Lessons and Activities* (Begum, 1996). Medications that improve impulsivity and moodiness, such as methylphenidate and clonidine, can work synergistically with therapy.

CASE HISTORY: JOAN

Joan is a 13-year-old girl with fragile X syndrome, and DNA testing has demonstrated a mosaic status with bands of 166, 210, and 296 CGG repeats. She was found to have an activation ratio of 0.65, and her FMRP level is 59%, which means that 59% of her lymphocytes stain positive for FMRP.

Joan was born after a normal pregnancy, and her weight was 8 lb. 8 oz. The Apgar scores were 8 and 9, and she did well in the newborn period. As an infant and preschooler, she had only occasional difficulties with tactile defensiveness, along with rare hand flapping. She did not have hand biting. She also has had problems with poor eye contact. Her early developmental milestones included sitting at 6½ months and walking at 12 months. She said words at 12 months and short phrases and sentences at 3 years of age. Her past medical history included a small ventricular septal defect (VSD), which closed on its own in the first 2 to 3 years of life and she has not had problems with seizures or otitis media infections.

She has been in special education programming since the preschool period, and attentional problems associated with hyperactivity have been an ongoing difficulty for her. She was started on dextroamphetamine (Dexedrine) tablets at age 3½, and this was helpful for her attentional problems and hyperactivity at preschool. At age 5, the Stanford Binet demonstrated a general cognitive index of 87, and distractibility and some oppositional behavior was noted during this testing. The Kaufman Assessment Battery for Children (K-ABC) was given at age 7. Her Mental Processing Composite was 71 with an Achievement Score of 89. Her Sequential IQ was 55, and her Simultaneous IQ was 86. The significant discrepancy between Sequential and Simultaneous IQ was thought to relate to her ADHD.

At age 10 years, Joan was switched to methylphenidate (Ritalin) at a dose of 20 mg slow release in the morning with 10 mg short acting at noon and also at 2 p.m. This appeared to give her better coverage throughout the day than the dextroamphetamine tablets.

Joan's educational program includes mainstreaming into the regular classroom, but she has a special education aide working with her. She does not want to be pulled out into a separate special education program, and her self-image has improved in the regular classroom. The aide works with her on a one-to-one basis four times a day for 20 minutes. The aide has targeted money concepts and practical aspects of math for more intensive remediation.

Joan started menstruating last year and has had an increase in boisterous behavior and mood swings now at age 13 years. Her present dose of methylphenidate includes 20 mg of the long-acting form in the morning and 10 mg of the short-acting form three times a day. She has not had side effects from the methylphenidate. Her height and weight growth percentile have increased appropriately, and she sleeps well. She has never shown aggression in school, but she has had outbursts, sometimes getting loud in school and yelling, "I have no friends." She gets along well with four or five other children in her special needs program at school, and all of the kids at the school know her.

To treat her mood swings and boisterous behavior, a Catapres TTS1 patch was added to her medication regimen, and this has made a significant difference in decreasing ADHD symptoms and moodiness. Her EKG in follow-up was normal. She is in a social skills building group at school, and she will have a more intensive program in the summer through a private therapist.

FUTURE DIRECTIONS

The future of treatment of patients with FXS will no doubt include either protein replacement therapy or gene therapy; however, several obstacles must be overcome before this type of intervention is a safe alternative (Rattazzi and Ioannou, 1996). It is important to remember that the *FMR1* gene is intact in the vast majority of individuals with FXS, and if one could remove the CGG expansion, activate the promoter, or eliminate the methylation which silences the *FMR1* gene, then significant levels of FMRP could be produced, perhaps leading to a cure for this disorder. Chiurazzi et al. (1998) recently reported reactivation of the *FMR1* gene in vitro by inducing DNA demethylation with 5-azadeoxycytidine. This is an exciting advance; however, it will be extremely difficult to target the demethylation of only one gene in vivo. The rapid pace of molecular biological advances in the fragile X field suggests that a molecular or protein intervention will be a safe alternative within the next 10 years. If FMRP is supplied to a child or adult with FXS, it is uncertain how significant the benefits would be. When possible, molecular interventions should be tried as early as possible and perhaps even in utero so that the significant structural changes of the brain in FXS can be avoided.

The most exciting area in educational intervention includes the use of computer technology to enhance development and learning in children with FXS. New approaches such as the computerized slowing of phonemic segments to improve auditory processing and comprehension in the Fast Forward program has been beneficial in children with language deficits and even with pervasive developmental disorders (Merzenich et al., 1996; Tallal et al., 1996). Such new technology may turn out to be helpful in patients with FXS, although controlled studies are necessary.

Advances in psychotropic medication which can counteract the effect of a deficiency in FMRP are promising. Although we have excellent medications which can enhance the functioning of the dopamine, norepinephrine, and serotonin systems, newer medications such as those which enhance the cholinergic system are likely to be helpful in patients with FXS (Capone, 1998; Hagerman, 1996b). Studies could take place in the fragile X knockout mouse initially, and those agents which are helpful can be advanced to human trials. The future appears bright, and significant advances will continue to occur to improve the treatment of children and adults with FXS.

ACKNOWLEDGMENTS   I thank the fragile X treatment team, including Louise Gane, Rebecca O'Connor, Jennifer Hills, Sarah Scharfenaker, Kristen Gray, Lisa Noble, Tracy Kovach, Tracy Stackhouse, Clare Summers, Lucy Miller, Marcia Braden, and Edward Goldson for teaching me about intervention and for helpful comments on the manuscript. We have all learned what we know about fragile X syndrome from the families, children, and adults who are affected by this disorder. A special thanks to Rachel Calvert and Amy Gleisher, whose words have greatly enhanced the meaning of this chapter. This work was partially supported by MCH training grant no. MCJ-089413, NICHD grant no. HD36071, March of Dimes grant no. M12-FY96-0492, the National Center for Research Resources NIH grant no. M01 RR00069 to the General Clinical Research Center, the Kenneth Kendal King Foundation, the Denver Foundation, the Kettering Family Foundation, the Wallace Genetic Foundation, the Developmental Psychobiology Research group, and the Children's Hospital Research Institute.

REFERENCES

Abbeduto, L., and Hagerman, R. J. (1997) Language and communication in fragile X syndrome. Mental Retardation and Developmental Disabilities Research Reviews 3 (4): 313–22.

Abitbol, M., Menini, C., Delezoide, A. L., Rhyner, T., Vekemans, M., Mallet, J. (1993) Nucleus basalis magnocellularis and hippocampus are the major sites of FMR-1 expression in the human fetal brain. Nature Genetics 4 (2): 147–53.

Abrams, M. T., Reiss, A. L., Freund, L. S., Baumgardner, T. L., Chase, G. A., Denckla, M. B. (1994) Molecular-neurobehavioral associations in females with the fragile X full mutation. American Journal of Medical Genetics 51 (4): 317–27.

Adcock, K. G., MacElroy, D. E., Wolford, E. T., Farrington, E. A. (1998) Pemoline therapy resulting in liver transplantation. Annals of Pharmacotherapy 32: 422–25.

Alderman, J., Wolkow, R., Chung, M., Johnston, H. F. (1998) Setraline treatment of children and adolescents with obsessive-compulsive disorder or depression: Pharmacokinetics, tolerability and efficacy. Journal of the American Academy of Child and Adolescent Psychiatry 37 (4): 386–94.

Allingham-Hawkins, D .J., Brown, C. A., Babul, R., Chitayat, D., Krekewich, K., Humphries, T., Ray, P. N., Teshima, I. E. (1996) Tissue-specific methylation differences and cognitive function in fragile X premutation females. American Journal of Medical Genetics 64 (2): 329–33.

Alvarez, N., Besag, F., Iivanainen, M. (1998) Use of antiepileptic drugs in the treatment of epilepsy in people with intellectual disability. Journal of Intellectual Disability Research 42 (Suppl. 1): 1–15.

Aman, M. G., Kern, R. A., McGhee, D. E., Arnold, L. E. (1993) Fenfluramine and methylphenidate in children with mental retardation and ADHD: Clinical and side effects. Journal of American Academy of Child and Adolescent Psychiatry 32: 851–59.

American Academy of Pediatrics Committee on Genetics (1996) Health supervision for children with fragile X syndrome. Pediatrics 98 (2, Pt. 1): 297–300.

Ashley, C. T., Sutcliffe, J. S., Kunst, C. B., Leiner, H. A., Eichler, E. E., Nelson, D. L., Warren, S. T. (1993) Human and murine FMR-1: Alternative splicing and translational initiation downstream of the CGG-repeat. Nature Genetics 4 (3): 244–51.

Bailey, D. B., Hatton, D. D., Skinner, M. (1998) Early developmental trajectories of males with fragile X syndrome. American Journal on Mental Retardation 103 (1): 29–39.

Bailey, D. B., Mesibov, G. B., Hatton, D. D., Clark, R. D., Roberts, J. E., Mayhew, L. (1998) Autistic behavior in young boys wtih fragile X syndrome. Journal of Autism and Developmental Disorders 28 (6): 499–508.

Bakker, C. E., Verheij, C., Willemsen, R., Vanderhelm, R., Oerlemans, F., Vermey, M., Bygrave, A., Hoogereen, A. T., Oostra, B. A., Reyniers, E., De Boulle, K., Dhooge, R., Cras, P., Van Velzen, D., Nagels, G., Martin, J. J., Dedeyn, P. P., Darby, J. K., Willems, P. J. (1994) FMR1 knockout mice: A model to study fragile X mental retardation. Cell 78: 23–33.

Barkley, R. A. (1990) Attention deficit hyperactivity disorder: A handbook for diagnosis and treatment. Guilford Press, New York.

Barkley, R. A., DuPaul, G. J., McMurray, M. B. (1991) Attention deficit disorder with and without hyperactivity: Clinical response to three dose levels of methylphenidate. Pediatrics 87: 519–31.

Baumgardner, T. L., Reiss, A. L., Freund, L. S., Abrams, M. T. (1995) Specification of the neurobehavioral phenotype in males with fragile X syndrome. Pediatrics 95 (5): 744–52.

Begum, R. W. (1996) Social skills lessons and activities. Center for Applied Research in Education, West Nyack, New York.

Bell, M. V., Hirst, M. C., Nakahori, Y., MacKinnon, R. N., Roche, A., Flint, T. J., Jacobs, P. A., Tommerup, N., Tranebjaerg, L., Froster Iskenius, U., et al. (1991) Physical mapping across the fragile X: Hypermethylation and clinical expression of the fragile X syndrome. Cell 64 (4): 861–6.

Belser, R. C., and Sudhalter, V. (1995) Arousal difficulties in males with Fragile X Syndrome: A preliminary report. Developmental Brain Dysfunction 8: 270–79.

Bennetto, L., and Pennington, B. F. (1996) The neuropsychology of fragile X syndrome. In: Fragile X syndrome: Diagnosis, treatment and research. Hagerman, R. J., and Cronister, A. (eds.). 2nd ed. Johns Hopkins University Press, Baltimore, pp. 210–48.

Berkovitz, G. D., Wilson, D. P., Carpenter, N. J., Brown, T. R., Migeon, C. J. (1986) Gonadal function in men with the Martin Bell (fragile X) syndrome. American Journal of Medical Genetics 23: 227–39.

Besag, F. M. C. (1998) Lamotrigine in the treatment of epilepsy in people with intellectual disability. Journal of

Intellectual Disability Research 42 (Suppl. 1): 50–56.

Birot, A. M., Delobel, B., Gronnier, P., Bonnet, V., Maire, I., Bozon, D. (1996) A 5-megabase familial deletion removes the IDS and FMR-1 genes in a male Hunter patient. Human Mutation 7 (3): 266–8.

Bowden, C. L., Brugger, A. M., Swann, A. C., Calabrese, J. R., Janicak, P. G., Petty, F., Dilsaver, S. C., Davis, J. M., Rush, A. J., Small, J. G., Garza-Trevino, E. S., Risch, S. C., Goodnick, P. J., Morris, D. D. (1994) Efficacy of divalproex vs. lithium and placebo in the treatment of mania. Journal of the American Medical Association 271: 918–24.

Braden, M. L. (1997) Fragile, handle with care: Understanding fragile X syndrome. 2nd ed. Avanta Publishing, Chapel Hill, N.C.

Bregman, J. D. (1991) Current developments in understanding mental retardation. Part II: Psychopathology. Journal of the American Academy of Child and Adolescent Psychiatry 30: 861–72.

Brown, J., Braden, M., Sobesky, W. (1991) The treatment of behavior and emotional problems. In: Fragile X syndrome: Diagnosis, treatment, and research. Hagerman, R. J., and Silverman, A. C. (eds.). Johns Hopkins University Press, Baltimore, pp. 311–26.

Brown, W. T. (1996a) The FRAXE syndrome: Is it time for routine screening? [Editorial]. American Journal of Human Genetics 58 (5): 903.

Brown, W. T. (1996b) The molecular biology of the fragile X mutation. In: Fragile X syndrome: Diagnosis, treatment, and research. Hagerman, R. J., and Cronister, A. (eds.). 2nd ed. Johns Hopkins University Press, Baltimore, pp. 88–113.

Brown, W. T., Nolin, S., Houck, G., Jr., Ding, X., Glicksman, A., Li, S. Y., Stark-Houck, S., Brophy, P., Duncan, C., Dobkin, C., Jenkins, E. (1996) Prenatal diagnosis and carrier screening for fragile X by PCR. American Journal of Medical Genetics 64: 191–5.

Butler, M. G., Allen, G. A., Haynes, J. L., Singh, D. N., Watson, M. S., Breg, W. R. (1991) Anthropometric comparison of mentally retarded males with and without the fragile X syndrome. American Journal of Medical Genetics 38 (2–3): 260–8.

Butler, M. G., Brunschwig, A., Miller, L. K., Hagerman, R. J. (1992) Standards for selected anthropometric measurements in males with the fragile X syndrome. Pediatrics 89 (6, Pt. 1): 1059–62.

Cantwell, D. P., Swanson, J., Connor, D. F. (1997) Case study: Adverse response to clonidine. Journal of American and Academic Child and Adolescence Psychiatry 36: 539–44.

Capone, G. T. (1998) Drugs that increase intelligence? Applications for childhood cognitive impairment. Mental Retardation and Developmental Disabilities Research Reviews 4: 36–49.

Chandran, K. S. K. (1994) ECG and clonidine. Journal of the American Academy of Child and Adolescent Psychiatry 33: 1351–2.

Chiurazzi, P., Pomponi, M. G., Willemsen, R., Oostra, B. A., Neri, G. (1998) In vitro reactivation of the FMR1 gene involved in fragile X syndrome. Human Molecular Genetics 7 (1): 109–13.

Clarke, A., Bradley, D., Gillespie, K., Rees, D., Holland, A., Thomas, N. S. (1992) Fragile X mental retardation and the iduronate sulphatase locus: Testing Laird's model of fra(X) inheritance. American Journal of Medical Genetics 43 (1–2): 299–306.

Comery, T. A., Harris, J. B., Willems, P. J., Oostra, B. A., Irwin, S. A., Weiler, I. J., Greenough, W. T. (1997) Abnormal dendritic spines in fragile X knockout mouse: Maturation and pruning deficits. Proceedings of the National Academy of Sciences of the United States of America 94: 5401–4.

Cook, E. H., Jr., Rowlett, R., Jaseiskis, C., Leventhal, B. L. (1992) Fluoxetine treatment of children and adults with autistic disorder and mental retardation. Journal of the American Academy of Child and Adolescent Psychiatry 31: 739–50.

Cook, E. H., Jr., Courchesne, R., Lord, C., Cox, N. J., Yan, S., Lincoln, A., Haas, R., Courchesne, E., Leventhal, B. L. (1997) Evidence of linkage between the serotonin transporter and autistic disorder. Molecular Psychiatry 2: 247–50.

Coy, J. F., Sedlacek, Z., Bachner, D., Hameister, H., Joos, S., Lichter, P., Delius, H., Poustka, A. (1995) Highly conserved 3'UTR and expression pattern of FXR1 points to a divergent gene regulation of FXR1 and FMR1. Human Molecular Genetics 4: 2209–18.

Crabbe, L. S., Bensky, A. S., Hornstein, L., Schwartz, D. C. (1993) Cardiovascular abnormalities in children with fragile X syndrome. Pediatrics 91 (4): 714–5.

Craft, A. (1994) Practice issues in sexuality and learning disabilities. Routledge, London and New York.

Crepeau-Hobson, F., and O'Connor, R. (1996) Appendix 4: Toilet training the child with fragile X syndrome. In: Fragile X syndrome: Diagnosis, treatment, and research, Hagerman, R. J., and Cronister, A. (eds.). 2nd ed. Johns Hopkins University Press, Baltimore, pp. 470–2.

Cronister, A. J. (1996) Genetic counseling. In Fragile X syndrome: Diagnosis, treatment, and research. Hagerman, R. J., and Cronister, A. (eds.). 2nd ed. Johns Hopkins University Press, Baltimore, pp. 251–82.

Davids, J. R., Hagerman, R. J., Eilert, R. E. (1990) Orthopaedic aspects of frag-

ile-X syndrome. Journal of Bone and Joint Surgery—American 72 (6): 889–96.

Dawson, P. M., VanderZander, J. A., Werkman, S. L., Washington, R. L., Tyma, T. A. (1989) Cardiac dysrhythmia with the use of clonidine in explosive disorder. Annals of Pharmacotherapy 23: 465–6.

de Boulle, K., Verkerk, A. J., Reyniers, E., Vits, L., Hendrickx, J., Van Roy, B., Van den Bos, F., de Graaff, E., Oostra, B. A., Willems, P. J. (1993) A point mutation in the FMR-1 gene associated with fragile X mental retardation. Nature Genetics 3 (1): 31–5.

de Graaff, E., Rouillard, P., Willems, P. J., Smits, A. P., Rousseau, F., Oostra, B. A. (1995) Hotspot for deletions in the CGG repeat region of FMR1 in fragile X patients. Human Molecular Genetics 4 (1): 45–9.

de Vries, B. B., Fryns, J. P., Butler, M. G., Canziani, F., Wesby-van Swaay, E., vanHemel, J. O., Oostra, B. A., Halley, D. J. J., Niermeyer, M. F. (1993) Clinical and molecular studies in fragile X patients with a Prader-Willi-like phenotype. Journal of Medical Genetics 30: 761–6.

de Vries, B. B., Robinson, H., Stolte Dijkstra, I., Tjon Pian Gi, C. V., Dijkstra, P. F., van Doorn, J., Halley, D. J., Oostra, B. A., Turner, G., Niermeijer, M. F. (1995) General overgrowth in the fragile X syndrome: Variability in the phenotypic expression of the FMR1 gene mutation. Journal of Medical Genetics 32 (10): 764–9.

de Vries, B. B., Jansen, C. C., Duits, A. A., Verheij, C., Willemsen, R., van Hemel, J. O., van den Ouweland, A. M., Niermeijer, M. F., Oostra, B. A., Halley, D. J. (1996a) Variable FMR1 gene methylation of large expansions leads to variable phenotype in three males from one fragile X family. Journal of Medical Genetics 33 (12): 1007–10.

de Vries, B. B., Wiegers, A. M., Smits, A. P., Mohkamsing, S., Duivenvoorden, H. J., Fryns, J. P., Curfs, L. M., Halley, D. J., Oostra, B. A., van den Ouweland, A. M., Niermeijer, M. F. (1996b) Mental status of females with an FMR1 gene full mutation. American Journal of Medical Genetics 58 (5): 1025–32.

de Vries, B. B., van den Ouweland, A. M., Mohkamsing, S., Duivenvoorden, H. J., Mol, E., Gelsema, K., van Rijn, M., Halley, D. J., Sandkuijl, L. A., Oostra, B. A., Tibben, A., Niermeijer, M. F. (1997) Screening and diagnosis for the fragile X syndrome among the mentally retarded: An epidemiological and psychological survey. American Journal of Human Genetics 61 (3): 660–7.

Delahunty, C., Schaffer, M., Logan, L., Blodgett, R. L., Burgess, D., Hagerman, R. (1999) Electrocardiographic changes in children treated with clonidine, alone or in combination wtih stimulant medications: A retrospective study. Manuscript submitted for publication.

Devys, D., Lutz, Y., Rouyer, N., Bellocq, J. P., Mandel, J. L. (1993) The FMR-1 protein is cytoplasmic, most abundant in neurons and appears normal in carriers of a fragile X premutation. Nature Genetics 4 (4): 335–40.

Dreifuss, F. E., and Langer, D. H. (1987) Hepatic considerations in the use of antiepileptic drugs. Epilepsia 28 (suppl. 2): S23.

Durack, D. T. (1995) Drug therapy. New England Journal of Medicine 332 (1): 38–44.

Dykens, E. M., Hodapp, R. M., Ort, S., Finucane, B., Shapiro, L. R., Leckman, J. F. (1989) The trajectory of cognitive development in males with fragile X syndrome. Journal of the American Academy of Child and Adolescent Psychiatry 28 (3): 422–6.

Dykens, E. M., Hodapp, R. M., Leckman, J. F. (1994) Behavior and development in fragile X syndrome. Sage, Thousand Oaks, CA.

Eichler, E. E., Holden, J. J., Popovich, B. W., Reiss, A. L., Snow, K., Thibodeau, S. N., Richards, C. S., Ward, P. A., Nelson, D. L. (1994) Length of uninterrupted CGG repeats determines instability in the FMR1 gene. Nature Genetics 8 (1): 88–94.

Erickson, K. A., and Koppenhaver, D. A. (1995) Developing a literacy program for children with severe disabilities. Reading Teacher 48 (8): 676–84.

Escalante, J. A., and Frota-Pessona, O. (1973) Retardamento mental. In Genetica Medica. Becak, W., and Frota-Pessoa, O. (eds.). Sarvier, São Paulo, pp. 300–8.

Fegan, L., Rauch, A., McCarthy, W. (1993) Sexuality and people with intellectual disability. Brookes, Baltimore.

Feng, Y., Absher, D., Eberhart, D. E., Brown, V., Malter, H. E., Warren, S. T. (1997a) FMRP associates with polyribosomes as an mRNP, and the I304N mutation of severe fragile X syndrome abolishes this association. Molecular Cell 1: 109–18.

Feng, Y., Gutekunst, C. A., Eberhart, D. E., Yi, H., Warren, S. T., Hersch, S. M. (1997b) Fragile X mental retardation protein: Nucleocytoplasmic shuttling and association with somatodendritic ribosomes. Journal of Neurosciences 17 (5): 1539–47.

Finelli, P. F., Pueschel, S. M., Padre-Mendoza, T., O'brien, M. M. (1985) Neurological findings in patients with the fragile-X syndrome. Journal of Neurology, Neurosurgery and Psychiatry 48 (2): 150–3.

Fisch, G. S., Shapiro, L. R., Simensen, R., Schwartz, C. E., Fryns, J. P., Borghgraef, M., Curfs, L. M., Howard Peebles, P. N., Arinami, T., Mavrou, A. (1992) Longitudinal changes in IQ among fragile X males: Clinical evidence of more than one mutation? American Journal of Medical Genetics 43 (1–2): 28–34.

Fishman, S., and Steele, M. (1996) Use of risperidone in pervasive developmental disorders: A case series. Journal of Child and Adolescent Psychopharmacology 6 (3): 177–90.

Franke, P., Maier, W., Hautzinger, M., Weiffenbach, O., Gansicke, M., Iwers, B., Poustka, F., Schwab, S. G., Froster, U. (1996) Fragile-X carrier females: Evidence for a distinct psychopathological phenotype? American Journal of Medical Genetics 64 (2): 334–9.

Franke, P., Leboyer, M., Gansicke, M., Weiffenbach, O., Biancalana, V., Cornillet-Lefebre, P., Croquette, M. F., Froster, U., Schwab, S. G., Poustka, F., Hautzinger, M., Maier, W. (1998) Genotype-phenotype relationship in female carriers of the premutation and full mutation of FMR-1. Psychiatry Research 80: 113–27.

Freeman, M. P., and Stoll, A. (1998) Mood stabilizer combinations: A review of safety and efficacy. American Journal of Psychiatry 155: 12–21.

Freund, L. S., and Reiss, A. L. (1991) Cognitive profiles associated with the fra(X) syndrome in males and females. American Journal of Medical Genetics 38 (4): 542–7.

Freund, L. S., Reiss, A. L., Abrams, M. T. (1993) Psychiatric disorders associated with fragile X in the young female. Pediatrics 91 (2): 321–9.

Freund, L., Peebles, C. A., Aylward, E., Reiss, A. L. (1995) Preliminary report on cognitive and adaptive behaviors of preschool-aged males with fragile X. Developmental Brain Dysfunction 8: 242–61.

Friis, M. L. (1998) Valproate in the treatment of epilepsy in people with intellectual disability. Journal of Intellectual Disability Research 42 (suppl. 1): 32–5.

Fryns, J. P. (1984) The fragile X syndrome: A study of 83 families. Clinical Genetics 26 (6): 497–528.

Fryns, J. P., Dereymaeker, A. M., Hoefnagels, M., Volcke, P., Van den Berghe, H. (1986) Partial fra(X) phenotype with megalotestes in fra(X) negative patients with acquired lesions of the central nervous system. American Journal of Medical Genetics 23: 213–9.

Fryns, J. P., Moerman, P., Gilis, F., d'Espallier, L., Van den Berghe, H. (1988) Suggestively increased rate of infant death in children of fra(X) positive mothers. American Journal of Medical Genetics 30 (1–2): 73–5.

Fu, Y. H., Kuhl, D. P., Pizzuti, A., Pieretti, M., Sutcliffe, J. S., Richards, S., Verkerk, A. J., Holden, J. J., Fenwick, R. G., Jr., Warren, S. T., et al. (1991) Variation of the CGG repeat at the fragile X site results in genetic instability: Resolution of the Sherman paradox. Cell 67 (6): 1047–58.

Gao, J., Parsons, L. M., Bower, J. M., Xiong, J., Li, J., Fox, P. T. (1996) Cerebellum implicated in sensory acquisition and discrimination rather than motor control. Science 272: 545–7.

Gedeon, A. K., Baker, E., Robinson, H., Partington, M. W., Gross, B., Manca, A., Korn, B., Poustka, A., Yu, S., Sutherland, G. R., et al. (1992) Fragile X syndrome without CCG amplification has an FMR1 deletion. Nature Genetics 1 (5): 341–4.

Giangreco, C. A., Steele, M. W., Aston, C. E., Cummins, J. H., Wenger, S. L. (1996) A simplified six-item checklist for screening for fragile X syndrome in the pediatric population. Journal of Pediatrics 129 (4): 611–4.

Gillberg, C., Melander, H., von Knorring, A. L., Janols, L. O., Thernlund, G., Hagglof, B., Eidevall-Wallin, L., Gustafsson, P., Kopp, S. (1997) Long-term stimulant treatment of children with attention-deficit hyperactivity disorder symptoms. A randomized, double-blind, placebo-controlled trial. Archives of General Psychiatry 54 (9): 857–64.

Giraud, F., Ayme, S., Mattei, M. G. (1976) Constitutional chromosomal breakage. Human Genetics 34: 125–36.

Gringras, P., and Barnicoat, A. (1998) Retesting for fragile X syndrome in cytogentically normal males. Developmental Medicine and Child Neurology 40: 62–4.

Grønskov, K., Hjalgrim, H., Bjerager, M. O., Brøndum-Nielsen, K. (1997) Deletion of all CGG repeats plus flanking sequences in FMR1 does not abolish gene expression. American Journal of Human Genetics 61 (4): 961–7.

Gu, Y., Lugenbeel, K. A., Vockley, J. G., Grody, W. W., Nelson, D. L. (1994) A de novo deletion in FMR1 in a patient with developmental delay. Human Molecular Genetics 3 (9): 1705–6.

Gualtieri, C. T. (1990) Neuropsychiatry and behavioral pharmacology. Springer Verlag, Berlin.

Gualtieri, C. T. (1992) Psychopharmacology and the fragile X syndrome. In: 1992 International Fragile X Conference Proceedings. Hagermah, R. J., and McKenzie, P. (eds.). National Fragile X Foundation and Spectra Publishing, Dillon, Colo., pp. 167–78.

Hagerman, R. J. (1984) Pediatric assessment of the learning disabled child. Journal of Developmental and Behavioral Pediatrics 5: 274–84.

Hagerman, R. J. (1992) Clinical conundrums in fragile X syndrome. Nature Genetics 1 (3): 157–8.

Hagerman, R. J. (1996a) Medical follow-up and pharmacotherapy. In: Fragile X syndrome: Diagnosis, treatment, and research. Hagerman, R. J., and Cronister, A. (eds.). 2nd ed. Johns Hopkins University Press, Baltimore, pp. 283–331.

Hagerman, R. J. (1996b) Physical and behavioral phenotype. In: Fragile X syndrome: Diagnosis, treatment and research. Hagerman, R. J., and Cronister, A. (eds.). 2nd ed. Johns Hopkins University Press, Baltimore, pp. 3–87.

Hagerman, R. J. (1997) Fragile X: Treatment of hyperactivity [Letter to the editor]. Pediatrics 99 (5): 753.

Hagerman, R. J., Van Housen, K., Smith, A. C., McGavran, L. (1984) Consideration of connective tissue dysfunction in the fragile X syndrome. American Journal of Medical Genetics 17 (1): 111–21.

Hagerman, R. J., Altshul-Stark, D., McBogg, P. (1987) Recurrent otitis media in boys with the fragile X syndrome. American Journal of Diseases in Childhood 141: 184–7.

Hagerman, R. J., Murphy, M. A., Wittenberger, M. D. (1988) A controlled trial of stimulant medication in children with the fragile X syndrome. American Journal of Medical Genetics 30 (1–2): 377–92.

Hagerman, R. J., Schreiner, R. A., Kemper, M. B., Wittenberger, M. D., Zahn, B., Habicht, K. (1989) Longitudinal IQ changes in fragile X males. American Journal of Medical Genetics 33 (4): 513–8.

Hagerman, R. J., Amiri, K., Cronister, A. (1991) Fragile X checklist. American Journal of Medical Genetics 38 (2–3): 283–7.

Hagerman, R. J., Jackson, C., Amiri, K., Silverman, A. C., O'Connor, R., Sobesky, W. (1992) Girls with fragile X syndrome: Physical and neurocognitive status and outcome. Pediatrics 89 (3): 395–400.

Hagerman, R. J., Hull, C. E., Safanda, J. F., Carpenter, I., Staley, L. W., O'Connor, R., Seydel, C., Mazzocco, M. M., Snow, K., Thibodeau, S. N., et al. (1994) High functioning fragile X males: Demonstration of an unmethylated fully expanded FMR-1 mutation associated with protein expression.

American Journal of Medical Genetics 51 (4): 298–308.

Hagerman, R. J., Fulton, M. J., Leaman, A., Riddle, J., Hagerman, K., Sobesky, W. (1994) Fluoxetine therapy in fragile X syndrome. Developmental Brain Dysfunction 7: 155–64.

Hagerman, R. J., Riddle, J. E., Roberts, L. S., Brease, K., Fulton, M. (1995) A survey of the efficacy of clonidine in fragile X syndrome. Developmental Brain Dysfunction 8: 336–44.

Hagerman, R. J., Staley, L. W., O'Connor, R., Lugenbeel, K., McLean, S. D., Taylor, A. (1996) Learning-disabled males with a fragile X CGG expansion in the upper premutation size range. Pediatrics 97: 8–12.

Hagerman, R. J., Bregman, J. D., Tirosh, E. (1998a) Clonidine. In: Psychotropic medication and developmental disabilities: The international consensus handbook. Reiss, S., and Aman, M. G. (eds.). Ohio State University Nisonger Center, Columbus, Ohio, pp. 259–69.

Hagerman, R. J., Hills, J., Scharfenaker, S., Lewis, H. (1999) Fragile X syndrome and Selective Mutism. American Journal of Medical Genetics 83: 313–17.

Hagerman, R. J., Kimbro, L. T., Taylor, A. K. (1998c) Fragile X syndrome: A common cause of mental retardation and premature menopause. Contemporary OB/GYN 43 (1): 47–70.

Handen, B. L., Janosky, J., McAuliffe, S., Breaux, A. M., Feldman, H. (1994) Prediction of response to methylphenidate among children with ADHD and mental retardation. Journal of American Academy of Child and Adolescent Psychiatry 33: 1185–93.

Hanson, D. M., Jackson, A. W., III, Hagerman, R. J. (1986) Speech disturbances (cluttering) in mildly impaired males with the Martin-Bell/fragile X syndrome. American Journal of Medical Genetics 7: 471–89.

Hart, P. S., Olson, S. M., Crandall, K., Tarleton, J. (1995) Fragile X syndrome resulting from a 400 base-pair deletion within the FMR1 gene. American Journal of Human Genetics Supplement 57: A1395.

Harvey, J., Judge, C., Weiner, S. (1977) Familial X-linked mental retardation with an X chromosome abnormality. Journal of Medical Genetics 14: 46–50.

Hatton, D. D., Buckley, E. G., Lachiewicz, A., Roberts, J. (1997) Ocular status of young boys with fragile X syndrome: A prospective study. Eighth International Conference on Fragile X Syndrome and X-linked Mental Retardation, Ontario, Canada.

Hilton, D. K., Martin, C. A., Heffron, W. M., Hall, B. D., Johnson, G. L. (1991) Imipramine treatment of ADHD in a fragile X child. Journal of American Academy of Child and Adolescent Psychiatry 30 (5): 831–4.

Hinds, H. L., Ashley, C. T., Sutcliffe, J. S., Nelson, D. L., Warren, S. T., Housman, D. E., Schalling, M. (1993) Tissue specific expression of FMR-1 provides evidence for a functional role in fragile X syndrome [see comments]. Nature Genetics 3 (1): 36–43.

Hirst, M., Grewal, P., Flannery, A., Slatter, R., Maher, E., Barton, D., Fryns, J. P., Davies, K. (1995) Two new cases of FMR1 deletion associated with mental impairment. American Journal of Human Genetics 56 (1): 67–74.

Hockey, A., and Crowhurst, J. (1988) Early manifestations of the Martin-Bell syndrome based on a series of both sexes from infancy. American Journal of Medical Genetics 30 (1–2): 61–71.

Hodapp, R. M., Dykens, E. M., Hagerman, R. J., Schreiner, R., Lachiewicz, A. M., Leckman, J. F. (1990) Developmental implications of changing trajectories of IQ in males with fragile X syndrome. Journal of the American

Academy of Child and Adolescent Psychiatry 29 (2): 214–9.

Hodapp, R. M., Leckman, J. F., Dykens, E. M., Sparrow, S. S., Zelinsky, D. G., Ort, S. I. (1992) K-ABC profiles in children with fragile X syndrome, Down syndrome, and nonspecific mental retardation. American Journal on Mental Retardation 97 (1): 39–46.

Holloway, S. L., Loesch, D., Hagerman, R. J. (in press) Temporal sleep characteristics of young boys with fragile X syndrome. American Journal on Mental Retardation.

Hull, C., and Hagerman, R. J. (1993) A study of the physical, behavioral, and medical phenotype, including anthropometric measures, of females with fragile X syndrome. American Journal of Diseases of Children 147 (11): 1236–41.

Hunt, R. D., Arnsten, A. F. T., Asbell, M. D. (1995) An open trial of guanfacine in treatment of attention deficit hyperactivity disorder. Journal of American Academy of Child and Adolescent Psychiatry 34: 50–54.

Imbert, G., Feng, Y., Nelson, D. L., Warren, S. T., Mandel, J.-L. (1998) FMR1 and mutations in fragile X syndrome: Molecular biology, biochemistry, and genetics. In Genetic instabilities and hereditary neurological diseases. Wells, R. D., Warren, S. T., Sarmiento, M. (eds.). Academic Press, San Diego, pp. 27–53.

Isojarvi, J. I., Laatikainen, T. J., Pakarinen, A. J., Juntunen, K. T., Myllyla, V. V. (1993) Polycystic ovaries and hyperandrogenism in women taking valproate for epilepsy. New England Journal of Medicine 329 (19): 1383–8.

Jacky, P. (1996) Cytogenetics. In: Fragile X syndrome: Diagnosis, treatment and research. Hagerman, R. J., and Cronister, A. (eds.). 2nd ed. Johns Hopkins University Press, Baltimore, pp. 114–64.

Jan, J. E., and O'Donnell, M. E. (1996) Use of melatonin in the treatment of paediatric sleep disorders. Journal of Pineal Research 21 (4): 193–9.

Johnson, G. E. (1897) Contribution to the psychology and pedagogy of feebleminded children. Journal of Psycho-asthenics 2: 26–32.

Kälviäinen, R. (1998) Tiagabine: A new therapeutic option for people with intellectual disability and partial epilepsy. Journal of Intellectual Disability Research 42 (suppl. 1): 63–7.

Kapur, S., and Remington, G. (1996) Serotonin-dopamine interaction and its relevance to schizophrenia. American Journal of Psychiatry 153 (4): 466–76.

Kaufmann, P. M., Leckman, J. F., Ort, S. I. (1990) Delayed response performance in males with fragile X syndrome. Journal of Clinical and Experimental Neuropsychology 12: 69.

Keck, P. E., McElroy, S. L., Strakowski, S. M. (1998) Anticonvulsants and antipsychotics in the treatment of bipolar disorder. Journal of Clinical Psychiatry 59 (suppl. 6): 74–81.

Kemper, M. B., Hagerman, R. J., Ahmad, R. S., Mariner, R. (1986) Cognitive profiles and the spectrum of clinical manifestations in heterozygous fragile (X) females. American Journal of Medical Genetics 23: 139–56.

Kemper, M. B., Hagerman, R. J., Altshul-Stark, D. (1988) Cognitive profiles of boys with the fragile X syndrome. American Journal of Medical Genetics 30: 191–200.

Keogh, M. (1992) Intervention to enhance attention skills in children with attention deficit hyperactivity disorder. In: International Fragile X Conference proceedings. Hagerman, R.J., and McKenzie, P. (eds.). Spectra, Dillon, Colo., pp. 251–9.

Kerr, M. P. (1998) Topiramate: Uses in people with an intellectual disability who have epilepsy. Journal of Intellectual Research 42 (suppl. 1): 74–9.

Khan, B. U. (1997) Brief report: Risperidone for severely disturbed behavior and tardive dyskinesia in developmentally disabled adults. Journal of Autism and Developmental Disorders 27 (4): 479–89.

Khandjian, E. W., Fortin, A., Thibodeau, A., Tremblay, S., Cote, F., Devys, D., Mandel, J. L., Rousseau, F. (1995) A heterogeneous set of FMR1 proteins is widely distributed in mouse tissues and is modulated in cell culture. Human Molecular Genetics 4 (5): 783–9.

Khin, N. A., Tarleton, J., Raghu, B., Park, S. K. (1998) Clinical description of an adult male with psychosis who showed FMR1 gene methylation mosaicism. American Journal of Medical Genetics (Neuropsychiatric Genetics) 81: 222–4.

King, R. A., Hagerman, R. J., Houghton, M. (1995) Ocular findings in fragile X syndrome. Developmental Brain Dysfunction 8: 223–9.

Koegel, L., Koegel, R., Parks, D. (1992) How to teach self-management to people with severe disabilities: A training manual. University of California, Santa Barbara.

Kowalczyk, C. L., Schroeder, E., Pratt, V., Conard, J., Wright, K., Feldman, G. L. (1996) An association between precocious puberty and fragile X syndrome? Journal of Pediatric and Adolescent Gynecology 9 (4): 199–202.

Kramer, P. D. (1993) Listening to Prozac. Viking/Penguin, New York.

Krishnamoorthy, J., and King, B. H. (1998) Open-label olanzapine treatment in five preadolescent children. Journal of Child and Adolescent Psychopharmacology 8 (2): 107–13.

Kumra, S., Jacobsen, L. K., Lenane, M., Karp, B. I., Frazier, J. A., Smith, A. K., Bedwell, J., Lee, P., Malanga, C. J., Hamburger, S., Rapoport, J. L. (1998) Childhood-onset schizophrenia: An open-label study of Olanzapine in adolescents. Journal of American Academy of Child and Adolescent Psychiatry 37 (4): 377–85.

Lachiewicz, A. (1995) Females with fragile X syndrome: A review of the effects of an abnormal gene. Mental Retardation and Developmental Disabilities Research Reviews 1: 292–7.

Lachiewicz, A. M., and Dawson, D. V. (1994a) Behavior problems of young girls with fragile X syndrome: Factor scores on the Conners' Parent's Questionnaire. American Journal of Medical Genetics 51 (4): 364–9.

Lachiewicz, A. M., and Dawson, D. V. (1994b) Do young boys with fragile X syndrome have macroorchidism? Pediatrics 93 (6, Pt. 1): 992–5.

Lachiewicz, A. M., Gullion, C., Spiridigliozzi, G., Aylsworth, A. (1987) Declining IQs of young males with the fragile X syndrome. American Journal of Mental Retardation 92: 272–8.

Lachiewicz, A. M., Hoegerman, S. F., Holmgren, G., Holmberg, E., Arinbjarnarson, K. (1991) Association of the Robin sequence with the fragile X syndrome. American Journal of Medical Genetics 41 (3): 275–8.

Lachiewicz, A. M., Spiridigliozzi, G. A., McConkie-Rosell, A., Burgess, D., Feng, Y., Warren, S. T., Tarleton, J. (1996) A fragile X male with a broad smear on Southern blot analysis representing 100–500 CGG repeats and no methylation at the EagI site of the FMR-1 gene. American Journal of Medical Genetics 64 (2): 278–82.

Landau, W. M., Batanian, J. R., Morris, J. C., Hagerman, R. J. (1999) Adult onset of movement disorder and dementia in a carrier of both fragile X and Werdnig-Hoffman mutations. Manuscript submitted for publication.

Lehrke, R. G. (1974) X-linked mental retardation and verbal disability. Birth defects: Original Article Series. In Bergsma, D. (ed.). National Foundation, March of Dimes, New York, pp. 1–100.

Liu, Q., Siomi, H., Siomi, M. C., Fischer, U., Zhang, Y., Wan, L., Dreyfuss, G. (1996) Molecular characteristics of the protein products of the fragile X syndrome gene and the survival of motor neurons gene. Cold Spring Harbor Symposia on Quantitative Biology LXI: 689–97.

Livingston, M. G. (1994) Risperidone. Lancet 343: 457–60.

Loehr, J. P., Synhorst, D. P., Wolfe, R. R., Hagerman, R. J. (1986) Aortic root dilatation and mitral valve prolapse in the fragile X syndrome. American Journal of Medical Genetics 23: 189–94.

Loesch, D. Z., and Hay, D. A. (1988) Clinical features and reproductive patterns in fragile X female heterozygotes. Journal of Medical Genetics 25: 407–14.

Loesch, D. Z., Hay, D. A., Sheffield, L. J. (1992) Fragile X family with unusual digital and facial abnormalities, cleft lip and palate, and epilepsy. American Journal of Medical Genetics 44 (5): 543–50.

Loesch, D. Z., Huggins, R., Hay, D. A., Gedeon, A. K., Mulley, J. C., Sutherland, G. R. (1993) Genotype-phenotype relationships in fragile X syndrome: A family study. American Journal of Human Genetics 53 (5): 1064–73.

Loesch, D. Z., Huggins, R. M., Hoang, N. H. (1995) Growth in stature in fragile X families: A mixed longitudinal study. American Journal of Medical Genetics 58 (3): 249–56.

Lubs, H. A. (1969) A marker X chromosome. American Journal of Human Genetics 21: 231–44.

Lubs, H. A., Schwartz, C. E., Stevenson, R. E., Arena, J. F. (1996) Study of X-linked mental retardation (XLMR): Summary of 61 families in the Miami/Greenwood Study. American Journal of Medical Genetics 64 (1): 169–75.

Lugenbeel, K. A., Peier, A. M., Carson, N. L., Chudley, A. E., Nelson, D. L. (1995) Intragenic loss of function mutations demonstrate the primary role of FMR1 in fragile X syndrome. Nature Genetics 10 (4): 483–5.

Luxem, M., and Christopherson, E. (1994) Behavioral toilet training in early childhood: Research practice and implications. Journal of Developmental and Behavioral Pediatrics 15: 370–8.

Maino, D. M., Wesson, M., Schlange, D., Cibis, G., Maino, J. H. (1991) Optometric findings in the fragile X syndrome. Optometry and Visual Sciences 68 (8): 634–40.

Malhotra, S., and Santosh, P. J. (1998) An open clinical trial of buspirone in children with attention deficit/hyperactivity disorder. Journal of the American Academy of Child and Adolescent Psychiatry 37 (4): 364–71.

Malter, H. E., Iber, J. C., Willemsen, R., de Graaff, E., Tarleton, J. C., Leisti, J., Warren, S. T., Oostra, B. A. (1997) Characterization of the full fragile X syndrome mutation in fetal gametes. Nature Genetics 15 (2): 165–9.

Martin, J. P., and Bell, J. (1943) A pedigree of mental defect showing sex linkage. Journal of Neurological Psychiatry 6: 154–7.

Mayes, S. D., Crites, D. L., Bixler, E. O., Humphrey, F. J., Mattison, R. E. (1994) Methylphenidate and ADHD: Influence of age, IQ and neurodevelopmental status. Developmental Medicine and Child Neurology 36: 1099–1107.

Mazzocco, M. M., Pennington, B. F., Hagerman, R. J. (1993) The neurocognitive phenotype of female carriers of fragile X: Additional evidence for specificity. Journal of Developmental and Behavioral Pediatrics 14 (5): 328–35.

Mazzocco, M. M., Kates, W. R., Baumgardner, T. L., Freund, L. S., Reiss, A. L. (1997a) Autistic behaviors among girls with fragile X syndrome. Journal of Autism and Developmental Disorders 27 (4): 415–35.

Mazzocco, M. M. M., Sonna, N. L., Teisl, J. T., Pinit, A., Shapiro, B. K., Shah, N., Reiss, A. L. (1997b) The FMR1 and FMR2 mutations are not common etiologies of academic difficulty among school-age children. Developmental and Behavioral Pediatrics 18 (6): 392–8.

Mazzocco, M., Baumgardner, T., Freund, L. S., Reiss, A. (1998) Social functioning amoung girls with fragile X or Turner syndrome. Journal of Autism and Developmental Disorders 28 (6): 509–17.

McConkie-Rosell, A., Lachiewicz, A. M., Spiridigliozzi, G. A., Tarleton, J., Schoenwald, S., Phelan, M. C., Goonewardena, P., Ding, X., Brown, W. T. (1993) Evidence that methylation of the FMR-I locus is responsible for variable phenotypic expression of the fragile X syndrome. American Journal of Human Genetics 53 (4): 800–9.

McConkie-Rosell, A., Robinson, H., Wake, S., Staley, L. W., Heller, K., Cronister, A. (1995) Dissemination of genetic risk information to relatives in the fragile X syndrome: Guidelines for genetic counselors. American Journal of Medical Genetics 59 (4): 426–30.

McConkie-Rosell, A., Spiridigliozzi, G. A., Iafolla, T., Tarleton, J., Lachiewicz, A. M. (1997) Carrier testing in the fragile X syndrome: Attitudes and opinions of obligate carriers. American Journal of Medical Genetics 68 (1): 62–9.

McDermott, A., Walters, R., Howell, R. T., Gardner, A. (1983) Fragile X chromosome: Clinical and cytogenetic studies on cases from seven families. Journal of Medical Genetics 20 (3): 169–78.

McDougle, C. J., Fleischmann, R. L., Epperson, C. N., Wasyling, S., Leckman, J. F., Price, L. H. (1995) Risperidone addition in fluvoxamine-refractory obsessive-compulsive disorder: Three cases. Journal of Clinical Psychiatry 56: 526–8.

Meijer, H., de Graaff, E., Merckx, D. M., Jongbloed, R. J., de Die Smulders, C. E., Engelen, J. J., Fryns, J. P., Curfs, P. M., Oostra, B. A. (1994) A deletion of 1.6 kb proximal to the CGG repeat of the FMR1 gene causes the clinical phenotype of the fragile X syndrome. Human Molecular Genetics 3 (4): 615–20.

Merenstein, S. A., Shyu, V., Sobesky, W. E., Staley, L., Berry Kravis, E., Nelson, D. L., Lugenbeel, K. A., Taylor, A. K., Pennington, B. F., Hagerman, R. J. (1994) Fragile X syndrome in a normal IQ male with learning and emotional problems. Journal of American Academy of Child and Adolescent Psychiatry 33 (9): 1316–21.

Merenstein, S. A., Sobesky, W. E., Taylor, A. K., Riddle, J. E., Tran, H. X., Hagerman, R. J. (1996) Molecular-clinical correlations in males with an expanded FMR1 mutation. American Journal of Medical Genetics 64 (2): 388–94.

Merzenich, M. M., Jenkins, W. M., Johnston, P., Schreiner, C., Miller, S. L., Tallal, P. (1996) Temporal processing deficits of language-learning impaired children ameliorated by training. Science 271 (5245): 77–81.

Miezejeski, C. M., and Hinton, V. J. (1992) Fragile X learning disability: Neurobehavioral research, diagnostic models and treatment options. In International Fragile X Conference proceedings. Hagerman, R. J., and McKenzie, P. (eds.). Spectra, Dillon, Colo., pp. 165–6.

Mikati, M. A., Choueri, R., Khurana, D. S., Riviello, J., Helmers, S., Holmes, G. (1998) Gabapentin in the treatment of refractory partial epilepsy in children with intellectual disability. Journal of Intellectual Disability Research 42 (suppl. 1): 57–62.

Míla, M., Kruyer, H., Glover, G., Sanchez, A., Carbonell, P., Castellvi-Bell,

S., Volpini, V., Rossell, J., Gabarron, J., Lopez, I., et al. (1994) Molecular analysis of the (CGG)n expansion in the FMR-1 gene in 59 Spanish fragile X syndrome families. Human Genetics 94 (4): 395–400.

Miller, L. J., McIntosh, D. N., McGrath, J., Shyu, V., Lampe, M., Taylor, A. K., Tassone, F., Neitzel, K., Stackhouse, T., Hagerman, R. J. (1999) Electrodermal responses to sensory stimuli in individuals with fragile X syndrome. American Journal of Medical Genetics 83: 268–79.

Mostofsky, S. H., Mazzocco, M. M. M., Aakalu, G., Warsofsky, I. S., Denckla, M. B., Reiss, A. L. (1998) Decreased cerebellar posterior vermis size in fragile X syndrome. American Academy of Neurology 50: 121–30.

Mulley, J. C., Yu, S., Loesch, D. Z., Hay, D. A., Donnelly, A., Gedeon, A. K., Carbonell, P., Lopez, I., Glover, G., Gabarron, I., et al. (1995) FRAXE and mental retardation. Journal of Medical Genetics 32 (3): 162–9.

Mundy, J. (1991) Let's talk. Western Psychological Services, Los Angeles.

Musumeci, S. A., Colognola, R. M., Ferri, R., Gigli, G. L., Petrella, M. A., Sanfilippo, S., Bergonzi, P., Tassinari, C. A. (1988a) Fragile-X syndrome: A particular epileptogenic EEG pattern. Epilepsia 29: 41–7.

Musumeci, S. A., Ferri, R., Colognola, R. M., Neri, G., Sanfilippo, S., Bergonzi, P. (1988b) Prevalence of a novel epileptogenic EEG pattern in the Martin-Bell syndrome. American Journal of Medical Genetics 30: 207–12.

Musumeci, S. A., Ferri, R., Elia, M., Del Gracco, S., Scuderi, C., Stefanini, M. C. (1996) Normal respiratory pattern during sleep in young fragile X-syndrome patients [Letter to the editor]. Journal of Sleep Research 5 (4): 272.

Musumeci, S. A., Hagerman, R. J., Ferri, R., Bosco, P., Bernardina, B. D., Tassinari, C. A., De Sarro, G. B., Elia, M.

(In press) Epilepsy and EEG findings in males with fragile X syndrome. Epilepsia.

Nelson, D. L. (1998) FRAXE mental retardation and other folate-sensitive fragile sites. In Genetic instabilities and hereditary neurological diseases. Wells, R. D., Warren, S. T., Sarmiento, M. (eds.). Academic Press, San Diego, pp. 65–74.

Nezu, C. M., and Nezu, A. M. (1994) Outpatient psychotherapy for adults with mental retardation and concomitant psychopathology: Research and clinical imperatives. Journal of Consulting and Clinical Psychology 62 (1): 34–42.

Nolin, S. L., Snider, D. A., Jenkins, E. C., Brown, W. T., Krawczun, M., Stetka, D., Houck, G., Jr., Dobkin, C. S., Strong, G., Smith Dobransky, G., et al. (1991) Fragile X screening program in New York State. American Journal of Medical Genetics 38 (2–3): 251–5.

Nolin, S. L., Lewis, F. A., III, Ye, L. L., Houck, G. E., Jr., Glicksman, A. E., Limprasert, P., Li, S. Y., Zhong, N., Ashley, A. E., Feingold, E., Sherman, S. L., Brown, W. T. (1996) Familial transmission of the FMR1 CGG repeat. American Journal of Human Genetics 59 (6): 1252–61.

O'Hare, J. P., O'Brien, I. A. D., Arendt, J., Astley, P., Ratcliffe, W., Andrews, H., Walters, R., Corrall, R. J. M. (1986) Does melatonin deficiency cause the enlarged genitalia of the fragile X syndrome? Clinical Endocrinology 24: 327–33.

Oostra, B. A. (1996) FMR1 protein studies and animal model for fragile X syndrome. In: Fragile X syndrome: Diagnosis, treatment, and research. Hagerman, R. J., and Cronister, A. (eds.). 2nd ed. Johns Hopkins University Press, Baltimore, pp. 193–209.

Oostra, B. A., and Willems, P. J. (1998) Murine model of fragile X syndrome.

In: Genetic instabilities and hereditary neurological diseases. Wells, R. D., Warren, S. T., Sarmiento, M. (eds.). Academic Press, San Diego, pp. 55–62.

Opitz, J. M., Westphal, J. M., Daniel, A. (1984) Discovery of a connective tissue dysplasia in the Martin-Bell syndrome. American Journal of Medical Genetics 17: 101–9.

Parrish, J. E., Oostra, B. A., Verkerk, A. J., Richards, C. S., Reynolds, J., Spikes, A. S., Shaffer, L. G., Nelson, D. L. (1994) Isolation of a GCC repeat showing expansion in FRAXF, a fragile site distal to FRAXA and FRAXE. Nature Genetics 8 (3): 229–35.

Partington, M. W. (1984) The fragile X syndrome II: Preliminary data on growth and development in males. American Journal of Medical Genetics 17 (1): 175–94.

Partington, M. W., Moore, D. Y., Turner, G. M. (1996) Confirmation of early menopause in fragile X carriers. American Journal of Medical Genetics 64 (2): 370–2.

Patzer, C. E., and Pettegrew, B. (1996) Finding a voice: Primary students with developmental disabilities express personal meanings through writing. Teaching Exceptional Children 29 (2): 22–7.

Pellock, J. M. (1987) Carbamazepine side effects in children and adults. Epilepsia 28 (suppl. 3): S64–S70.

Penrose, L. S. (1938) A clinical and genetic study of 1,280 cases of mental defect. Mental Research Council Special Report Series 229. Medical Research Council, London.

Pippenger, C. E. (1987) Clinically significant carbamazepine drug interactions: An overview. Epilepsia 28 (suppl. 3): S71–S76.

Piussan, C., Mathieu, M., Berquin, P., Fryns, J. P. (1996) Fragile X mutation and FG syndrome-like phenotype. American Journal of Medical Genetics 64 (2): 395–8.

Purdon, S. E., Lit, W., Labelle, A., Jones, B. D. W. (1994) Risperidone in the treatment of pervasive developmental disorder. Canadian Journal of Psychiatry 39 (7): 400–5.

Puzzo, A., Fiamma, G., Rubino, V. E., Gagliano, P. A., Giordano, G., Russo, L., Aloisi, B., Manzoli, U. (1990) Cardiovascular aspects of Martin-Bell syndrome. Cardiologia 35 (10): 857–62.

Quan, F., Grompe, M., Jakobs, P., Popovich, B. W. (1995a) Spontaneous deletion in the FMR1 gene in a patient with fragile X syndrome and cherubism. Human Molecular Genetics 4 (9): 1681–4.

Quan, F., Zonana, J., Gunter, K., Peterson, K. L., Magenis, R. E., Popovich, B. W. (1995b) An atypical case of fragile X syndrome caused by a deletion that includes the FMR1 gene. American Journal of Human Genetics 56 (5): 1042–51.

Rattazzi, M. C., and Ioannou, Y. A. (1996) Molecular approaches to therapy. In: Fragile X syndrome: Diagnosis, treatment, and research. Hagerman, R. J., and Cronister, A. (eds.). 2nd ed. Johns Hopkins University Press, Baltimore, pp. 412–52.

Raymond, J. L., Lisberger, S. G., Mauk, M. D. (1996) The cerebellum: A neuronal learning machine? Science 272: 1126–31.

Reinhartsen, D. B., Edmondson, R., Crais, E. R. (1997) Developing assistive technology strategies for infants and toddlers wtih communication difficulties. Seminars in Speech and Language 18 (3): 283–301.

Reiss, A. L., Aylward, E., Freund, L. S., Joshi, P. K., Bryan, R. N. (1991a) Neuroanatomy of fragile X syndrome: The posterior fossa. Annals of Neurology 29 (1): 26–32.

Reiss, A. L., Freund, L., Tseng, J. E., Joshi, P. K. (1991b) Neuroanatomy in fragile X females: The posterior fossa.

American Journal of Human Genetics 49 (2): 279–88.

Reiss, A. L., Freund, L., Abrams, M. T., Boehm, C., Kazazian, H. (1993) Neurobehavioral effects of the fragile X premutation in adult women: A controlled study. American Journal of Human Genetics 52 (5): 884–94.

Reiss, A. L., Lee, J., Freund, L. (1994) Neuroanatomy of fragile X syndrome: The temporal lobe. Neurology 44 (7): 1317–24.

Reiss, A. L., Abrams, M. T., Greenlaw, R., Freund, L., Denckla, M. B. (1995a) Neurodevelopmental effects of the FMR-1 full mutation in humans. Nature Medicine 1 (2): 159–67.

Reiss, A. L., Freund, L. S., Baumgardner, T. L., Abrams, M. T., Denckla, M. B. (1995b) Contribution of the FMR1 gene mutation to human intellectual dysfunction. Nature Genetics 11 (3): 331–4.

Reus, V. I. (1997) Olanzapine: A novel atypical neuroleptic agent. Lancet 349: 1264–65.

Reyniers, E., Vits, L., De Boulle, K., Van Roy, B., Van Velzen, D., de Graaff, E., Verkerk, A. J., Jorens, H.Z., Darby, J. K., Oostra, B., et al. (1993) The full mutation in the FMR-1 gene of male fragile X patients is absent in their sperm. Nature Genetics 4 (2): 143–6.

Richards, B. W., and Webb, T. (1982) The Martin-Bell-Renpenning syndrome. Journal of Medical Genetics 19: 79.

Riddle, J. E., Cheema, A., Sobesky, W. E., Gardner, S. C., Taylor, A. K., Pennington, B. F., Hagerman, R. J. (1998) Phenotypic involvement in females with the FMR1 gene mutation. American Journal on Mental Retardation 102 (6): 590–601.

Riddle, M. A., Claghorn, J., Gaffney, G. (1996) A controlled trial of fluvoxamine for OCD in children and adolescents. Biological Psychiatry 39 (7): 568.

Roberts, J. E. (1998) Bio-behavioral regulation in boys with fragile X. Thirty-first Annual Gatlinburg Conference on Research and Theory in Mental Retardation and Developmental Disabilities, Charleston, South Carolina.

Robinson, H., Wake, S., Wright, F., Laing, S., Turner, G. (1996) Informed choice in fragile X syndrome and its effects on prevalence. American Journal of Medical Genetics 64: 198–202.

Rosh, J. R., Dellert, S. F., Narkewicz, M., Birnbaum, A., Whitington, G. (1998) Four cases of severe hepatotoxicity associated with pemoline: Possible autoimmune pathogenesis. Pediatrics 101 (5): 921–3.

Rousseau, F., Heitz, D., Tarleton, J., MacPherson, J., Malmgren, H., Dahl, N., Barnicoat, A., Mathew, C., Mornet, E., Tejada, I., et al. (1994a) A multicenter study on genotype-phenotype correlations in the fragile X syndrome, using direct diagnosis with probe StB12.3: The first 2,253 cases. American Journal of Human Genetics 55 (2): 225–37.

Rousseau, F., Robb, L. J., Rouillard, P., Der Kaloustian, V. M. (1994b) No mental retardation in a man with 40% abnormal methylation at the FMR-1 locus and transmission of sperm cell mutations as premutations. Human Molecular Genetics 3 (6): 927–30.

Rousseau, F., Rouillard, P., Morel, M. L., Khandjian, E. W., Morgan, K. (1995) Prevalence of carriers of premutation-size alleles of the FMRI gene—and implications for the population genetics of the fragile X syndrome. American Journal of Human Genetics 57 (5): 1006–18.

Rousseau, F., Morel, M.-L., Rouillard, P., Khandjian, E. W., Morgan, K. (1996) Surprisingly low prevalance of FMR1 premutation among males from the general population. American Journal of Human Genetics 59 (suppl): A188.

Rowe, W., and Savage, S. (1987) Sexuality and the developmentally handicapped: A guidebook for health care professionals. Edwin Mellen Press, Lewiston and Queenston, London.

Russo, S., Selicorni, A., Bedeschi, M. F., Natacci, F., Viziello, P., Fortuna, R., Pagani, G., Dalpra, L., Larizza, L. (1998) Molecular characterization of FRAXE-positive subjects with mental impairment in two unrelated Italian families. American Journal of Medical Genetics 75: 304–8.

Ruvalcaba, R. H., Myhre, S. A., Roosen-Runge, E. C., Beckwith, J. B. (1977) X-linked mental deficiency megalotestes syndrome. Journal of the American Medical Association 238: 1646–50.

Ryan, G., and Rodeck, C. H. (1993) Fetal blood sampling. In: Essentials of prenatal diagnosis. Simpson, J. L., and Elias, S. (eds.). Churchill Livingston, New York, pp. 63–75.

Salee, F. R., Richman, H., Sethuraman, G., Dougherty, D., Sine, L., Altman-Hamamdzic, S. (1998) Clonidine challenge in childhood anxiety disorder. Journal of the American Academy of Child and Adolescent Psychiatry 37 (6): 655–62.

Saxena, S., Want, D., Bystritsky, A., Baxter, L. R. (1996) Risperidone augmentation of SRI treatment for refractory obsessive-compulsive disorder. Journal of Clinical Psychiatry 57: 303–6.

Scharfenaker, S., O'Connor, R., Stackhouse, T., Braden, M., Hickman, L., Gray, K. (1996) An integrated approach to intervention. In: Fragile X syndrome: Diagnosis, treatment, and research. Hagerman, R. J., and Cronister, A. (eds.). 2nd ed. Johns Hopkins University Press, Baltimore, pp. 349–411.

Schapiro, M. B., Murphy, D. G. M., Hagerman, R. J., Azari, N. P., Alexander, G. E., Miezejeski, C. M., Hinton, V. J., Hozwitz, B., Haxby, J. V., Kumar, A., White, B., Grady, C. L. (1995) Adult fragile X syndrome: Neuropsychology, bioinanatomy, and metabolism. American Journal of Medical Genetics 60: 480–93.

Schinzel, A., and Largo, R. H. (1985) The fragile X syndrome (Martin-Bell syndrome). Clinical and cytogenetic findings in 16 prepubertal boys and in 4 of their 5 families. Helvetica Paediatrica Acta 40 (2–3): 133–52.

Schmidt, M. (1992) Do sequences in Xq27.3 play a role in X inactivation? [Letter to the editor]. American Journal of Medical Genetics 43 (1–2): 279–81.

Schopmeyer, B. B., and Lowe, F. (1992) The fragile X child. Singular, San Diego.

Schrander-Stumple, C., Gerver, W.-T., Meyer, H., Engelen, J., Mulder, H., Fryns, J.-P. (1994) Prader-Willi-like phenotype in fragile X syndrome. Clinical Genetics 45: 175–80.

Schwartz, C. E., Dean, J., Howard-Peebles, P. N., Bugge, M., Mikkelsen, M., Tommerup, N., Hull, C., Hagerman, R., Holden, J. J., Stevenson, R. E. (1994) Obstetrical and gynecological complications in fragile X carriers: A multicenter study. American Journal of Medical Genetics 51 (4): 400–2.

Sherman, S. (1996) Epidemiology. In Fragile X syndrome: Diagnosis, treatment, and research. Hagerman, R. J., and Cronister, A. (eds.). 2nd ed. Johns Hopkins University Press, Balitmore, pp. 165–92.

Simko, A., Hornstein, L., Soukup, S., Bagamery, N. (1989) Fragile X syndrome: Recognition in young children. Pediatrics 83 (4): 547–52.

Simon, E. W., and Finucane, B. M. (1996) Facial emotion identification in males with fragile X syndrome. American Journal of Medical Genetics 67: 77–80.

Siomi, H., Siomi, M. C., Nussbaum, R. L., Dreyfuss, G. (1993) The protein product of the fragile X gene, FMR1, has characteristics of an RNA-binding protein. Cell 74 (2): 291–8.

Siomi, M. C., Siomi, H., Sauer, W. H., Srinivasan, S., Nussbaum, R. L., Dreyfuss, G. (1995) FXR1, an autosomal homolog of the fragile X mental retardation gene. EMBO Journal 14 (11): 2401–8.

Slaney, S. F., Wilkie, A. O., Hirst, M. C., Charlton, R., McKinley, M., Pointon, J., Christodoulou, Z., Huson, S. M., Davies, K. E. (1995) DNA testing for fragile X syndrome in schools for learning difficulties [see comments]. Archives of Diseases in Childhood 72 (1): 33–7.

Smeets, H. J., Smits, A. P., Verheij, C. E., Theelen, J. P., Willemsen, R., van de Burgt, I., Hoogeveen, A. T., Oosterwijk, J. C., Oostra, B. A. (1995) Normal phenotype in two brothers with a full FMR1 mutation. Human Molecular Genetics 4 (11): 2103–8.

Smith, T., Eikeseth, S., Klevstrand, M., Lovaas, O. I. (1997) Intensive behavioral treatment for preschoolers with severe mental retardation and pervasive developmental disorder. American Journal on Mental Retardation 102 (3): 238–49.

Snow, K., Doud, L. K., Hagerman, R., Pergolizzi, R. G., Erster, S. H., Thibodeau, S. N. (1993) Analysis of a CGG sequence at the FMR-1 locus in fragile X families and in the general population. American Journal of Human Genetics 53 (6): 1217–28.

Sobesky, W. E. (1996) The treatment of emotional and behavioral problems. In Fragile X syndrome: Diagnosis, treatment, and research. Hagerman, R. J., and Cronister, A. (eds.). 2nd ed. Johns Hopkins University Press, Baltimore, pp. 332–48.

Sobesky, W. E., Hull, C. E., Hagerman, R. J. (1994a) Symptoms of schizotypal personality disorder in fragile X women. Journal of the American Academy of Child and Adolescent Psychiatry 33 (2): 247–55.

Sobesky, W. E., Pennington, B. F., Porter, D., Hull, C. E., Hagerman, R. J. (1994b) Emotional and neurocognitive deficits in fragile X. American Journal of Medical Genetics 51 (4): 378–85.

Sobesky, W. E., Porter, D., Pennington, B. F., Hagerman, R. J. (1995) Dimensions of shyness in fragile X females. Developmental Brain Dysfunction 8: 280–92.

Sobesky, W. E., Taylor, A. K., Pennington, B. F., Bennetto, L., Porter, D., Riddle, J., Hagerman, R. J. (1996) Molecular/clinical correlations in females with fragile X. American Journal of Medical Genetics 64 (2): 340–5.

Sondheimer, J. M. (1994) Gastroesophageal reflux in children: Clinical presentation and diagnostic evaluation. Gastrointestinal Endoscopy Clinics of North America 4: 55–74.

Spence, W. C., Black, S. H., Fallon, L., Maddalena, A., Cummings, E., Menapace-Drew, G., Bick, D. P., Levinson, G., Schulman, J. D., Howard-Peebles, P. N. (1996) Molecular fragile X screening in normal populations. American Journal of Medical Genetics 64 (1): 181–3.

Spiridigliozzi, G., Lachiewicz, A., MacMordo, C., Vizoso, A., O'Donnell, C., McConkie-Rosell, A., Burgess, D. (1994) Educating boys with fragile X syndrome: A guide for parents and professionals. Duke University Medical Center, Durham, N.C.

Sreeram, N., Wren, C., Bhate, M., Robertson, P., Hunter, S. (1989) Cardiac abnormalities in the fragile X syndrome. British Heart Journal 61 (3): 289–91.

Staley Gane, L., Flynn, L., Neitzel, K., Cronister, A., Hagerman, R. J. (1996) Expanding the role of the genetic counselor. American Journal of Medical Genetics 64 (2): 382–7.

Steiner, M., Steinberg, S., Stewart, D., Carter, D., Berger, C., Reid, R., Grover, D., Streiner, D. (1995) Fluoxetine in the treatment of premenstrual dysphoria. New England Journal of Medicine 332: 1529–34.

Steyaert, J., Borghgraef, M., Legius, E., Fryns, J. P. (1996) Molecular-intelligence correlations in young fragile X males with a mild CGG repeat expansion in the FMR1 gene. American Journal of Medical Genetics 64 (2): 274–7.

Storm, R. L., PeBenito, R., Ferretti, C. (1987) Opthalmologic findings in the fragile X syndrome. Archives of Opthalmology 105: 1099–102.

Sudhalter, V., Cohen, I. L., Silverman, W., Wolf-Schein, E. G. (1990) Conversational analyses of males with fragile X, Down syndrome, and autism: Comparison of the emergence of deviant language. American Journal of Mental Retardation 94 (4): 431–41.

Sudhalter, V., Scarborough, H. S., Cohen, I. L. (1991) Syntactic delay and pragmatic deviance in the language of fragile X males. American Journal of Medical Genetics 38 (2–3): 493–7.

Sutcliffe, J. S., Nelson, D. L., Zhang, F., Pieretti, M., Caskey, C. T., Saxe, D., Warren, S. T. (1992) DNA methylation represses FMR-1 transcription in fragile X syndrome. Human Molecular Genetics 1 (6): 397–400.

Sutherland, G. R. (1977) Fragile sites on human chromosomes: Demonstration of their dependence of the type of tissue culture medium. Science 197: 265–6.

Sutherland, G. R. (1979) Heritable fragile sites on human chromosomes I: Factors affecting expression in lymphocyte culture. American Journal of Human Genetics 31 (2): 125–35.

Sutherland, G. R., and Hecht, F. (1985) Fragile sites on human chromosomes. Oxford University Press, New York.

Sutherland, G. R., Baker, E., Fratini, A. (1985) Excess thymidine induces folate sensitive fragile sites. American Journal of Medical Genetics 22 (2): 433–43.

Swanson, J. M., Flockhart, D., Udrea, D., Cantwell, D., Connor, D., Williams, L. (1995) Clonidine and the treatment of ADHD: Questions about safety and efficacy. Journal of Child and Adolescent Psychopharmacology 5: 301–4.

Swanson, J., Wigal, S., Greenhill, L., Browne, R., Waslick, B., Lerner, M., Williams, L., Flynn, D., Agler, D., Crowley, K. L., Fineberg, E., Regino, R., Baren, M., Cantwell, D. (1998a) Objective and subjective measures of the pharmacodynamic effects of Adderall in the treatment of children with ADHD in a controlled laboratory classroom setting. Psychopharmacology Bulletin 34 (1): 55–60.

Swanson, J. M., Wigal, S., Greenhill, L. L., Browne, R., Waslik, B., Lerner, M., Williams, L., Flynn, D., Agler, D., Crowley, K., Fineberg, E., Baren, M., Cantwell, D. P. (1998b) Analog classroom assessment of Adderall in children with ADHD. Journal of American Academy of Child and Adolescent Psychiatry 37 (5): 519–26.

Tallal, P., Miller, S. L., Bedi, G., Byma, G., Wang, X., Nagarajan, S. S., Schreiner, C., Jenkins, W. M., Merzenich, M. M. (1996) Language comprehension in language-learning impaired children improved with acoustically modified speech [see comments]. Science 271 (5245): 81–4.

Tarleton, J., Richie, R., Schwartz, C., Rao, K., Aylsworth, A. S., Lachiewicz, A. (1993) An extensive de novo deletion removing FMR1 in a patient with mental retardation and the fragile X syndrome phenotype. Human Molecular Genetics 2 (11): 1973–4.

Tassone, F., Hagerman, R. J., Ikle, D., Dyer, P. N., Lampe, M., Willemsen, R., Oostra, B. A., Taylor, A. K. (1999) FMRP expression as a potential prognostic indicator in fragile X syndrome.

American Journal of Medical Genetics 84: 250–261.

Tassone, F., Hagerman, R. J., Taylor, A., Gane, F., Wood, S., Mills, J., Hagerman, P. J. (1999) Clinical involvement and protein expression in individuals with the FMR1 premutation. Manuscript submitted for publication.

Taylor, A. K., Safanda, J. F., Lugenbeel, K. A., Nelson, D. L., Hagerman, R. J. (1994) Molecular and phenotypic studies of fragile X males with variant methylation of the FMR1 gene reveal that the degree of methylation influences clinical severity. American Journal of Human Genetics 55: 85.

Taylor, A. K., Tassone, F., Dyer, P. N., Hersch, S. M., Harris, J. B., Greenough, W. T., Hagerman, R. J. (1999) Tissue heterogeneity of the FMR1 mutation in a high functioning male with fragile X syndrome. American Journal of Medical Genetics 84: 233–239.

Taylor, R., Scharfenaker, S., O'Connor, R., Lampe, M., Kovach, T., Hills, J., Taylor, A. K., Tassone, F., Hagerman, R. J. (1998) Severe language impairment in fragile X syndrome: Clinical correlates and treatment approaches. Paper presented at the fifth International Conference of Fragile X and X -linked Mental Retardation, Asheville, North Carolina, July 26–29.

Thompson, N. M., Gulley, M. L., Rogeness, G. A., Clayton, R. J., Johnson, C., Hazelton, B., Cho, C. G., Zellmer, V. T. (1994) Neurobehavioral characteristics of CGG amplification status in fragile X females. American Journal of Medical Genetics 54 (4): 378–83.

Thompson, N. M., Rogeness, G. A., McClure, E., Clayton, R., Johnson, C. (1996) Influence of depression on cognitive functioning in fragile X females. Psychiatry Research 64: 97–104.

Tirosh, E., and Borochowitz, Z. (1992) Sleep apnea in fragile X syndrome. American Journal of Medical Genetics 43: 124–7.

Tranfaglia, M. R. (1996) A parent's guide to drug treatment of fragile X syndrome. FRAXA Research Foundation, West Newbury, Mass.

Trottier, Y., Imbert, G., Poustka, A., Fryns, J. P., Mandel, J. L. (1994) Male with typical fragile X phenotype is deleted for part of the FMR1 gene and for about 100 kb of upstream region. American Journal of Medical Genetics 51 (4): 454–7.

Turk, J. (1992) The fragile-X syndrome. On the way to a behavioural phenotype. British Journal of Psychiatry 160: 24–35.

Turk, J., and Graham, P. (1997) Fragile X syndrome, autism, and autistic features. Autism 1 (2): 175–197.

Turk, J., and Cornish, K. (1998) Face recognition and emotional perception in boys with fragile-X syndrome. Journal of Intellectual Disability Research 42 (6): 490–9.

Turnbull, H. R., Turnbull, A. P., Bronicki, G. J., Summers, J. A., Roeder-Gordon, D. (1989) Disability and the family: A guide to decisions for adulthood. Brookes, Baltimore.

Turner, G. (1983) Historical overview of X-linked mental retardation. In: The fragile X syndrome: Diagnosis, biochemistry, and intervention. Hagerman, R. J., and McBogg, P. M. (eds.). Spectra, Dillon, Colo., pp. 1–16.

Turner, G., Eastman, C., Casey, J., McLeay, A., Procopis, P., Turner, B. (1975) X-linked mental retardation associated with macro-orchidism. Journal of Medical Genetics 12: 367–71.

Turner, G., Till, R., Daniel, A. (1978) Marker X chromosomes, mental retardation and macro-orchidism. New England Journal of Medicine 299: 1472.

Turner, G., Daniel, A., Frost, M. (1980) X-linked mental retardation, macroorchidism, and the Xq27 fragile site. Journal of Pediatrics 96: 837–41.

Turner, G., Robinson, H., Wake, S., Martin, N. (1994) Dizygous twinning and premature menopause in fragile X syndrome [Letter to the editor]. Lancet 344: 1500.

Turner, G., Webb, T., Wake, S., Robinson, H. (1996) Prevalence of fragile X syndrome. American Journal of Medical Genetics 64 (1): 196–7.

Verkerk, A. J., Pieretti, M., Sutcliffe, J. S., Fu, Y. H., Kuhl, D. P., Pizzuti, A., Reiner, O., Richards, S., Victoria, M. F., Zhang, F. P., et al. (1991) Identification of a gene (FMR-1) containing a CGG repeat coincident with a breakpoint cluster region exhibiting length variation in fragile X syndrome. Cell 65 (5): 905–14.

Verkerk, A. J., de Graaff, E., De Boulle, K., Eichler, E. E., Konecki, D. S., Reyniers, E., Manca, A., Poustka, A., Willems, P. J., Nelson, D. L., et al. (1993) Alternative splicing in the fragile X gene FMR1. Human Molecular Genetics 2 (8): 1348.

Vincent, A., Heitz, D., Petit, C., Kretz, C., Oberle, I., Mandel, J. L. (1991) Abnormal pattern detected in fragile-X patients by pulsed-field gel electrophoresis. Nature 349 (6310): 624–6.

Waldstein, G., and Hagerman, R. (1988) Aortic hypoplasia and cardiac valvular abnormalities in a boy with fragile X syndrome. American Journal of Medical Genetics 30 (1–2): 83–98.

Waldstein, G., Mierau, G., Ahmad, R., Thibodeau, S. N., Hagerman, R. J., Caldwell, S. (1987) Fragile X syndrome: Skin elastin abnormalities. Birth Defects: Original Article Series 23: 103–114.

Wang, Y.-C., Lin, M.-L., Lin, S. J., Li, Y.-C., Li, S.-Y. (1997) Novel point mutation within intron 10 of FMR1 gene causing fragile X syndrome. Human Mutation 10: 393–9.

Wang, Z., Taylor, A. K., Bridge, J. A. (1996) FMR1 fully expanded mutation with minimal methylation in a high

functioning fragile X male. Journal of Medical Genetics 33 (5): 376–8.

Ward, R. M., Lemons, J. A., Molteni, R. A. (1999) Cisapride: A survey of the frequency of use and adverse events in premature newborns. Pediatrics 103 (2): 469–72.

Warren, S. T. (1996) The expanding world of trinucleotide repeats [comment]. Science 271 (5254): 1374–5.

Warren, S. T. (1997) Trinucleotide repetition and fragile X syndrome. Hospital Practice 32 (4): 73–6, 81–5, 90–2.

Webb, T. P., Bundey, S., Thake, A., Todd, J. (1986) The frequency of the fragile X chromosome among school children in Coventry. Journal of Medical Genetics 23: 396–9.

Weiler, I. J., Irwin, S. A., Klintsova, A. Y., Spencer, C. M., Brazelton, A. D., Miyashiro, K., Comery, T. A., Patel, B., Eberwine, J., Greenough, W. T. (1997) Fragile X mental retardation protein is translated near synapses in response to neurotransmitter activation. Proceedings of the National Academy of Sciences of the United States of America 94: 5395–400.

Wershing, A., and Symington, L. (1995) High tech and small folks: Learning and growing with technology. LTVEC, Loudon, Tenn.

Wildhagen, M. F., van Os, T. A. M., Polder, J. J., ten Kate, L. P., Habbema, J. D. F. (1998) Explorative study of costs, effects and savings of screening for female fragile X premutation and full mutation carriers in the general population. Community Genetics 1: 36–47.

Wilens, T. E., Biederman, J., Spencer, T. (1994) Clonidine for sleep disturbances associated with attention deficit hyperactivity disorder. Journal of American Academy of Child and Adolescent Psychiatry 33: 424–6.

Willemsen, R., Mohkamsing, S., de Vries, B., Devys, D., van den Ouweland, A., Mandel, J. L., Galjaard, H., Oostra, B.

(1995) Rapid antibody test for fragile X syndrome. Lancet 345 (8958): 1147–8.

Willemsen, R., Los, F., Mohkamsing, S., van den Ouweland, A., Deelen, W., Galjaard, H., Oostra, B. (1997) Rapid antibody test for prenatal diagnosis of fragile X syndrome on amniotic fluid cells: A new appraisal. Journal of Medical Genetics 34 (3): 250–1.

Wilson, D. P., Carpenter, N. J., Berkovitz, G. (1988) Thyroid function in men with fragile X-linked MR [Letter to the editor]. American Journal of Medical Genetics 31 (4): 733–4.

Wilson, P. G. (1992) Educational strategies for children with fragile X. International Fragile X Conference proceedings. Spectra, Dillon, Colo.

Wilson, P., Stackhouse, T., O'Connor, R., Scharfenaker, S., Hagerman, R. J. (1994) Issues and strategies for educating children with fragile X syndrome: A monograph. Spectra and the National Fragile X Foundation, Denver, Colo.

Wisniewski, K. E., Segan, S. M., Miezejeski, C. M., Sersen, E. A., Rudelli, R. D. (1991) The Fra(X) syndrome: Neurological, electrophysiological, and neuropathological abnormalities. American Journal of Medical Genetics 38 (2–3): 476–80.

Wöhrle, D., Hirst, M. C., Kennerknecht, I., Davies, K. E., Steinbach, P. (1992) Genotype mosaicism in fragile X fetal tissues. Human Genetics 89 (1): 114–6.

Wohrle, D., Salat, U., Gläser, D., Mücke, J., Meisel-Stosiek, M., Schindler, D., Vogel, W., Steinbach, P. (1998) Unusual mutations in high functioning fragile X males: Apparent instability of expanded, unmethylated CGG repeats. Journal of Medical Genetics 35: 103–11.

Wright Talamante, C., Cheema, A., Riddle, J. E., Luckey, D. W., Taylor, A. K., Hagerman, R. J. (1996) A controlled study of longitudinal IQ changes in females and males with fragile X syndrome. American Journal of Medical Genetics 64 (2): 350–5.

Ylinen, A. (1998) Antiepileptic efficacy of vigabatrin in people with severe epilepsy and intellectual disability. Journal of Intellectual Disability Research 42 (suppl. 1): 46–9.

Yu, S., Pritchard, M., Kremer, E., Lynch, M., Nancarrow, J., Baker, E., Holman, K., Mulley, J. C., Warren, S. T., Schlessinger, D., et al. (1991) Fragile X genotype characterized by an unstable region of DNA. Science 252 (5010): 1179–81.

Zhang, Y., O'Connor, J. P., Siomi, M. C., Srinivasan, S., Dutra, A., Nussbaum, R. L., Dreyfuss, G. (1995) The fragile X mental retardation syndrome protein interacts with novel homologs FXR1 and FXR2. EMBO Journal 14 (21): 5358–66.

RESOURCES

Foundations

National Fragile X Foundation
1441 York Street, Suite 303
Denver, CO 80206
telephone: (303) 333-6155; toll free: 1-800-688-8765

fax: (303) 333-4369
e-mail: natlfx@sprintmail.com
http://www.nfxf.org

FRAXA Research Foundation
P.O. Box 935
West Newbury, MA 01985-0935

telephone: (978) 462-1866
fax: (978) 463-9985
e-mail: info@fraxa.org
http://www.fraxa.org

Fragile X syndrome listserv sponsored by FRAXA—to be added to the listserv, e-mail "subscribe fragilex-l" to listserv@listserv.cc.emory.edu

Fragile X Research Foundation of Canada
167 Queen Street West
Brampton, Ontario, Canada L6Y 1M5
telephone: (905) 453-9366
e-mail: FXRFC@ibm.net
http://dante.med.utoronto.ca/Fragile-X/linksto.htm

The Fragile X Society (England)
53 Winchelsea Lane
Hastings, East Sussex, England
TN35 4LG
telephone: 011-424-813147

The International Fragile X Alliance (Australia)
263 Glen Elra Road
North Caulfield 3161
Melbourne, Australia
telephone: (03) 9528-1910
fax: (03) 9532-9555
e-mail: jcohen@netspace.net.au

Fragile X Association of Australia, Inc.
15 Bowen Close
Cherrybrook, NSW Australia
telephone: (019) 987012
e-mail: fragilex@oze-mail.com.au

Reading for Families

Braden, M. (1997) Fragile, handle with care: Understanding fragile X syndrome. Chapel Hill, NC: Avanta.

Dillworth, W. (ed.) (1998) Fragile X: A to Z, a guide for families. FRAXA Research Foundation: West Newbury, Mass.

Dykens, E. M., Hodapp, R. M., Leckman, J. F. (1994) Behavior and development in fragile X syndrome. Thousand Oaks, CA: Sage.

Finucane, B., McConkie-Rosell, A., and Cronister-Silverman, A. (1993) The fragile X syndrome: A handbook for parents and professionals. National Fragile X Foundation.

Hagerman, R. J., and Cronister, A. (eds.). (1996) Fragile X syndrome: Diagnosis, treatment and research, 2nd ed. Baltimore: Johns Hopkins University Press.

Schopmeyer, B. B., and Lowe, F. (1992) The fragile X child. San Diego: Singular.

Spiridigliozzi, G., et al. (1994) Educating boys with fragile X syndrome: A guide for parents and professionals. Duke University Medical Center, Durham, N.C. (919-684-5513)

Tranfaglia, M. R. (1996) A parent's guide to drug treatment of fragile X syndrome. FRAXA Research Foundation, West Newbury, Mass.

Weber, J. D. (1994) Transitioning 'special' children into elementary school. (Available from Books Beyond Borders, Inc., 1881 4th Street, #108, Boulder, CO 80302, (800) 347-6440)

Wilson, P., Stackhouse, T., O'Connor, R., Scharfenaker, S., Hagerman, R. (1994) Issues and strategies for educating children with fragile X syndrome: A monograph. National Fragile X Foundation.

Newsletters

National Fragile X Foundation Newsletter. (Available from the National Fragile X Foundation, at (800) 688-8765)

FRAXA Research Foundation Newsletter. (Available through FRAXA, P.O. Box 935, West Newbury, MA 01985)

Reading for Children

O'Connor, R. (1995) Boys with fragile X syndrome. (Available from the National Fragile X Foundation. (800) 688-8765)

Steiger, C. (1998) My brother has fragile X syndrome. Chapel Hill: Avanta. (800) 434-0322.

Internet Resources

The National Fragile X Foundation
http://www.nfxf.org

FRAXA Research Foundation Home Page
http://www.fraxa.org

Descriptions of fragile X syndrome issues
http://TheArc.org/faqs/fragqa.html

Molecular Genetic Testing (DNA): Frequently asked questions http://www.givf.com/molgen1.html

Assistive Technology Devices

VOCAs
BIGMac   Abelnet 1-800-3220956

CheapTalk   Enabeling Devices: 1-800-832-8697

Talk Back Mirror   Crestwood: 414-352-5678

Audio/Visual Aids

Fragile X Syndrome: Medical and Educational Approaches to Intervention. Cassette. This 90-minute audiocassette is a tool for families and educators as they develop appropriate educational programs for children with fragile X syndrome. Speakers include Lois Hickman, Sarah Scharfenaker, Tracy Stackhouse, Randi Hagerman, and Phil Wilson. Available from the National Fragile X Foundation.

Educational Strategies and Issues for Children with Fragile X Syndrome. Video. In this 59-minute video, Randi Hagerman, Elizabeth Holder, Sarah Scharfenaker, Tracy Stackhouse, and numerous teachers present tactics for educating children with fragile X syndrome. The video, which includes molecular information and medication therapies, follows one child through a multidisciplinary evaluation. It then looks into the school day of a kindergartner, a fifth grader, and a freshman in high school, all of whom have fragile X. Available from the National Fragile X Foundation.

The National Fragile X Foundation Medical Video. "Diagnostic and Treatment." This concise video explains the medical diagnosis and treatments in a very informative way for professionals and families. Available from the National Fragile X Foundation.

Toilet Training Video: Developed by Duke University to train children with pervasive developmental delays to use the toilet: 1-800-23POTTY.

3

Tourette Syndrome

In 1885, George Gilles de la Tourette, an energetic, impatient, and brilliant young intern of the famous French neurologist, Jean-Martin Charcot, published a description of nine patients in Paris who suffered from a movement disorder (Gilles de la Tourette, 1885). In his paper titled "A study of a neurologic condition characterized by motor incoordination accompanied by echolalia and coprolalia," he described abrupt, involuntary movements which most often started in the face before proceeding gradually lower on the body, although he never used the word *tic*. He also described inarticulate sounds, echolalia, coprolalia (vocalizations of obscenities), and echopraxia (imitation of the movements of another person), with onset in childhood and a male predominance. He noted that sensory abilities and intelligence were normal in his patients and that there was a hereditary nature to the disorder. One of his patients was originally described by Jean Itard in 1925 and another by Armand Trousseau in 1873, but Gilles de la Tourette is credited with describing this neurological condition in multiple patients and differentiating it from hysteria. Subsequent lectures by Charcot described this condition as *le maladie de Gilles de la Tourette* (Lajonchere et al., 1996).

Today the diagnosis of Tourette syndrome (TS) is spelled out in the *DSM-IV* (American Psychiatric Association [APA], 1994) and includes the presence of both motor and vocal tics with onset before 18 years of age. The tics can be simple, meaning the involvement of one muscle group, such as an eye blink, head jerk, sniffing, coughing, grunting or squeaking, or complex, meaning the involvement of multiple muscle groups in a sequential movement, such as touching, kicking, imitating gestures (echopraxia), verbalizations, or repetition of some-

Neurodevelopmental Disorders: Diagnosis and Treatment, by Randi Jenssen Hagerman. New York: Oxford University Press, 1999. © Oxford University Press, Inc.

one else's phrases (echolalia) or one's own phrases (palilalia). Vocal tics are actually motor tics that involve respiratory, laryngeal, oral, or nasal muscles.

Although tics are the hallmark of TS, they represent only part of the syndrome. Patients with TS usually have obsessive and compulsive behaviors (OCB) and often have attention-deficit hyperactivity disorder (ADHD). Obsessions are intrusive, recurrent, and persistent ideas, thoughts, images, or impulses which can be thought of as mental tics. Compulsions are repetitive and intentional actions which are performed in response to an obsession and are usually associated with reducing discomfort. For instance, a patient may have the obsession to even things out or to maintain symmetry, and if he bumps his side on a doorway there is a compulsive action to bump the other side of his body and to go back and forth from one side to the other perhaps four or five times to maintain symmetry. The patient often feels relieved from the uncomfortable pressure of the obsession after carrying out a compulsive act.

Strictly speaking, TS is not a true neurodevelopmental disorder, because significant developmental delays or mental retardation are not typically part of the syndrome. Dysmorphic features are not seen in TS (Figure 3.1). However, it is included in this book because learning disabilities and emotional problems, in addition to school and family difficulties, are part of the syndrome, and a coordinated multiprofessional treatment approach is necessary and is described herein. Tourette syndrome is a fascinating disorder because it not only includes features which we label as OCB or ADHD or tics but it also characterizes a personality that has intense drive, enthusiastic interests, and volatility of mood, which can be explosive and abrupt. I believe individuals with TS experience the ups and downs of life far more intensely than any other patient group with whom I have worked. Although these personality features are associated with problems, they can also lead to great achievements because of the drive and enthusiasm which is part of TS. It is worthwhile to consider these strengths in two great men from history who suffered from TS.

Both Dr. Samuel Johnson and Peter the Great were geniuses, but the personality features of TS from which they suffered throughout their lives had an influence on their productivity and accomplishments. Samuel Johnson (1709–1784) is best known for compiling the first great dictionary of the English language, along with writing novels and poems. He is also considered "the greatest talker who ever lived, with the most varied talk and varied audience of any man in history" (Norman, 1951). He had motor and vocal tics which were documented from adolescence and continued throughout his life. There are numerous descriptions by his biographers of repetitive sudden jerking of his face, lips, head, neck, shoulders, arms, and legs (Murray, 1979). His vocal tics included moaning, grunting, whistling, and talking to himself. He also frequently surprised his companions by blurting out unintelligible sounds (Murray, 1979). One of his biographers describes his vocal tics as follows:

> In the intervals of articulating he made various sounds with his mouth, sometimes as if ruminating, or what is called chewing the cud, sometimes giving

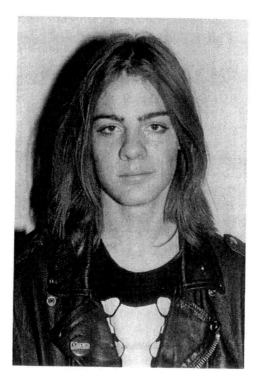

FIGURE 3.1: This 17-year-old male with Tourette syndrome experienced motor and vocal tics and ADHD throughout childhood and adolescence, but these problems have resolved gradually over the last 2 years. Also note lack of dysmorphic features in this young man.

a half whistle, sometimes making his tongue play backwards from the roof of his mouth, as if clucking like a hen, and sometimes protruding it against his upper gums in front, as if pronouncing quickly under his breath too, too, too: all this accompanied sometimes with a thoughtful look, but more frequently with a smile. Generally when he had concluded a period, in the course of a dispute, by which time he was a good deal exhausted by violence and vociferation, he used to blow out his breath like a whale. (Boswell, 1791/1949)

He was also hampered by obsessive-compulsive behavior, but perhaps only an obsessive personality could have compiled the first English dictionary. His movements and compulsive behavior are described here by another biographer:

He walked slowly, weaving ponderously from side to side, now against the wall, now at the pavement's edge, muttering to himself, whistling and clucking, his hands jerking out in involuntary gestures to startle other pedestrians in the London gloom. He came at length to the west side of Leicester Square, and paused before No. 47 to do a kind of mysterious jig in order to ascend the steps with the proper foot put forward first. Again, at the threshold, he repeated the strange jig, like a man hesitating to enter, drawing back and going forward; but enter at last he did, and found himself in the midst of a celebrated company. (Norman, 1951)

Clearly his genius, particularly his verbal abilities, facilitated his great achievements, but his personality, his energy, and his obsessions, all part of TS, made sure these accomplishments took place.

Peter the Great, the seventeenth-century Russian tsar who brought his country into the modern age, is also thought to have suffered from TS. He was extremely hyperactive in childhood and adulthood:

His most extraordinary quality, even more remarkable than his height, was his titanic energy. He could not sit still or stay long in the same place. He walked so quickly with his long, loose-limbed stride that those in his company had to trot to keep up with him. When forced to do paperwork he paced around a stand-up desk. Seated at a banquet, he would eat for a few minutes, then spring up to see what was happening in the next room or to take a walk outdoors. Needing movement, he liked to burn off his energy in dancing. When he had been in one place for a while, he wanted to leave, to move along, to see new people and new scenery, to form new impressions. The most accurate image of Peter the Great is of a man who throughout his life was perpetually curious, perpetually restless, perpetually in movement. (Massie, 1980, p. 134)

He began to have tics as a young tsar, and when he was agitated or under stress his face would twitch (Massie, 1980). One lady of the court described him by saying; "His grimaces and facial contortion were not as bad as they had expected and, Sophia Charlotte added sympathetically, some are not in his power to correct" (Massie, 1980, p. 176). He was described by a cardinal who met him as having constant movement of his arm and leg, and, to hide this, he accompanied the involuntary motion with continual movements of his entire body (Massie, 1980). Although many historians considered his movement disorder to be convulsive in nature, his symptoms are more consistent with TS (Berecz, 1992). His hyperactivity is also consistent with this diagnosis. His intense interests, particularly in Western culture, appeared to be obsessional at times, but this led to his greatness and his ability to forcibly bring Western culture to Russia.

EPIDEMIOLOGY, GENETICS, AND COMORBID DIAGNOSES

Although the genetic defect has not yet been discovered, family studies have documented the hereditary nature of TS and the broad spectrum of involvement in this disorder. The *DSM-IV* diagnostic criteria for TS is as follows (APA, 1994, p. 103):

1. Both multiple motor and one or more vocal tics have been present at some time during the illness, although not necessarily concurrently. (A tic is a sudden, rapid, recurrent, nonrhythmic, stereotyped motor movement or vocalization.)
2. The tics occur many times a day (usually in bouts) nearly every day or intermittently throughout a period of more than 1 year, and during this period there was never a tic-free period of more than 3 consecutive months.
3. The disturbance causes marked distress or significant impairment in social, occupational, or other important areas of functioning
4. The onset is before age 18 years.
5. The disturbance is not due to the direct physiological effects of a substance (e.g., stimulants) or a general medical condition (e.g., Huntington's disease or postviral encephalitis).

Although the *DSM-IV* separates the diagnoses of transient tic disorder, meaning motor or vocal tics for less than 1 year; chronic tic disorder, meaning motor or vocal tics for longer than 1 year; TS; and obsessive-compulsive disorder, the family studies demonstrate that these diagnoses are all part of the same biologic continuum related to the genetic etiology. The *DSM-IV* diagnostic criteria for OCD is as follows (APA, 1994, pp. 422–3):

A. Either obsessions or compulsions:
   Obsessions as defined by (1), (2), (3), and (4):
   (1) Recurrent and persistent thoughts, impulses, or images that are experienced, at some time during the disturbance, as intrusive and inappropriate and that cause marked anxiety or distress.
   (2) The thoughts, impulses, or images are not simply excessive worries about real-life problems.
   (3) The person attempts to ignore or suppress such thoughts, impulses, or images, or to neutralize them with some other thought or action.
   (4) The person recognizes that the obsessional thoughts, impulses, or images are a product of his or her own mind (not imposed from without as in thought insertion).

   Compulsions as defined by (1) and (2):
   (1) Repetitive behaviors (e.g., hand washing, ordering, checking) or mental acts (e.g., praying, counting, repeating words silently) that the person feels driven to perform in response to an obsession, or according to rules that must be applied rigidly.
   (2) The behaviors or mental acts are aimed at preventing or reducing distress or preventing some dreaded event or situation; however, these behaviors or mental acts either are not connected in a realistic way with what they are designed to neutralize or prevent or are clearly excessive.

B. At some point during the course of the disorder, the person has recognized that the obsessions or compulsions are excessive or unreasonable. *Note*: This does not apply to children.

C. The obsessions or compulsions cause marked distress, are time consuming (take more than 1 hour a day), or significantly interfere with the person's normal routine, occupational (or academic) functioning, or usual social activities or relationships.

In a recent family study of 53 child probands with TS, 35.3% of the families had another member affected with TS, and 70.6% of the families had another member affected with either TS, chronic tic disorder (CT), or obsessive-compulsive disorder (OCD) (Walkup et al., 1996). When the 154 first-degree relatives were carefully assessed, 13.6% received a lifetime diagnosis of TS, 7.8% received a lifetime diagnosis of CT, and 22.7% received a lifetime diagnosis of OCD. Genetic modeling of this data supports a mixed model with a major locus that accounts for over half of the phenotypic variance; the authors estimate that 0.01% of individuals in the general population are homozygous for this susceptibility allele (Walkup et al., 1996). In addition, a multifactorial background accounts for 40–45% of the phenotypic variance. In this study, 19% of the families had two parents with the broader TS phenotype, demonstrating bilineal inheritance and assortative mating (Walkup et al., 1996). Bilineal transmission was also reported in a large pedigree with 175 descendants, of whom 36% had TS; 31% of married-in spouses also had TS, which lead to increased morbidity in their offspring (McMahon et al., 1996).

The Yale family study of TS has demonstrated a sex difference in the manifestation of the broader spectrum of TS. Female relatives are three times more likely to be affected with OCD than with CT and nine times more likely to be affected with OCD than with TS (Santangelo et al., 1996). Males are at higher risk for TS than females, and the sex ratio is approximately 3 : 1. However, if the broader spectrum of TS is used, including CT and OCD, then the sex ratio reduces to 1.6 : 1 (Santangelo et al., 1996). Male probands were four times more likely to experience rage episodes, that is, sudden and explosive anger, irritability, temper tantrums, and aggression, than female probands at the onset of their TS. Rage at onset of TS in the proband also increased the risk 1.75 times that a relative would develop a TS spectrum disorder compared with relatives who did not have a proband with rage symptoms (Santangelo et al., 1996). Also, the younger the proband was at first tic symptom, the greater the risk for becoming ill for the proband's family members (Santangelo et al., 1996).

Obsessive-compulsive symptoms are seen in almost all patients with TS, although approximately 60% will meet diagnostic criteria for OCD (Coffey and Park, 1997). Sometimes it is difficult to differentiate complex motor tics from compulsive behavior, such as repetitive tapping, rubbing, or touching that is repeated again and again until the patient feels better. If it is carried out because of an obsession, that is, to even things out or for symmetry, then it is considered a compulsion. For some individuals, the OCD symptoms are far more debilitating than the tics. Patients with just OCD have a 7% lifetime risk of developing TS and a 20% risk of developing tics (Coffey and Park, 1997). When patients having OCD are compared with patients having TS, contamination concerns and washing rituals are found to be more common in patients with OCD alone, whereas sensorimotor experiences that were generalized or local body sensations occur more commonly in patients with TS in association with their repetitive compulsions (Coffey and Park, 1997).

In addition to OCD, other anxiety and mood disorders are common in patients with TS. In a study of the first 100 children and adolescents with TS who presented to a specialty clinic, 76% met *DSM-III-R* (APA, 1987) criteria for a mood disorder, 25% met criteria for OCD, 52% met criteria for subthreshold OCD, and 64% met criteria for an anxiety disorder, including 6% with panic disorder, 50% with agoraphobia, 20% with social phobia, 30% with simple phobia, 22% with overanxious disorder, and 26% with separation anxiety disorder (Coffey and Park, 1997). Other investigators have also found a higher incidence of mood disorders, including anxiety, depression, and bipolar disorder, in patients with TS than in controls (Coffey et al., 1992; Comings and Comings, 1987a; Kerbeshian and Burd, 1989; Kerbeshian et al., 1995).

Attention Deficit Hyperactivity Disorder

The association of ADHD with TS is controversial, with rates of co-occurrence ranging from 8 to 80% (Freeman, 1997). Clearly, problems with impulse control and attention occur in the majority of individuals affected by TS, but the frequency of ADHD depends on how it is defined, particularly for family studies (Freeman, 1997). In a careful analysis of the co-occurrence of ADHD and TS using *DSM-III* (APA, 1980) criteria, 54.1% of probands with TS met criteria for a diagnosis of ADHD, 30.6% of probands had a diagnosis of learning disabilities, and 15.3% of probands stuttered (Pauls et al., 1993). An increased incidence of ADHD in relatives occurred only for the probands who had both ADHD and TS (Pauls et al., 1993). ADHD symptoms often begin before the onset of tics; therefore, the attentional problems are not caused by the tic manifestations themselves. Comings has been a long term supporter of the concept that there is a pleiotrophic effect of the TS genes because they cause an underlying disturbance in the balance of serotonin and dopamine, which leads to an increased susceptibility to a wide range of impulsive, compulsive, affective, and anxiety disorders (Comings, 1995a, 1995b, 1995c). Comings urges physicians to recognize and appropriately treat all of the problems associated with TS, including the tics and a variety of behavioral problems, such as ADHD, OCD, mood disturbances, anxiety, and sleep difficulties.

Epidemiology

Epidemiology studies have demonstrated a prevalence range of 0.5 to 299 per 10,000 for TS (Tanner and Goldman, 1997; Mason et al. 1998). The variability depends on the methodology used and the age and sex of the population because TS usually improves with age and is less common in women. A high prevalence (50 per 10,000) was found in a questionnaire survey of 1321 parents of children attending kindergarten or primary school in Japan (Nomoto and Machiyama, 1990). A subsequent study in Los Angeles involved the surveillance of 3034 elementary and intermediate school children for the presence of tics and a thorough evaluation of the children, who were referred for problems by the teacher or psychologist (Comings et al., 1990). The overall prevalence of TS was 1 per 95 boys and 1 in 759 girls. Seventy percent of the children diagnosed with TS were in special education classes, and 12% of children in special education classes had TS (Comings et al., 1990). Similar results were found in New York, where 8.6% of special education students had TS (Kurlan et al., 1994). The highest prevalence figures come from a recent study in England which evaluated all ninth-graders ($n = 167$) at a regular school with a two-stage screening involving questionnaires and classroom observation followed by a clinical interview for students with possible tics (Mason et al. 1998). Five students fulfilled criteria for TS, yielding an overall prevalence of 299 per 10,000, or 3%, which is three times higher than reported by Comings et al. (1990). Other tic disorders are also common in the general population, and the mildest form of tics, transient tic disorder, is estimated to occur in up to 24% of school-aged children (Jankovic, 1997).

Clearly, TS is no longer considered a rare disorder, and it is relatively commonly diagnosed in boys who are in special education or who present to the clinic with ADHD if the appropriate questions regarding tics and OCB are asked. The majority of the children who are now diagnosed have a mild form of the disorder, and fewer than one-third experience coprolalia (Bruun and Budman, 1997).

LIFE COURSE

Before tics develop, many children present with hyperactivity, tantrums, rigidity in behavior, and impulsivity. Approximately 20% of patients have an exaggerated startle response which may fail to habituate with repetition of stimuli and may be noticeable in infancy (Stell et al., 1995); see the case study later in this chapter. Rage episodes may also occur in early childhood, and the presence of rage episodes in patients with TS is strongly correlated with the combination of OCD and ADHD (Coffey and Park, 1997). Young children are often medicated with stimulants because of the ADHD symptoms, and they later develop tics. This sequence of events led to the concept that the tics were simply side effects of the stimulant medication. Now we know that the children who develop TS are genetically predisposed to this disorder and that stimulants may worsen tics in approximately 30% but that they can also improve tics in 10% (see the section on treatment and the case history).

The onset of tics occurs at a mean age of 6 to 7 years, and 75% of patients have tics by the age of 11 years (Bruun and Budman, 1997). The first tics are usually facial, followed by involuntary movements of the upper extremities. Motor tics can be described as clonic tics, which are fast and brief; dystonic tics, which involve twisting, squeezing, or stretching movements; or tonic tics, which have sustained isometric contractions without movement, such as abdominal muscle tensing or limb tensing (Jankovic, 1997). In a study of 156 patients with TS, 57% exhibited dystonic tics, including oculogyric deviations (28%) and neck stretching or twisting movements (7%; Jankovic, 1997).

Vocal tics usually come after 1 or more years of motor tics, and they initially usually involve noises rather than words (Bruun and Budman, 1997). The most common vocal tic is throat clearing (Jankovic, 1997). Both motor and vocal tics are usually preceded by premonitory feelings, which are sensations, such as a burning feeling, a crick in the neck, or a feeling of tightness or itching that is relieved by the tic, such as stretching the neck or arm, throat clearing, or other movement or sound. Sometimes the premonitory feeling is a general psychic sensation such as anxiety, anger, or an urge. In a study of 132 patients with TS, 83% described the premonitory sensations as either partly or completely physical in nature, and tics of the head, neck, and shoulder were most frequently associated with these sensations (Leckman et al., 1993). There is typically a 3-year lag between the onset of tics and the development of premonitory sensations (Leckman et al., 1993). In a sense, the tics have a compulsive quality because of the premonitory feelings or urges. In a study of 60 patients with TS, 93% of the tics were perceived by the patient to be "irresistibly but purposefully executed" (Jankovic, 1997). In a study of compulsive behavior such as checking, evening up, or rearranging, 44% reported the urge to repeat these behaviors until it looked, felt, or sounded "just right" (Leckman et al., 1994). Patients are able to distinguish the premonitory feelings from the "just right" feelings. There is a 7-year delay between the onset of tics and the development of the "just right" feelings, but this is probably related to the later onset of complex tics and compulsive behavior in the natural history of TS (Leckman et al., 1994).

Although the premonitory sensations have been called sensory tics, unusual sensory experiences can occur in isolation, without the urge for subsequent motor or vocal tics (Scahill et al., 1995). Such a sensory tic is described later in this chapter in the case history. It is also possible to experience extracorporeal or out-of-body sensations. For instance, one patient was reported to experience a "feel" at the end of the pencil he was holding which was associated with the need to press the pencil down hard while writing (Karp and Hallett, 1996). External sensations can arise in angles, corners, at the edge of tables, or even at the edge of a computer screen (Karp and Hallett, 1996).

Kane, who has TS, reports somatic hyperattention as a continual state in TS (Kane, 1994). He is always supersensitive to sensory input; for instance, when seated he is continually aware of the tactile sensation of the seat against his body, and he experiences "enduring sensory bombardment" (Kane, 1994). He hypothesizes that patients with TS have an inability to suppress the preconscious processing of somatosensory stimulation (Kane, 1994). Once attention is drawn to an area of the body by external stimulation, there is somatic hyperawareness (the premonitory sensation) which leads to tics. For example, a cough tic may develop after a cold, or throat clearing may develop after wearing a tight tie. For Kane, concern about overeating led to touching his stomach to check for stomach protrusion after meals. Subsequently, somatosensory hyperawareness became entangled with cognitive and emotional hyperattention, as he developed excessive worries about weight (Kane, 1994). An inability to inhibit somatic attention coupled with an inability to inhibit thought (obsessions) suggest a deficit of inhibition in TS, which is consistent with neurophysiological studies described subsequently and with the enhanced startle response reported in some patients with TS.

Tics usually wax and wane, although anxiety, stress, fatigue, heat, or even boredom will often increase tics (Jankovic, 1997). The clinician will notice that the onset of school after a summer vacation is usually associated with tic exacerbation in many patients because of the stress and anxiety associated with school anticipation. Most patients have multiple tics at a single period in time, but many tics disappear after a few weeks and are replaced by others. Usually one or two tics are consistently seen in an individual; they may be continuous tics, or they may be present periodically during the day. Motor and vocal tics may persist during all stages of sleep (Jankovic, 1997). Tics can be temporarily suppressed, so they may not be noticeable in the office or during tasks that require concentration, particularly in the patient with a mild form of TS. Some children and even adults may not be aware of their tics or may deny their presence even when the tics are obvious to the clinician. Tics can often cause sore muscles, and many children with head or shoulder jerking complain of a sore neck. A secondary effect of tics may be a decline in self-image caused by the patient's feelings of helplessness in controlling these disturbing movements.

Usually tics reach their maximum intensity in early adolescence, and they often improve subsequently. Approximately one-third of patients with TS will experience complete remission of their tics by late adolescence, and another one-third will experience significant improvements such that their tics will be mild and unimpairing (Bruun and Budman, 1997; Figure 3.1). The remaining one-third of patients will continue to experience tics throughout their lives; the cases of Dr. Samuel Johnson and Peter the Great are in this category. ADHD symptoms usually improve in adolescence and become more manageable, although approximately half of the patients continue to have limited symptoms, such as impulsivity, a high energy level, or inattention in adulthood (Bruun and Budman, 1997).

NEUROIMMUNOLOGY AND PANDAS

In the 1990s a subgroup of patients with movement disorders, including TS and OCD, and who have acute exacerbation of their symptoms related to group A beta-hemolytic streptococcal infections, was identified. This subgroup is designated by the acronym PANDAS (pediatric autoimmune neuropsychiatric disorders associated with streptococcal infections; Swedo et al., 1997). During a strep infection, which is most often a sore throat, antibodies are produced, particularly to the M protein of the strep, which cross react to basal ganglion areas of the brain. The strep infection is documented by a positive throat culture and elevation of antistrep antibodies, such as antistreptolysin O and antistreptococcal DNAse B titers. Antineuronal antibodies directed against the caudate and or the putamen have been shown to be significantly higher in children with tics or OCD than in controls with ADHD (Kiessling et al., 1994). Although the controls demonstrated antibodies to either the caudate or putamen in 37% of cases, the study patients had these antibodies in 63% of cases. These antineuronal antibodies were also seen in 10 of 11 patients with Sydenham's chorea, which occurs after a strep infection that causes rheumatic fever (Swedo et al., 1993). Sydenham's chorea is also included in the PANDAS disease category because of the psychological dysfunction that has been documented, which includes obsessive compulsive behavior in 82% and emotional lability, irritability, decreased attentiveness, and anxiety in the majority of patients (Swedo et al., 1993).

Since antibodies do not typically cross the blood-brain barrier, it is thought that activated B lymphocytes migrate through the blood-brain barrier to the CNS, where they differentiate into plasma cells and begin to secrete antigen-specific antibodies. In an animal model, sera from patients with TS was infused into the caudate nuclei of rats, and an increase in licking, paw licking, head and paw shaking, and phonic utterances was documented over the controls (Hallett and Kiessling, 1997). These abnormal behaviors waxed and waned, but they persisted for 7 days after the infusion stopped.

The identification of PANDAS has prompted novel treatment approaches to eliminate antibody production. A few cases of abrupt obsessive-compulsive behavior or severe tics after strep infections have been reported to improve after undergoing several plasma exchanges (plasmapheresis) (Allen et al., 1995). One case demonstrated a 24% decrease in the size of the caudate, a 12% decrease in the putamen, and a 28% decrease in the globus pallidus on MRI after plasmapheresis compared with sizes before treatment (Allen et al., 1995; Giedd et al., 1996). Acute inflammation of the basal ganglia causes edema and an initial increase in the size of the structure; however, prolonged edema leads to a vascular compromise in this area, with eventual necrosis which reduces the size of the structure (Giedd et al., 1996). Another patient experienced improvement in tics after intravenous immunoglobulin (1 mg/kg/day for 2 days), and an additional patient improved with immunosuppressive doses of prednisone after experiencing severe exacerbation of his tics with a flu-like viral illness 6 months prior to treatment (Allen et al., 1995).

Many questions remain unanswered, including whether an immune reaction can occur with infections other than strep, such as viruses, and what the treatment efficacy is of prophylactic penicillin and other more expensive interventions, such as plasmapheresis. It is unclear how many patients with TS are experiencing an antineuronal antibody effect and whether other areas of the brain, such as frontal regions, could also be affected. It is imperative that the physician is diligent in monitoring for strep infections, using frequent throat cultures and aggressive antibiotic treatment when strep is found (Allen et al., 1995; Swedo et al., 1994). The genetic predisposition to TS may involve differences in antibody formation or the ease with which activated lymphocytes enter the CNS. A recent report documented that 85% of children with PANDAS and 89% of children with Sydenham's chorea were positive for a cell surface marker DR+ that is recognized by a monoclonal antibody D8/17 compared with only 17% of healthy children (Swedo et al., 1997). This cell surface marker is highly sensitive in identifying children who are at high risk for developing rheumatic fever.

NEUROANATOMICAL AND NEUROIMAGING STUDIES

Very few reports exist of thorough autopsy studies in individuals with TS (reviewed by Leckman et al., 1997). The only significant finding is a report of an increased packing density of neurons in the caudate and putamen in a 42-year-old patient with TS compared with controls (Leckman et al., 1997). Several neuroimaging studies have been carried out in patients with TS, and they show evidence of volume reduction of the basal ganglia (Leckman et al., 1997). In both children and adults with TS, MRI volumetric studies have shown a significant reduction in the size of the left striatum, particularly the putamen, and the globus pallidus compared with controls (Leckman et al., 1997; Singer et al., 1993). Therefore, patients with TS may not demonstrate the normal left-greater-than-right volumetric asymmetry in this area that is seen in the controls.

Studies in patients with OCD but without TS have also demonstrated reduced volumes of the striatum, particularly the putamen, which receives more projections from the amygdala than the caudate does (Rosenberg et al., 1997). Increased metabolic rates have been seen in the orbital prefrontal area and in the caudate on functional neuroimaging in patients with OCD than in controls (Baxter, 1992). Metabolic studies using PET scanning in patients with TS demonstrate metabolic increases in lateral premotor and supplementary motor association areas (both are associated with movement) and metabolic decreases in left caudate and both thalamic areas compared with controls (Eidelberg et al., 1997). The enhanced frontal metabolic activity is also consistent with a recent report that the corpus callosum is more enlarged in 16 patients with TS than in controls (Baumgardner et al., 1996). The most consistent enlargement was seen in the rostral corpus callosum, which provides interhemispheric connections for regions of the frontal cortex.

The metabolic and volumetric findings in TS are consistent with dysfunction in the cortico-striato-thalamo-cortical (CSTC) neuronal circuits that modulate psychomotor behavior (reviewed in Leckman et al., 1997). The CSTC circuit begins with excitatory projections from the cortex to the striatum, involving excitatory amino acids such as glutamate. From the striatum, both direct and indirect inhibitory projections (GABA) go to the globus pallidus and the substantia nigra, with subsequent inhibitory connections to the reticular nucleus of the thalamus. The thalamus subsequently feeds back to the cortex with excitatory (glutamate) projections. Hyperinnervation of the striatum by dopaminergic neurons has been proposed in TS, leading to enhanced inhibition of the globus pallidus and subsequently less inhibition of the thalamus that in turn leads to enhanced thalamus-cortical stimulation (Leckman et al., 1997). Both postmortem studies and the effects of medications that block dopamine support the theory that dopamine hypersensitivity or hyperinnervation exists in TS and modulates the output of the basal ganglia. In addition, single-photon emission computed tomography (SPECT) studies of identical twins who are discordant for TS symptoms found that binding to D2 receptors in the caudate nucleus was increased in all of the twins who were more affected by TS (Wolf et al., 1996). This is consistent with a hypothesis of D2 receptor supersensitivity, either secondary to increased receptor density or affinity or a combination of factors (Wolf et al., 1996). In addition, a recent positron emission tomography study found higher DOPA decarboxylase activity in the left candate and right midbrain in patients with TS compared to controls (Ernst et al., 1999). This finding suggests either a greater number of dopaminergic synapses or an up regulation of the enzyme, but both possibilities support a model of abnormal presynaptic dopaminergic activity in TS (Ernst et al., 1999).

Recent linkage studies have demonstrated an association between an allele of the dopamine D4 receptor gene, *DRD4*7R*, and TS (Grice et al., 1996). The protein product of this allele has a reduced ability to inhibit forskolin-induced cAMP formation, perhaps because this allele has seven repeat units, so it is a longer form of the gene. In addition, the *DRD4*7R* allele has been associated with novelty seeking in personality measures. Although this allele does not cause TS, it may be an additive factor to the overall phenotype.

To further characterize the motor inhibition problem that is present in TS, transcranial magnetic stimulation of the left motor cortex and surface electromyography of a right-hand muscle was carried out on 20 patients with TS and on controls (Ziemann et al., 1997). The motor threshold and peripheral motor excitability were normal, suggesting that the neuronal membrane and ion permeability are normal, but the cortical silent period was shortened and intracortical inhibition was reduced compared with controls. These findings are consistent with the CSTC abnormalities already described.

SCHOOL PROBLEMS AND LEARNING DISABILITIES

Children with TS are five times more likely to end up in special education than their peers, and, as noted, a significant percentage of children in special education have TS (Comings and Comings, 1987b; Comings et al., 1990). The cause of the learning problems relates to several factors. It may be hard to keep up with the class if significant obsessions disrupt thinking and attention. Severe tics that involve the arms may interfere with handwriting and concentration. However, in a study of 138 children with TS, the most significant predictor for placement into special education was the comorbid diagnosis of ADHD (Abwender et al., 1996). ADHD was present in 75% of children with TS who had academic problems and in 44% of those who had no academic problems (Abwender et al., 1996). In children with TS who present to a child development clinic, ADHD was present in 85% (Singer et al., 1995b).

In addition to a diagnosis of ADHD, 46% of 138 children with TS experienced school difficulties and 38% were in a nonstandard classroom at least part time (Abwender et al., 1996). Repetition of school grades was not uncommon, with 12% repeating one grade and 3% repeating two grades. Although a diagnosis of a specific learning disability was made in 22%, 33% of those who were not diagnosed as learning disabled were experiencing academic difficulties. Common school problems or learning disabilities in children with TS are as follows:

1. *Written language deficits:* Visual motor coordination problems are common in TS and may relate to the basal ganglia pathology and the associated ADHD symptoms. Impulsivity and the tendency to rush through work may further impair the quality of written language. Stimulant medication can directly improve visual-motor coordination, in addition to improving ADHD symptoms that have a secondary effect on the quality of handwriting.

2. *Visual perceptual deficits:* Approximately 35% of children with TS have a significantly higher Verbal IQ (15-point significant discrepancy) than Performance IQ, suggesting a tendency for nonverbal learning disabilities related to visual perceptual deficits (Hagin and Kugler, 1988). In neuropsychological studies of visuospatial priming, individuals with TS demonstrated reduced inhibition in visual spatial processing tasks (Swerdlow et al. 1996).

3. *Reading comprehension and spelling deficits:* Although oral reading and word attack skills are considered a strength in TS, reading comprehension is below expectations for IQ in 40% of patients on individual reading comprehension tasks and in 68% in group reading comprehension tasks (Hagin et al., 1988). The latter academic testing requires prolonged concentration in a group setting which can be influenced by ADHD symptoms. Spelling was below IQ expectations in 52% and perhaps this is related to visual perceptual deficits or auditory processing deficits (Hagin and Kugler, 1988; Packer, 1997).

4. *Written math problems:* Mathematics was below expectations for IQ in 56% of children with TS (Hagin et al., 1988). The visual motor coordination problems in TS can interfere with written aspects of math. Visual spatial deficits, in addition to organizational problems, may confuse the sequence that is needed to carry out long division problems or carrying and borrowing.

5. *Executive function deficits:* Deficits in attention, impulse control, organization, and set shifting and problems with perseveration are all considered to be related to executive function deficits which are the neuropsychological underpinnings of ADHD. These problems interfere remarkably with school performance because the ability to listen in class attentively and to remember when to turn in what assignment is related to these functions. Deficits in executive function associated with a timed output or cognitive slowing was problematic in children with TS only, but children with TS plus ADHD had more significant difficulties in maintaining attention and a preparedness to act on neuropsycho-

logical testing (Singer et al., 1995b). Children with TS but without ADHD did not demonstrate executive function deficits on neuropsychological testing (Ozonoff et al. 1994).

Pervasive Developmental Disorder and TS

IQ deficits below the normal range are not part of TS; however, over the last decade an increasing number of patients have been reported with both TS and pervasive developmental disorder (PDD). Over 90 patients have been reported in the literature with both disorders (Stern and Robertson, 1997). In a series of 59 patients with autism or PDD, 12 demonstrated features of TS (Burd et al., 1987). These patients had a higher IQ and language abilities than the overall sample, suggesting a better prognosis for the combination of TS and autism compared to autism alone. Problems with obsessive-compulsive behavior are commonly seen in both individuals with Asperger syndrome and individuals with autism, which suggests that similar pathology involving the basal ganglia occurs in all three disorders. The incidence of MRI abnormalities is higher in patients with TS and Asperger syndrome together, compared with TS alone. Four of seven patients with both diagnoses demonstrated cortical abnormalities, including incomplete formation of the superior temporal gyrus, defects in the frontal region, hypoplasia of the temporo-occipital cortex, and small gyri in the parietal lobes, and a fifth patient had abnormal signal density of the striatum (Berthier et al., 1993). TS has also been diagnosed in some patients with fragile X syndrome who also suffer from frontal deficits, obsessive-compulsive behavior, perseveration, coprolalia, and ADHD (Hagerman, 1996). Approximately 10 to 20% of children with fragile X syndrome also have motor tics, but this is not significantly different from IQ-matched control patients (Baumgardner et al., 1995).

Peer Problems

Part of the school difficulties in TS relates to peer problems. As a group, patients with TS are significantly more withdrawn, aggressive and less popular than their classmates (Stokes et al., 1991). Almost half of 29 children with TS scored greater than 1 SD above the mean for withdrawal, and 28% scored greater than 1 SD above the mean for aggression. These problems did not correlate with the severity of the tics or the severity of neuropsychological deficits; however, the presence of ADHD correlated significantly with aggression (Stokes et al., 1991). Such problems suggest that peer relations training would be helpful for children with TS, in addition to the traditional interventions described in the next section.

TREATMENT

The treatment of individuals with TS involves a multiprofessional approach because of the combination of behavioral, emotional, physical, and learning problems that affect performance at school, home, and in the workplace. It is important for the professional to help parents set appropriate expectations for their child that facilitate growth and the development of a good self-image but also protect the child from excessive demands or unreachable goals. Most children with TS get better in adolescence, so expectations need to be readjusted with age. With patience and support, most children do well. The best medicine is tolerance. An overview of treatment approaches ordered by age of the patient is presented here.

Infants, Toddlers, and Preschoolers

Approximately 20% of children with TS have an increased startle response, and this may be noticed in infancy (see the case history). Otherwise, infants with TS have normal developmental milestones. In the toddler or preschool years, hyperactivity or ADHD may become apparent with moodiness or tantrums. The most severe cases may present with rage outbursts in the preschool period. If ADHD symptoms are present, low doses of stimulant medication, such as methylphenidate or Adderall, can be used, preferably after the child turns 4, and control of the impulsivity and hyperactivity often leads to improvement in rage reactions. The use of a selective serotonin reuptake inhibitor (SSRI) may also be helpful in reducing aggressive behavior or rage reactions (Bruun and Budman, 1998). Sometimes rages are associated with obsessive-compulsive behavior and rigidity or anxiety, which are usually improved with an SSRI such as fluoxetine (Prozac), fluvoxamine (Luvox), or paroxetine (Paxil). Usually these interventions take place before the diagnosis of TS is made because the child often has not begun to display tics in the preschool period.

It is important to refer a child with significant behavior problems to a psychologist who can work with the whole family and the child on a behavior management program (Bloomquist, 1996; Howard, 1996). The use of positive reinforcement, structure, consistency, time-out, and helping the child with transitions to avoid outbursts are very helpful to the child and family. Weekly guidance in how to deal with new behaviors is usually necessary.

Problems in the motor area are often diagnosed in the preschool period, including clumsiness; poor motor planning; frustrations with motor tasks that require fine motor coordination, such as drawing or early handwriting; and excessive sensitivity to various sensory stimuli, such as sounds or clothing textures (Kane, 1994; Packer, 1997). Referral to an occupational therapist (OT) can lead to appropriate intervention in the motor and sensory-motor areas, which may also have a positive impact on behavior.

School-Aged Children

By this age the child usually has a combination of problems, including tics, ADHD, OCB, and perhaps other difficulties, such as anxiety and mood lability or outburst behavior. When the diagnosis of TS is made, it is important to discuss the full spectrum of problems which occur and their biological and genetic basis.

A detailed family history for problems with tics, OCD, ADHD, anxiety, and other emotional difficulties is essential at the initial evaluation. Sometimes a parent or relative becomes aware of the problem in themselves when the child is diagnosed. It is also essential to refer families to a nearby support group for TS where they can talk comfortably with other parents and hear practical solutions to many problems. The Tourette Syndrome Association (TSA) has a list of support groups around the country (see Resources at the end of this chapter). The education of the patient and family is primary, but it may also be important to educate school personnel and peers about TS, particularly if the child is being ridiculed by peers or if the child is disruptive in the classroom. An educational presentation can be given at the school by the parent, teacher, or school nurse with the help of videos put out by the TSA, such as "A Regular Kid—That's Me" or "Stop It—I Can't." Packer (1997) reports on the reaction of a 7-year-old child whose class had been severely disrupted by the tics and behavior of a student with TS. After seeing the video "Stop It—I Can't," the student remarked, "Why didn't you tell us before?" (Packer, 1997).

Treatment of Tics

The philosophy behind psychopharmacologic management of tics is to treat only if they are bothersome to the patient and to accept the fact that the tics will not disappear with treatment. Therefore, the target is decreasing the severity of the tics with the least amount of medication possible. It is also important to use the least toxic medications first and avoid neuroleptics if possible because of their side effects (described herein).

Patients usually present with a combination of tics and ADHD together, so an appropriate initial medication is clonidine, which improves both problems (Leckman et al., 1988). Although clonidine is not as effective for improving attention and concentration as the stimulants, it has an overall calming effect and helps to decrease hyperactivity, overarousal, and tantrums, and it improves tics in approximately 60–70% of patients (Hagerman et al., 1998; Lichter and Jackson, 1996). In a double-blind crossover trial, clonidine was superior to placebo in the treatment of some TS symptoms, including impulsivity, hyperactivity, and motor tics (Leckman et al., 1991). Clonidine is an α_2-adrenergic presynaptic agonist which lowers the amount of norepinephrine released from the synapse both centrally and peripherally. Clonidine comes in a 0.1-mg tablet, in addition to a Catapres patch which can deliver 0.1 mg (TTS-1), 0.2 mg (TTS-2), or 0.3 mg (TTS-3) of clonidine per day for a period of approximately 5 days before the patch needs to be changed. The main side effect of clonidine is sedation, so the use of a low dose initially is essential or else the child will fall asleep in class. In preschool children, beginning with one-fourth or even one-eighth of a tablet once or twice a day will usually avoid sedation. For the school-aged child one-half of a tablet once or twice a day is an initial dose. The dose can be gradually increased depending on side effects, particularly sedation, which usually improves after the first week or two. The dose can be given up to four times a day, and the standard dose for TS is 3 to 4 micrograms/kg/day, which translates to one-half to one tablet (0.1 mg) three times a day for the school-aged child. The sedation side effect is helpful for children who have difficulty going to sleep at night, so the last dose is often given at bedtime.

Clonidine is also an antihypertensive agent, so another side effect is low blood pressure, which can present as dizziness or fainting. It is important not to abruptly discontinue clonidine because a rebound increase in blood pressure will occur that leads to headache, agitation, and on rare occasion chest pain (Hagerman et al., 1998). Patients and their families should be directly told not to abruptly discontinue this medication. Removal of the Catapres patch allows for a slow withdrawal because of skin stores.

Use of the patch causes less sedation than the pill, but skin irritation underneath the patch is seen in approximately 40% of patients. The skin irritation usually responds to the use of hydrocortisone cream after the patch is removed and placed in a new location on the back or buttocks. However, if the skin irritation is severe, an aqueous-based steroid spray, such as Vancenase double strength AQ or Beconase AQ nasal spray, can be sprayed on the back and allowed to dry before placing the patch on that area (Hagerman et al., 1998). This technique usually significantly decreases skin irritation, although some children are unable to tolerate the patch. The patch is usually placed on the back where young children cannot reach it, because eating the patch causes an overdose which may lead to coma and respiratory suppression.

Clonidine lowers cardiac output by 20% and slows nodal conduction by 4 to 6% (Hagerman et al., 1998). Although this is not as severe an interference with cardiac conduction as that caused by tricyclics, recent reports regarding rare arrhythmias and four cases of sudden death in children using clonidine combined with other medications, particularly methylphenidate, have prompted caution (Cantwell et al., 1997; Swanson et al., 1995). Review of these three cases has shown that clonidine was not the cause of death, but caution is advocated nevertheless, and EKG monitoring is recommended (Blackman et al., 1996; Cantwell et al., 1997; Hagerman et al., 1998; Popper, 1995).

Although clonidine is helpful for the majority of patients with TS, the presence of ADHD, the presence of vocal tics, and an older age are all positive predictors of a good therapeutic response to clonidine (Lichter and Jackson, 1996). Younger children tend to have more sedation with clonidine, but again this can be avoided with the use of a lower dose, as previously described. If sedation is excessive, guanfacine (Tenex) can be tried instead of clonidine. Guanfacine is a more specific α_2-adrenergic agonist which preferentially binds α_{2A}-adrenergic receptors that are concentrated in prefrontal cortical regions (Chappell et al., 1995). Guanfacine therefore causes less sedation and hypotension than clonidine, although there has been less experience with use of guanfacine in childhood. The dose of guanfacine is 10 times the dose of clonidine, and it comes in 1-mg tablets. The plasma half-life of guanfacine in adults is 17 hours (range 10 to 30 hours), whereas the plasma half-life of clonidine is 8 to 12 hours in children and 12 to 16 hours in adults (Chappell et al., 1995; Hagerman et al., 1998). Therefore, the dosing of guanfacine can often be twice a day. An open trial of guanfacine was carried out in 10 children with TS, and improvements in motor and vocal tics were documented, along with improvements in a continuous performance task, but improvements in hyperactivity were not seen (Chappell et al., 1995). Improvement with guanfacine in another child with TS was also reported, and the vocal tics responded to a dose of 2.5 mg/day, whereas motor tics responded to a dose of 4.0 mg/day (Fras, 1996). Side effects of fatigue and headaches may also occur with guanfacine. Until more experience is obtained regarding the use of guanfacine in childhood and controlled efficacy studies are carried out in TS, this medication is not the first choice of treatment for tics or ADHD.

The adjunctive use of clonazepam (Klonopin), a benzodiazepine, with clonidine has been studied in an open trial of seven children with TS who showed improvement in ADHD symptoms with clonidine but required an additional agent to further improve their tics (Steingard et al., 1994). All seven patients experienced additional improvements in their tics on a combination of clonidine and clonazepam without worsening of their ADHD symptoms. Clonazepam was given either at bedtime or twice a day, with a mean dose of 0.96 mg/day. Side effects included mild sedation, but none of the patients experienced behavioral disinhibition. Treatment with benzodiazepines can cause behavioral disinhibition in approximately 2% of patients, so careful monitoring of behavior is necessary (Steingard et al., 1994). Clonazepam has also been used to treat OCD symptoms in several cases. In one 20-year-old with OCD who was unresponsive to high doses of SSRIs, a dramatic improvement was seen with 4 mg of clonazepam combined with 60 mg of fluoxetine per day (Leonard et al., 1994). Clonazapam is considered unique among the benzodiazepines because of its up-regulation of serotonin binding sites (Wagner et al., 1985). In general, benzodiazepines are not commonly used in pediatrics because of their addictive potential; however, there is experience in pediatrics with clonazepam because it is used as an anticonvulsant.

A recent double-blind placebo-controlled trial of clonidine (0.05 mg four times daily), desipramine (25 mg four times daily), and placebo was carried out in 34 children with TS and ADHD between the ages of 7 and 13 years (Singer et al., 1995a). Desipramine (Norpramin) was found to be superior to clonidine in the treatment of both ADHD symptoms and tics. Although desipramine may be more efficacious than clonidine, it is a more dangerous medication because of cardiac toxicity, including prolongation of conduction and delay in repolarization leading to arrhythmia and often death in overdose (Werry et al., 1995). Four cases of sudden death have also occurred in children who were taking therapeutic doses of desipramine (Riddle et al., 1993). Desipramine should therefore not be the first choice of treatment for tics or ADHD, and a discussion of its cardiotoxicity should be carried out with the family before its use. Baseline and follow-up EKGs should also be done.

Nortriptyline (Pamelor, Aventyl), another tricyclic antidepressant, has also been studied regarding benefits in children with TS or ADHD with chronic tics. A retrospective chart review of 12 children treated with nortriptyline (mean dose

106 mg/day) demonstrated improvement in tics in all but two patients (Spencer et al., 1993). A few of the patients had an unsuccessful trial of desipramine, and 7 of the 12 patients were concurrently treated with clonidine (Spencer et al., 1993). Although nortriptyline is not associated with sudden death, it is a trycyclic, and significant cardiac toxicity necessitates monitoring its use with EKGs. One patient in this study was treated with buproprion (Wellbutrin) prior to the treatment trial with nortriptyline but experienced significant exacerbation of tics on bupro-prion (Spencer et al., 1993). Case reports also document improvement in TS with the use of imipramine (Tofranil), another tricyclic which is commonly used for bed-wetting in childhood; however, controlled trials have not been carried out (Dillon et al., 1985).

Perhaps the most well studied and efficacious treatment of tics is the use of neuroleptic medication, including haloperidol (Haldol) and pimozide (Orap). The use of haloperidol was first reported in 1961 in France (Seignot, 1961), but the report by Shapiro and Shapiro in 1968 regarding the use of haloperidol brought the world's attention to the fact that TS was a biological disorder which deserved further study (Shapiro and Shapiro, 1968). For years haloperidol was the treatment of choice for tics because the response rate approaches 80%. How-ever, the side effects are significant and include sedation; acute dystonic reactions, such as opisthotonic posturing; tardive dyskinesias (late onset involuntary move-ments) that may include choreic or dystonic movements that do not wax and wane like tics; Parkinsonian symptoms, such as tremor, muscular rigidity, masked face, abnormal gait, and drooling; motor restlessness or akathisia; depression, including tearfulness, sadness, and decreased energy; school and social phobias; and weight gain (Kurlan, 1997). The motor side effects are called extrapyramidal symptoms (EPS) and arise because of the dopamine D_2 receptor blockade of neuroleptics. Patients report these side effects as "zombie-like" (Sallee et al., 1997). It is because of these side effects that haloperidol is no longer the treatment of choice for tics, particularly for mild cases.

A recent study compared the efficacy of haloperidol and pimozide in equiva-lent doses (3.5 mg/day) in a double-blind placebo-controlled triple-crossover 24-week trial in 22 patients aged 7 to 16 years with TS (Sallee et al., 1997). Pimozide was shown to be significantly different from placebo in improving tics but haloperi-dol was not. In addition, 41% of patients experienced moderate to severe adverse events (e.g., depression, anxiety, or severe dyskinesias) while taking haloperidol, a rate that was three times the rate of adverse events while on pimozide (14%). Although adult studies suggest that haloperidol may be more effective than pimoz-ide for treatment of tics in TS, this is not the case for children and adolescents (Sallee et al., 1997).

Pimozide comes in a 2-mg tablet, and it is usually initiated with one-half tablet at bedtime. The dose can be gradually increased and given two to three times per day with a maximum recommended dose of 0.2 mg/kg/day (Kurlan, 1997). Side effects increase at higher doses, so it is preferable to stay under 10 mg/day. Pimozide can prolong conduction, so a baseline and follow-up EKGs are recommended to make sure the Q–T interval is not prolonged. A rare case of sudden death has been documented at high doses (60 to 70 mg/day) (Kurlan, 1997).

An interesting report studied the effects of a transdermal nicotine patch (TNP), Nicoderm, to augment neuroleptic medication in the treatment of 16 children with TS between the ages of 9 and 15 years (Silver et al., 1996). The TNP released 7 mg of nicotine in a 24-hour period. The patch was removed after 24 hours but reapplied after 2 weeks for a second 24-hour period. There was a significant improvement in both motor and vocal tics and in overall behavior in 13 of the 16 patients. Fourteen of the patients experienced nausea, although this was mild in eight patients. Six patients experienced vomiting, and four of these six had headache and sedation (Silver et al., 1996). Because of these side effects, the nicotine patch is not widely used to treat tics. Nicotine gum has also been used to treat tics, but the effects are short-term (Silver et al., 1996).

Relatively new atypical neuroleptic medications block both dopamine D_2 receptors (with greater affinity for the mesolimbic dopamine systems than the nigrostriatal dopamine systems, which are associated with the Parkinsonian problems) and serotonin $5-HT_{2A}$ receptors, leading to a lower risk for EPS side effects (Chappell et al., 1997). Risperidone (Risperdal) is a new atypical neuroleptic that has been studied for the treatment of TS in three published open label trials. The first involved 11 patients with TS aged 19 to 52 years, who were given an average dose of 3.9 mg/day (Van der Linden et al., 1994). Nine of the eleven patients showed substantial decreases in both motor and vocal tics without EPS. The second study involved seven children with TS aged 11 to 16 years who were given an average dose of 1.5 mg/day of risperidone (Lombroso et al., 1995). There was a significant reduction in tics for the group, although one patient experienced an acute dystonic reaction when the dose was increased too quickly. A third study treated 38 patients with TS aged 8 to 53 years who had severe tics that were refractory to other treatments (Bruun and Budman, 1996). The average dose of risperidone was 2.7 mg/day divided twice daily. Fifty-eight percent improved significantly on risperidone, but eight dropped out of the study because of side effects, including sedation, akathesia, and dystonic reactions. Although the risk of EPS is lower in risperidone compared to haloperidol, the lower risk is only seen in low doses of risperidone (under 8 mg/day). When higher doses of risperidone are used, the risk for EPS is just as substantial as with other neuroleptics. Risperidone may also cause significant weight gain.

Risperidone has also been used to augment the effect of SSRIs in the treatment of OCD in patients with or without TS (Chappell et al., 1997; McDougle et al., 1994). In an open trial of eight patients with OCD alone, five patients with trichotillomania, and three patients with OCD and TS, risperidone was added to an SSRI. Significant improvement of obsessive-compulsive behavior was seen in 50% of the OCD patients, in 80% of the patients with trichotillomania, and in one patient with TS (Stein et al., 1997). In the other two patients with TS, risperidone was given to replace pimozide, and no change occurred in OCD symptoms, although one patient noted an improvement in tics. Although risperidone may often improve OCB, on occasion it may worsen this behavior. Controlled trials of risperidone are needed in children and adults with TS to evaluate the improvement in tics and obsessive-compulsive behavior.

Treatment of ADHD

The treatment of ADHD symptoms in TS has been problematic because of concern that stimulants will worsen the tics, and yet for many patients the stimulants work best for severe hyperactivity or attentional problems (Freeman, 1997; Riddle et al., 1995). A recent study has helped to clarify these concerns. In a double-blind placebo-controlled crossover study comparing low, medium, and high doses of methylphenidate and dextroamphetamine in 22 boys with ADHD and TS or chronic tic disorder, only 30% demonstrated worsening of their tics on medication overall, and the low dose of stimulants did not worsen tics for the group as a whole (Castellanos et al., 1997). Higher doses of stimulants tended to worsen tics, and dextroamphetamine had a greater effect in this regard than methylphenidate. At completion of the study, 17 of the 22 patients continued on stimulants, and 65% continued on methylphenidate. One patient was removed from the study because of severe exacerbation of his tics, but he was on placebo. Some patients experienced improved tics on stimulants and exacerbation in tics when stimulants were stopped (Castellanos et al., 1997). This effect has also been observed by others (Riddle et al., 1995). What is clear is that stimulants are very effective for ADHD symptoms in patients with TS and that only a subgroup of patients experience a worsening of their tics at higher doses. Stimulants can be used cautiously in TS, and they are definitely not contraindicated. Stimulants can also be combined with other medication, such as clonidine or risperidone, as discussed here, and with SSRIs as addressed later in this chapter.

Second-line medications for the treatment of ADHD include the tricyclics, such as desipramine, which was discussed previously, buspirone (Buspar), buproprion (Wellbutrin), mentioned previously, and deprenyl. A recent open trial of buspirone, an anxiolytic agent, for the treatment of ADHD demonstrated significant improvement in hyperactivity, impulsivity, inattention, and disruptive behavior in all 12 children studied (Malhotra et al., 1998). Buspirone is a partial agonist at some serotonin receptors ($5\text{-}HT_{1A}$ & $5\text{-}HT_2$). It also has a modest effect on the dopamine system and enhances dopamine synthesis and release, and it is a partial agonist of α-adrenergic receptors (Malhotra and Santosh, 1998). The dopaminergic and adrenergic effects of buspirone are likely responsible for the improvement of ADHD symptoms, but only one case of TS has been reported with a positive response to buspirone (Dursun et al., 1995). Further studies are needed to judge the efficacy of buspirone in TS. Both an open trial (Jankovic, 1993) and a controlled trial (Feigin et al., 1996) suggest that deprenyl, a type-B monoamine oxidase (MAO-B) inhibitor, is effective for ADHD in children and adolescents with TS. However, there was a high dropout rate in the controlled study, and further research is necessary to sort out side effects, including a possible worsening of tics.

Treatment of Obsessive-Compulsive Behavior

In the 1990s the use of SSRIs has dramatically helped the OCD symptoms of patients with TS. Fluoxetine (Prozac) was the first agent to be used, and it significantly improves not only obsessive-compulsive behavior but also depression and anxiety symptoms in both children and adults (King et al., 1992). The SSRIs are far less toxic than tricyclics because they are not deadly in overdose and they do not prolong cardiac conduction. Blood levels and liver function do not need to be monitored. SSRIs interfere with the cytochrome P_{450} metabolic system, so concurrent use of anticonvulsants requires careful monitoring of the anticonvulsant blood levels to avoid toxicity. Other medications which also interfere with the P_{450} system, such as erythromycin, antifungals, and nonsedating antihistamines such as terfenidine, should also be avoided. Sertraline (Zoloft) will interfere least with the P_{450} system, so it would be the SSRI of choice when treating a patient on anticonvulsants (Preskorn, 1996). Sertraline has been shown to be efficacious and safe for use in children and adolescents for treatment of OCD and depression (Alderman et al., 1998). The side effects of SSRIs include nausea, gastric distress, diarrhea, activation or hyperactivity, somnolence, and insomnia. Fluoxetine appears to have the highest rate of activation in children, which may present as nervousness, restlessness, hyperactivity, anxiety, insomnia, or even mania in rare cases. In adults, 10 to 25% may experience this activation, but in children the rate is higher (30 to 50%) (King et al., 1992). Three of nine children with TS experienced this side effect when treated with fluoxetine, although this problem disappeared when the dose was lowered or discontinued (King et al., 1992).

A recently approved SSRI for children who suffer from OCD is fluvoxamine (Luvox). In a double-blind placebo-controlled study of 120 children and adolescents with OCD, fluvoxamine was found to be effective and well tolerated (Riddle et al., 1996). In comparison to clomipramine, a tricyclic which is also effective for OCD, fluvoxamine does not cause EKG changes, and blood levels do not need to be followed (Goodman et al., 1997). Therefore, fluvoxamine is a relatively safe choice for treatment of OCD associated with TS. There has been one case, however, of a 14-year-old with OCD who developed TS while taking fluvoxamine and whose symptoms resolved when fluvoxamine was discontinued but reappeared when fluvoxamine was reintroduced (Fennig et al., 1994).

A recent report documented the neurochemical changes in the brain of a 9-year-old boy with OCD treated with paroxetine (Paxil), an SSRI (Moore et al., 1998). Magnetic resonance spectroscopy (MRS) carried out before and during a 12-week treatment with paroxetine showed a significant (40%) drop in glutamate concentrations in the caudate compared with controls. The patient showed a dramatic decrease in OCD symptoms on paroxetine, and the authors hypothesize that the increase in serotonin levels with paroxetine has an inhibitory effect on the excess release of the excitatory neurotransmitter glutamate (Moore et al., 1998).

Paroxetine has also been used for the treatment of rage attacks that may occur in up to 30% of children and adults with TS (Bruun and Budman, 1998). In an open 8-week trial of paroxetine, 76% of 38 patients reported significant improvement in the frequency and severity of rage episodes (Bruun and Budman, 1998). The mean age was 16 years, and the dosage ranged from 15 to 60 mg/day. Nine patients were also taking risperidone, and they appeared to make the most improvement of the study group. Only one patient became hypomanic, but four experienced a worsening of rage episodes on paroxetine.

CASE HISTORY: D.J.

D.J. is a 9½-year-old gifted boy with TS. His mother had a normal full-term pregnancy, except for a drop in fetal heart tones and an emergency C-section delivery. His Apgar scores were 9 and 9, and he subsequently did well in the nursery. At home he was noted to be a colicky baby who had a dramatic startle response to stimuli. He cried frequently during the day and slept very little day or night. He was treated with phenobarbital for his colic, but this caused excessive sedation, so it was discontinued.

D.J.'s developmental milestones were normal, including walking at 14 months and riding a tricycle at 3 years of age. He was precocious in his speech, with five words by 8 months, 25 words by 1 year, and sentences by 1½ years of age. He has always had remarkable verbal abilities and an excellent memory. By 1½ years he repeated questions over and over again, and by 3 years he was constantly talking. At 5½, he was referred to a psychiatrist because of behavior problems, which included hyperactivity, frequent rage episodes, bad dreams, poor sleeping, and a tendency to be "stuck on certain ideas." He was also sad and distraught about his behavior, saying, "I will never have a friend again." A diagnosis of depression, in addition to OCD and ADHD, was made. He was treated with fluoxetine (Prozac) after a medical work-up, including an EEG that was normal. With a gradually increasing dose up to 20 mg per day, there was improvement in his behavior and his obsessions, but his impulsivity and disruptive behavior, in addition to sleeping problems, continued. Clonidine was added to improve his sleep and hyperactivity at 6 years of age. He subsequently developed motor tics, such as shoulder shrugging and eye and facial grimacing, and to vocal tics, including episodes of coprolalia. He was tried on the clonidine patch, but it was discontinued because of skin irritation.

Although clonidine helped his disruptive behavior somewhat, D.J.'s hyperactivity and short attention span continued in school. He responded well to a trial of methylphenidate (Ritalin) beginning at a dose of 5 mg three times a day. There was no worsening of his tics, and in fact there appeared to be some improvement in his tic frequency on methylphenidate. His vocal tics include frequent singing, with occasional moans and blurting out of repetitive phrases and questions. He will also rock frequently, poke people, and spit. His aggressive behavior has improved with an increase in his clonidine to three times a day.

When D.J. was 6½ years old, his family moved to Denver, and he was reevaluated through the Child Development Unit at the Children's Hospital. He is being educated at a school for the gifted, and his cognitive testing in the past demonstrated a 23-point difference between his verbal comprehension at 134 and his Performance IQ of 111. His Verbal IQ on this testing was 126. He continues to have problems with distractibility, and his Freedom from Distractibility score on the WISC-III was 98. His cognitive testing also demonstrated significant problems with visual-spatial perception, visual-sequential memory, and visual-motor coordination. On the Kaufman Test of Educational Achievement, his math score was 122, reading 160, and spelling 106 (the mean for this test is 100). He enjoys reading on a regular basis, and he uses a computer word processor with a spell checker to enhance the quality of his written assignments. He is a very intense young man who is fidgety and on the go most of the time. He has had problems with aggression, both with peers and with family members.

His tics presently include sniffing, pulling up his leg with occasional kicking, and barking. He also has throat clicking and frequent verbalizations that include slogans and comical voices. His clonidine had been discontinued prior to moving to Denver because of concern regarding clonidine's use with methylphenidate. His sleep was more problematic without clonidine, and he was given Benedryl at bedtime in an effort to improve sleep, but it was not successful. Obsessive thinking continues to be a problem for him.

In Denver, D.J. was switched from fluoxetine to fluvoxamine (Luvox), starting with 25 mg and gradually increasing to a dose of 100 mg each evening. This improved his OCD considerably. An EKG was normal, so clonidine was reinstituted at bedtime, which improved his sleep. Clonidine was also increased to three-times-a-day dosing, presently at three-fourths of a tablet in the morning, one-half tablet midday, and one tablet at bedtime. He also continues on his methylphenidate at 10 mg in the morning, at noon, and in midafternoon. His follow-up EKGs have been normal.

Now at age 9½ D.J. sleeps well, he is not depressed, and his obsessive-compulsive behavior is minimal. He continues with daily tics, including eye grimacing, and vocal tics that include spitting, singing, constant verbalizations, and moaning. Although these tics interfere with peer interactions, his psychotherapy is helping him with peer conflicts and social skills. He has been in counseling since his first encounter with a psychiatrist at age 5, and he is presently followed by a child psychologist on a weekly basis. His mother is not interested in a trial of antipsychotic medications to further improve his tics. His visual motor coordination problems are treated by an occupational therapist who works with him once per week on his dysgraphia and his sensory integration difficulties.

His tics and OCD behaviors are exacerbated by group A beta-hemolytic streptococcal infections, which were common in his early childhood and have only rarely occurred over the last few years. His family history is positive for ADHD on both sides of the family, in addition to obsessive-compulsive behavior in both parents. The maternal grandfather has an eye tic, but there is no other family history of motor or vocal tics. Depression has been a problem for his mother and other members of her family, and his mother has responded well to fluvoxamine.

Educational Intervention

Many of the manifestations of TS can interfere with school progress and learning. The tics can be exacerbated during stressful experiences, such as class changes, test taking, or increased pressure to turn in assignments. It is important for school personnel to be knowledgeable about TS, either through reading or videos that can be obtained from the Tourette Syndrome Association (TSA) (see the Resource section). If the teacher does not understand this syndrome, the child is usually blamed for the tics and labeled as a problematic child because of additional ADHD behaviors that may lead to detentions or even expulsion from school. Once the diagnosis is known and understood, and if the behavior problems are significant, the school psychologist can usually be mobilized to develop a positive behavior modification program. Such a program should be utilized by all of the teachers involved with the patient so that there is consistency throughout the day. Parent and family participation should also take place if the behaviors are also problematic at home. The school can also make general accommodations, as noted in Table 3.1 to reduce the stress that leads to an increase in tics and OCD behaviors (Packer, 1997).

ADHD behaviors associated with TS cause the greatest interference with schoolwork. There is a mood lability and abruptness in these behaviors that usually place the patient on the most problematic end of the ADHD spectrum. General principles of structure, positive reinforcement, auditory and visual input, and repetition are helpful for patients with TS. More specific examples of intervention to help with ADHD symptoms are outlined in Table 3.2 (Packer, 1997). The organizational difficulties become very important when the child begins middle school and has multiple teachers and classrooms to contend with. Often tutoring support to teach study skills and organizational strategies can be beneficial for the adolescent. The Tourette Syndrome Association has regional support groups throughout the country and provides in-service programs for teachers and therapists regarding educational and behavioral interventions for children and adolescents with TS.

A positive aspect of TS is the lack of significant cognitive deficits, although learning problems are common, as noted. Individual tutoring can improve specific academic deficits, and computer software can be used to strengthen math, spelling, reading, and concept formation (see Appendix 2 to this volume). Problems with visual-motor coordination that interfere with handwriting can be circumvented by the use of a computer word processor. The modifications of word processors described in other chapters are usually not needed here because these children have normal cognitive abilities. In fact, many patients with TS are gifted, so additional stimulation is needed. Giving the child challenging school projects

TABLE 3.1: School-based Accommodations

Factors affecting tic severity	Ways to reduce tic-related stress	Ways to reduce OCD-related stress
Time pressure (including timed tests).	Extend time limit on tests.	Allow more time for completing tasks and tests.
Programs that do not provide opportunities to discharge symptoms or dissipate extra energy.	Allow the child to leave the room to discharge tics in a private location.	Consider limiting amount of handwritten work if the child has compulsive writing rituals. Teach word processing skills. If there are significant writing rituals, consider alternative testing techniques.
Holiday anticipation, birthdays, school and family vacations.	Modify task demands, as needed, to "work around" the tics. Allow alternative ways to produce work sample.	Consider limiting amount of reading if the child has significant reading rituals; use books on tape.
School reopening in September.	Consider cutting down task demands.	Agree on how much checking and rechecking will be permitted before work must be turned in.
Specific school settings if child has severe phonic tics (library, assembly, study hall).	Provide hard copies of any notes or assignments so that the child does not have the stress of missing important notes or work if he or she leaves the room.	Attempt to gently refocus the child to the task at hand.
Fatigue	Allow a larger "buffer zone" around the child who has tics that might impose on others.	Provide hard copies of notes or assignments so that the child does not miss important material while obsessing internally.
Peer ridicule or rejection.	Provide added adult supervision if the child is being teased or taunted.	
Unstructured or less structured settings such as cafeteria, recess, gym, school bus.	Provide peer education program if student consents.	
Tasks in which tics interfere directly (e.g., handwriting if arm tics, reading if eye tics).	Provide remediation, as needed, for any learning disabilities.	

From L. E. Packer (1997), Social and educational resources for patients with Tourette syndrome, Neurologic Clinics 15: 457–73; reprinted with permission.

TABLE 3.2: Strategies for Managing ADHD-related Stressors in School

Reducing Stress Associated with Attentional Problems
Seat the child near the teacher to help focus attention, but not "front and center" if the child is embarrassed by tics. Some children prefer to sit near the door so that they can leave unobtrusively to discharge tics.
Use concrete, short, simple instructions and review them with the student.
Break large tasks into smaller "chunks" and conference with the student between chunks.
Allow extra time to complete class work.
Provide a written or hard copy of all assignments. Negotiate intermediate deadlines with the child for larger assignments.
Teach the child how to use a day planner or electronic organizer.
Use hands-on multisensory approaches to teaching.
Avoid cluttered desks and cluttered worksheets: use blocking, folding, or cutting worksheets so that the student does not feel overwhelmed when he/she tries to start the task.
Allow the child extra time at the end of the day to pack up materials and papers. Allow older students to leave class a few minutes early to get to their next class.
Provide an extra set of books to keep at home. Have the younger student bring in an extra supply of pens and pencils that the teacher will hold for them when they cannot find one.

Managing Hyperactivity or Impulsivity
Allow the student flexibility in terms of how and where he or she completes work. Let the student change seats occasionally or even complete some work standing up.
Allow the child to leave the room occasionally to discharge extra energy; use a discrete signal.
Allow extra time for tasks and tests.
Give the younger child something to keep his or her hands acceptably occupied. Some children find soft "koosh" balls helpful.
Supervise the child closely during transitions; consider added adult supervision on the playground or school bus for younger children.
Provide immediate feedback about behavior. Use reprimands sparingly but be lavish with praise.
Ignore minor impulsive infractions.
Develop a behavior management system in collaboration with parents, teachers, and outside treating professionals.

Organizational Deficits
Color coordinate (code) textbooks and materials (e.g., cover all math books and notebooks in blue, all science books and notebooks in yellow, etc.)
Help the student develop an effective day planner, electronic organizer, or notebook with organized sections. Teach time management skills, including "chunking." Use intermediate deadlines for bigger projects.
Establish a daily routine in school (and home) and stick to it with respect to when homework gets done and turned in, when assignments get recorded, and so forth.
Arrange for an extra set of books to be left at home.
Praise progress rather than reprimand disorganization. Consider a behavioral contract for work completed or turned in on time.
Teach word processing skills.

From L. E. Packer (1997), Social and educational resources for patients with Tourette syndrome. Neurologic Clinics 15: 457–73; reprinted with permission.

related to their interest areas can often improve attention, focus, and motivation. Additional remediation suggestions can be found in Hagin and Kugler (1988) and Packer (1997).

Behavior Therapy and Psychotherapy

Emotional problems in TS can be related to the neurochemical features of the disorder which predispose the child to anxiety, phobias, obsessive-compulsive thinking, mood lability, depression, and ADHD. They can also be related to the secondary effects of TS, including peer rejection, negative reinforcement from parents and teachers, isolation, poor self-image, and feelings of inadequacy in controlling tics and thoughts. A detailed emotional assessment should be carried out in the child with TS who appears to be experiencing these difficulties. Often psychotherapeutic intervention in the form of counseling with a mental health provider is necessary. This intervention is usually on a weekly basis and may involve both individual work and family work.

Several studies have reported on the efficacy of cognitive-behavioral treatment of pediatric OCD (Franklin et al., 1998; March, 1995; March et al., 1994). Usually such therapy involves education of the patient and family; anxiety management training, including relaxation, constructive self-talk, breathing techniques, and positive coping strategies; and the gradual increase of exposure to feared situations or objects through exercises until distress decreases noticeably, combined with prevention of rituals that helped the patient avoid exposure to the object of fear. A recent study suggests that exposure and prevention of rituals is more efficacious than anxiety management training and that the results of this therapy alone are commensurate with the effects of therapy combined with SSRI medication (Franklin et al., 1998). Wolff (1988) has described further examples of psychotherapeutic intervention in TS. The combined use of behavioral and pharmacological approaches for a variety of tic and habit disorders, such as trichotillomania (compulsive pulling out of hair) or self-injurious behavior, is described in detail in Peterson et al. (1994).

Counseling through the school usually focuses on behavior in school and is often not adequate for more significant emotional problems that require family work in treatment. A social-skills group, however, can be helpful in school to teach the child appropriate social interactional skills (Begum, 1996; Bloomquist, 1996).

Specific behavior interventions have also been developed over the years to target improvement in tics. Some examples are outlined below; these are described in more detail in Azrin and Peterson (1988):

> *Massed negative practice:* The patient must deliberately perform the tic over and over again for a specified period of time (e.g., 30 minutes). Such work is supposed to make the patient "tired" of carrying out the tic and therefore subsequently decrease its frequency. Approximately half of the studies involving this technique have shown limited efficacy in decreasing a particular tic frequency (Azrin and Peterson, 1988).

Contingency management: The patient receives positive reinforcement for not carrying out a tic or for performing an alternative behavior. This intervention has not been studied well in isolation because additional interventions are usually given, so its efficacy alone is unclear (Azrin and Peterson, 1988). Negative reinforcement has also been given when tics occur, but this is not recommended because of the negative emotional consequences, such as poor self-image.

Relaxation training: Several techniques have been used to induce relaxation, such as visual imagery, deep breathing, muscular tensing and relaxing, and verbalizations to facilitate relaxation (Azrin and Peterson, 1988). Tics tend to decrease when the patient is relaxed, although not always. Relaxation techniques can be combined with self-monitoring, that is, having the patient write down the number of tics he or she has and when they occur. This procedure improves the patient's awareness of his or her tics and may often lead to a decrease in tic frequency (Azrin and Peterson, 1988).

Habit reversal: The patient carries out a competing response whenever he or she anticipates a tic. The opposing muscles to the tic are contracted for approximately 2 minutes or as long as the urge continues. Case studies have shown efficacy, but controlled studies have not been carried out (Azrin and Peterson, 1988).

Adolescence and Adulthood

As mentioned in the section on life course, two-thirds of patients will experience significant improvements or disappearance of their tics in adolescence (Bruun and Budman, 1997). In a follow-up questionnaire survey of 99 patients with TS in late adolescence or adulthood, 73% indicated that their tics had decreased markedly or disappeared (Erenberg et al., 1987). The majority of these patients felt that they were coping well with the associated learning or behavioral problems. Although obsessive-compulsive behavior may continue to be a problem in adulthood, many adults utilize these behaviors to excel in their field of interest, such as sports, science, literature, and so forth. The intensity of their interests combined with compulsive activity, such as compulsive exercising in an athlete, can be beneficial for a career.

Usually ADHD symptoms are improved in adolescence or adulthood, but the risk for bipolar disorder emerging at that time in individuals with TS is increased 4.6 to 5.5 times over that of the general population of adults and adolescents, respectively (Kerbeshian et al., 1995). Of 205 patients in North Dakota with TS who were followed, 15 (7%) were diagnosed with bipolar disorder. Seven of these patients were 18 or older, but six of the seven had an IQ of 70 or lower (Kerbeshian et al., 1995). Therefore, the co-occurrence of cognitive deficits, PDD, or autistic disorder appears to predispose a person with TS to bipolar disorder, likely because of the enhanced degree of brain dysfunction or brain damage. If bipolar disorder or severe mood instability occurs, treatment with a mood stabilizer, such as carbamazepine, valproic acid, lithium, or risperidone can be helpful, as previously discussed. Kerbeshian and Burd (1988) have found that TS patients with bipolar disorder who also have grandiose delusions usually do well with lithium in treatment. Psychotherapy, as previously discussed, may also facilitate coping for the adolescent or adult with TS.

Unusual Treatments and Future Directions

In very severe cases of TS that have been unresponsive to medical interventions, neurosurgery has been an option. Case reports are reviewed by Rauch et al. (1995). Surgery has involved the thalamus, cerebellum, and multisite lesions that affect the cortico-striato-thalmo-cortical (CSTC) circuits. Although some of the cases have improved significantly with surgery, it should be considered a last resort to be used only in patients who are severely disabled.

Another unusual intervention is the use of botulinum toxin (BoTox), which inhibits acetylcholine release at the neuromuscular junction and decreases muscle activity. An IM injection of BoTox in the muscles involved has been used to treat painful dystonic tics and decrease premonitory urges or sensations (Jankovic, 1994). In one case, injection of BoTox into one vocal cord successfully treated intractable coprolalia in a patient with TS (Scott et al., 1996).

The future will bring more innovations in medical approaches to TS as our understanding of the complex neurobiological processes which cause TS improves. Manipulations of hormonal systems and excitatory amino acid systems (glutamate) may lead to significant treatment modalities (Chappell et al., 1997).

The immunological aspects of TS in response to streptococcus infections are intriguing, and as studies expand in this area, immunological interventions, such as plasmapheresis, may be more widely used. Controlled trials are being carried out now regarding penicillin prophylaxis to decrease streptococcal infections in patients with TS. The genetic studies may link to immunological subtypes that are predisposed to antibody production in the cerebrospinal fluid (CSF). Eventually, identification of gene mutations which cause TS may lead to gene therapies or transgenes that can act on neural circuits more specifically than traditional drugs.

ACKNOWLEDGMENTS   I thank William McMahon, Edward Goldson, Teresa Binstock, Judy Selle, Michael Selle, and Mary Wolf for their thoughtful review and helpful comments. This work was partially supported by MCH training grant no. MCJ-089413. I also thank the Developmental Psychobiology Research group for helpful discussions.

REFERENCES

Abwender, D. A., Como, P. G., Kurlan, R., Parry, K., Fett, K. A., Cui, L., Plumb, S., Deeley, C. (1996) School problems in Tourette's syndrome. Archives of Neurology 53 (6): 509–11.

Alderman, J., Wolkow, R., Chung, M.,

Johnston, H. F. (1998) Sertraline treatment of children and adolescents with obsessive-compulsive disorder or depression: Pharmacokinetics, tolerability, and efficacy. Journal of the American Academy of Child and Adolescent Psychiatry 37 (4): 386–94.

Allen, A. J., Leonard, H. L., Swedo, S. E. (1995) Case study: A new infection-triggered, autoimmune subtype of pediatric OCD and Tourette's syndrome. Journal of the American Academy of Child and Adolescent Psychiatry 34 (3): 307–11.

American Psychiatric Association (1994) Diagnostic and statistical manual of mental disorders. 4th ed. (DSM-IV). American Psychiatric Association, Washington, D.C.

American Psychiatric Association (1987) Diagnostic and statistical manual of mental disorders. 3rd ed. (DSM-III-R). American Psychiatric Association, Washington, D.C.

American Psychiatric Association (1980) Diagnostic and statistical manual of mental disorders. 2nd ed. (DSM-III). American Psychiatric Association, Washington, D.C.

Azrin, N. H., and Peterson, A. L. (1988) Behavior therapy for Tourette's syndrome and tic disorders. In: Tourette's syndrome and tic disorders: Clinical understanding and treatment. Cohen, D. J., Bruun, R. D., Leckman, J. F. (eds.). Wiley, New York, pp. 237–56.

Baumgardner, T. L., Reiss, A. L., Freund, L. S., Abrams, M. T. (1995) Specification of the neurobehavioral phenotype in males with fragile X syndrome. Pediatrics 95 (5): 744–52.

Baumgardner, T. L., Singer, H. S., Denckla, M. B., Rubin, M. A., Abrams, M. T., Colli, M. J., Reiss, A. L. (1996) Corpus callosum morphology in children with Tourette syndrome and attention deficit hyperactivity disorder. Neurology 47 (2): 477–82.

Baxter, L. R. (1992) Neuroimaging studies of obsessive-compulsive disorders. Psychiatry Clinics of North America 15: 871–84.

Begum, R. W. (1996) Social skills lessons and activities. Center for Applied Research in Education, West Nyack, New York.

Berecz, J. M. (1992) Understanding Tourette syndrome, obsessive compulsive disorder, and related problems. Springer, New York.

Berthier, M. L., Bayes, A., Tolosa, E. S. (1993) Magnetic resonance imaging in patients with concurrent Tourette's disorder and Asperger's syndrome. Journal of the American Academy of Child and Adolescent Psychiatry 32 (3): 633–9.

Blackman, J. A., Samson-Fang, L., Gutgesell, H. (1996) Clonidine and electrocardiograms. Pediatrics 98: 1223–4.

Bloomquist, M. L. (1996) Skills training for children with behavior disorders: A parent and therapist guide book. Guilford, New York.

Boswell, J. (1791/1949) The Life of Samuel Johnson. Dent, London. (Original work published 1791)

Bruun, R. D., and Budman, C. L. (1996) Risperidone as a treatment for Tourette's syndrome. Journal of Clinical Psychiatry 57 (1): 29–31.

Bruun, R. D., and Budman, C. L. (1997) The course and prognosis of Tourette syndrome. Neurologic Clinics 15 (2): 291–8.

Bruun, R. D., and Budman, C. L. (1998) Paroxetine treatment of episodic rages associated with Tourette Disorder. Journal of Clinical Psychiatry 59 (11): 581–4.

Burd, L., Fisher, W. W., Kerbeshian, J., Arnold, M. E. (1987) Is development of Tourette disorder a marker for improvement in patients with autism and other pervasive developmental disorders? Journal of the American Academy of Child and Adolescent Psychiatry 26 (2): 162–5.

Cantwell, D. P., Swanson, J., Connor, D. F. (1997) Case study: Adverse response to clonidine. Journal of American and Academic Child and Adolescence Psychiatry 36: 539–44.

Castellanos, F. X., Giedd, J. N., Elia, J., Marsh, W. L., Ritchie, G. F., Hamburger, S. D., Rapoport, J. L. (1997) Controlled stimulant treatment of ADHD and comorbid Tourette's syndrome: Effects of stimulant and dose. Journal of the American Academy of Child and Adolescent Psychiatry 36 (5): 589–96.

Chappell, P. B., Riddle, M. A., Scahill, L., Lynch, K. A., Schultz, R., Arnsten, A., Leckman, J. F., Cohen, D. J. (1995) Guanfacine treatment of comorbid attention-deficit hyperactivity disorder and Tourette's syndrome: Preliminary clinical experience. Journal of the American Academy of Child and Adolescent Psychiatry 34 (9): 1140–6.

Chappell, P. B., Scahill, L. D., Leckman, J. F. (1997) Future therapies of Tourette syndrome. Neurologic Clinics 15 (2): 429–50.

Coffey, B. J., and Park, K. S. (1997) Behavioral and emotional aspects of Tourette syndrome. Neurologic Clinics 15 (2): 277–89.

Coffey, B. J., Frazier, J., Chen, S. (1992) Comorbidity, Tourette syndrome, and anxiety disorders [Review]. Advances in Neurology 58: 95–104.

Comings, D. E. (1995a) The role of genetic factors in conduct disorder based on studies of Tourette syndrome and attention-deficit hyperactivity disorder probands and their relatives. Journal of Developmental and Behavioral Pediatrics 16 (3): 142–57.

Comings, D. E. (1995b) Role of genetic factors in depression based on studies of Tourette syndrome and ADHD probands and their relatives. American

Journal of Medical Genetics 60 (2): 111–21.

Comings, D. E. (1995c) Tourette's syndrome: A behavioral spectrum disorder. Advances in Neurology 65: 293–303.

Comings, B. G., and Comings, D. E. (1987a) A controlled study of Tourette syndrome: V. Depression and mania. American Journal of Human Genetics 41: 804–21.

Comings, D. E., and Comings, B. G. (1987b) A controlled study of Tourette syndrome: I. American Journal of Human Genetics 41: 701–4.

Comings, D. E., Himes, J. A., Comings, B. G. (1990) An epidemiologic study of Tourette's syndrome in a single school district. Journal of Clinical Psychiatry 51 (11): 463–9.

Dillon, D. C., Salzman, I. J., Schulsinger, D. A. (1985) The use of imipramine in Tourette's syndrome and attention deficit disorder: Case report. Journal of Clinical Psychiatry 46: 348–9.

Dursun, S. M., Burke, J. G., Reveley, M. A. (1995) Buspirone treatment of Tourette's syndrome [Letter to the editor]. Lancet 345 (8961): 1366–7.

Eidelberg, D., Moeller, J. R., Antonini, A., Kazumata, K., Dhawan, V., Budman, C., Feigin, A. (1997) The metabolic anatomy of Tourette's syndrome. Neurology 48 (4): 927–34.

Erenberg, G., Cruse, R. P., Rothner, A. D. (1987) The natural history of Tourette syndrome: A follow-up study. Annals of Neurology 22 (3): 383–5.

Ernst, M., Zametkin, A. J., Jons, P. H., Matochik, J. A., Pascualvaca, D., Cohen, R. M. (1999) High presynaptic dopaminergic activity in children with Tourette's Disorder. Journal of the American Academy of Child and Adolescent Psychiatry 38 (1): 86–94.

Feigin, A., Kurlan, R., McDermott, M. P., Beach, J., Dimitsopulos, T., Brower, C. A., Chapieski, L., Trinidad, K., Como, P., Jankovic, J. (1996) A controlled trial of deprenyl in children with Tourette's syndrome and attention deficit hyperactivity disorder. Neurology 46 (4): 965–8.

Fennig, S., Fennig, S. N., Pato, M., Weitzman, A. (1994) Emergence of symptoms of Tourette's syndrome during fluvoxamine treatment of obsessive-compulsive disorder. British Journal of Psychiatry 164: 839–41.

Franklin, M. E., Kozak, M. J., Cashman, L. A., Coles, M. E., Rheingold, A. A., Foa, E. B. (1998) Cognitive-behavioral treatment of pediatric obsessive-compulsive disorder: An open clinical trial. Journal of the American Academy of Child and Adolescent Psychiatry 37 (4): 412–9.

Fras, I. (1996) Guanfacine for Tourette's disorder [Letter to the editor]. Journal of the American Academy of Child and Adolescent Psychiatry 35 (1): 3–4.

Freeman, R. D. (1997) Attention deficit hyperactivity disorder in the presence of Tourette syndrome. Neurologic Clinics 15 (2): 411–20.

Giedd, J. N., Rapoport, J. L., Leonard, H. L., Richter, D., Swedo, S. E. (1996) Case study: Acute basal ganglia enlargement and obsessive-compulsive symptoms in an adolescent boy. Journal of the American Academy of Child and Adolescent Psychiatry 35 (7): 913–5.

Gilles de la Tourette, G. (1885) Etude sur une affection nerveuse caractérisée par de l'incoordination motrice, accompagnée d'echolalie et de coprolalie (jumping, latah, myriachit). Archives de Neurologie (Paris) 9: 158–200.

Goodman, W. K., Ward, H., Kablinger, A., Murphy, T. (1997) Fluvoxamine in the treatment of obsessive-compulsive disorder and related conditions. Journal of Clinical Psychiatry 58 (Suppl 5): 32–49.

Grice, D. E., Leckman, J. F., Pauls, D. L., Kurlan, R., Kidd, K. K., Pakstis, A. J., Chang, F. M., Buxbaum, J. D., Cohen, D. J., Gelernter, J. (1996) Linkage disequilibrium between an allele at the dopamine D4 receptor locus and Tourette syndrome, by the transmission-disequilibrium test. American Journal of Human Genetics 59 (3): 644–52.

Hagerman, R. J. (1996) Physical and behavioral phenotype. In: Fragile X syndrome: Diagnosis, treatment and research. Hagerman, R. J., and Cronister, A. (eds.) 2nd ed. Johns Hopkins Universtiy Press, Baltimore, pp. 3–87.

Hagerman, R. J., Bregman, J. D., Tirosh, E. (1998) Clonidine. In: Psychotropic medication and developmental disabilities: The international consensus handbook. Reiss, S., and Aman, M. G. (eds.). Ohio State University Nisonger Center, Columbus, Ohio, pp. 259–69.

Hagin, R. A., and Kugler, J. (1988) School problems associated with Tourette's syndrome. In: Tourette's syndrome and tic disorders: Clinical understanding and treatment. Cohen, D. J., Bruun, R. D., Leckman, J. F. (eds.). Wiley, New York, pp. 223–36.

Hallett, J. J., and Kiessling, L. S. (1997) Neuroimmunology of tics and other childhood hyperkinesias. Neurologic Clinics 15 (2): 333–44.

Howard, B. J. (1996) Advising parents on discipline: What works. Pediatrics 98 (4, Pt. 2): 809–15.

Jankovic, J. (1993) Deprenyl in attention deficit associated with Tourette's syndrome. Archives of Neurology 50 (3): 286–8.

Jankovic, J. (1994) Botulinum toxin in the treatment of dystonic tics. Movement Disorders 9: 347–9.

Jankovic, J. (1997) Tourette syndrome. Phenomenology and classification of tics. Neurologic Clinics 15 (2): 267–75.

Kane, M. J. (1994) Premonitory urges as "attentional tics" in Tourette's syndrome. Journal of the American Academy of Child and Adolescent Psychiatry 33 (6): 805–8.

Karp, B. I., and Hallett, M. (1996) Extracorporeal 'phantom' tics in Tourette's syndrome. Neurology 46 (1): 38–40.

Kerbeshian, J., and Burd, L. (1988) Differential responsiveness to lithium in patients with Tourette disorder. Neuroscience and Biobehavioral Reviews 12 (3–4): 247–50.

Kerbeshian, J., and Burd, L. (1989) Tourette disorder and bipolar symptomatology in childhood and adolescence. Canadian Journal of Psychiatry—Revue Canadienne de Psychiatrie 34 (3): 230–3.

Kerbeshian, J., Burd, L., Klug, M. G. (1995) Comorbid Tourette's disorder and bipolar disorder: An etiologic perspective. American Journal of Psychiatry 152 (11): 1646–51.

Kiessling, L. S., Marcotte, A. C., Culpepper, L. (1994) Antineuronal antibodies: Tics and obsessive-compulsive symptoms. Journal of Developmental and Behavioral Pediatrics 15 (6): 421–5.

King, R. A., Riddle, M. A., Goodman, W. K. (1992) Psychopharmacology of obsessive-compulsive disorder in Tourette syndrome. Advances in Neurology 58: 283–91.

Kurlan, R. (1997) Treatment of tics. Neurologic Clinics of North America 15 (2): 403–9.

Kurlan, R., Whitmore, D., Irvine, C., et al. (1994) Tourette's syndrome in a special education population: A pilot study involving a single school district. Neurology 44: 699.

Lajonchere, C., Nortz, M., Finger, S. (1996) Gilles de la Tourette and the discovery of Tourette syndrome. Archives of Neurology 53 (6): 567–74.

Leckman, J. F., Walkup, J. T., Cohen, D. J. (1988) Clonidine treatment of Tourette's syndrome. In: Tourette's syndrome and tic disorders: Clinical understanding and treatment. Cohen, D.

J., Bruun, R. D., Leckman, J. F. (eds.). Wiley, New York, pp. 292–301.

Leckman, J. F., Hardin, M. T., Riddle, M. A., Stevenson, J., Ort, S. I., Cohen, D. J. (1991) Clonidine treatment of Gilles de la Tourette syndrome. Archives of General Psychiatry 48: 324–8.

Leckman, J. F., Walker, D. E., Cohen, D. J. (1993) Premonitory urges in Tourette's syndrome. American Journal of Psychiatry 150: 98–102.

Leckman, J. F., Walker, D. E., Goodman, W. K., Pauls, D. L., Cohen, D. J. (1994) "Just right" perceptions associated with compulsive behaviors in Tourette's syndrome. American Journal of Psychiatry 151 (5): 675–80.

Leckman, J. F., Peterson, B. S., Anderson, G. M., Arnsten, A. F., Pauls, D. L., Cohen, D. J. (1997) Pathogenesis of Tourette's syndrome. Journal of Child Psychology and Psychiatry and Allied Disciplines 38 (1): 119–42.

Leonard, H. L., Topol, D., Bukstein, O., Hindmarsh, D., Allen, A. J., Swedo, S. E. (1994) Clonazepam as an augmenting agent in the treatment of childhood-onset obsessive-compulsive disorder. Journal of the American Academy of Child and Adolescent Psychiatry 33 (6): 792–4.

Lichter, D. G., and Jackson, L. A. (1996) Predictors of clonidine response in Tourette syndrome: Implications and inferences. Journal of Child Neurology 11 (2): 93–7.

Lombroso, P. J., Scahill, L., King, R. A., Lynch, K. A., Chappell, P. B., Peterson, B. S., McDougle, C. J., Leckman, J. F. (1995) Risperidone treatment of children and adolescents with chronic tic disorders: A preliminary report. Journal of the American Academy of Child and Adolescent Psychiatry 34 (9): 1147–52.

Malhotra, S., and Santosh, P. J. (1998) An open clinical trial of buspirone in children with attention deficit/hyperactivity disorder. Journal of the American Academy of Child and Adolescent Psychiatry 37 (4): 364–71.

March, J. S. (1995) Cognitive-behavioral psychotherapy for children and adolescents with OCD: A review and recommendations for treatment. Journal of the American Academy of Child and Adolescent Psychiatry 34: 7–18.

March, J. S., Mulle, K., Herbel, B. (1994) Behavioral psychotherapy for children and adolescents with obsessive-compulsive disorder: An open trial of a new protocol-driven treatment package. Journal of the American Academy of Child and Adolescent Psychiatry 33 (3): 333–41.

Mason, A., Banerjee, S., Espen, V., Zeitlin, H., Robertson, M. M. (1998) The prevalence of Tourette syndrome in a mainstream school population. Developmental Medicine and Child Neurology, 40: 292–6.

Massie, R. K. (1980) Peter the Great: His life and world. Ballantine Books, New York.

McDougle, C. J., Goodman, W. K., Price, L. H. (1994) Dopamine antagonists in tic-related and psychotic spectrum obsessive compulsive disorder. Journal of Clinical Psychiatry 55 (Suppl): 24–31.

McMahon, W. M., van de Wetering, B. J., Filloux, F., Betit, K., Coon, H., Leppert, M. (1996) Bilineal transmission and phenotypic variation of Tourette's disorder in a large pedigree. Journal of the American Academy of Child and Adolescent Psychiatry 35 (5): 672–80.

Moore, G. J., MacMaster, F. P., Stewart, C., Rosenberg, D. R. (1998) Case study: Caudate glutamatergic changes with paroxetine therapy for pediatric obsessive-compulsive disorder. Journal of the American Academy of Child and Adolescent Psychiatry 37 (6): 663–7.

Murray, T. J. (1979) Dr. Samuel Johnson's movement disorder. British Medical Journal 1: 1610–4.

Nomoto, F., and Machiyama, Y. (1990) An epidemiological study of tics. Japanese Journal of Psychiatry and Neurology 44 (4): 649–55.

Norman, C. (1951) Mr. oddity, Samuel Johnson, LL.D. Bell, Drexel Hill, Pa.

Ozonoff, S., Strayer, D. L., McMahon, W. M., Filloux, F. (1994) Executive function abilities in autism and Tourette syndrome: An information processing approach. Journal of Psychology and Psychiatry 35 (6): 1015–32.

Packer, L. E. (1997) Social and educational resources for patients with Tourette syndrome. Neurologic Clinics 15 (2): 457–73.

Pauls, D. L., Leckman, J. F., Cohen, D. J. (1993) Familial relationship between Gilles de la Tourette's syndrome, attention deficit disorder, learning disabilities, speech disorders, and stuttering [see comments]. Journal of the American Academy of Child and Adolescent Psychiatry 32 (5): 1044–50.

Peterson, A. L., Campise, R. L., Azrin, N. H. (1994) Behavioral and pharmacological treatments for tic and habit disorders: A review. Journal of Developmental and Behavioral Pediatrics 15 (6): 430–41.

Popper, C. W. (1995) Combining methylphenidate and clonidine: Pharmacological questions and new reports about sudden death. Journal of Child and Adolescent Psychopharmacology 5: 157–66.

Preskorn, S. H. (1996) Clinical pharmacology of selective serotonin reuptake inhibitors. Professional Communications, Caddo, Okla.

Rauch, S. L., Baer, L., Cosgrove, G. R., Jenike, M. A. (1995) Neurosurgical treatment of Tourette's syndrome: A critical review. Comprehensive Psychiatry 36 (2): 141–56.

Riddle, M., Geller, B., Ryan, N. (1993) Case study: Another sudden death in a child treated with desipramine. Journal of the American Academy of Child and Adolescent Psychiatry 32: 792–7.

Riddle, M. A., Lynch, K. A., Scahill, L., deVries, A., Cohen, D. J., Lechman, J. F. (1995) Methylphenidate discontinuation and reinitiation during long-term treatment of children with Tourette's disorder and attention deficit hyperactivity disorder: A pilot study. Journal of Child and Adolescent Psychopharmacology 5: 205–14.

Riddle, M. A., Claghorn, J., Gaffney, G. (1996) A controlled trial of fluvoxamine for OCD in children and adolescents. Biological Psychiatry 39 (7): 568.

Rosenberg, D. R., Keshavan, M. S., O'Hearn, K. M., Dick, E. L., Bagwell, W. W., Seymour, A. B., Montrose, D. M., Pierri, J. N., Birmaher, B. (1997) Frontostriatal measurement in treatment-naive children with obsessive-compulsive disorder. Archives of General Psychiatry 54: 824–30.

Sallee, F. R., Nesbitt, L., Jackson, C., Sine, L., Sethuraman, G. (1997) Relative efficacy of haloperidol and pimozide in children and adolescents with Tourette's disorder. American Journal of Psychiatry 154 (9): 1057–62.

Santangelo, S. L., Pauls, D. L., Lavori, P. W., Goldstein, J. M., Faraone, S. V., Tsuang, M. T. (1996) Assessing risk for the Tourette spectrum of disorders among first-degree relatives of probands with Tourette syndrome. American Journal of Medical Genetics 67 (1): 107–16.

Scahill, L. D., Lechman, J. F., Marek, K. L. (1995) Sensory phenomena in Tourette's syndrome. In: Behavioral neurology of movement disorders. Weiner, W. J., and Lang, A. E. (eds.). Raven Press, New York, pp. 273–80.

Scott, B. L., Jankovic, J., Donovan, D. T. (1996) Botulinum toxin injection into vocal cord in the treatment of malignant coprolalia associated with Tourette's syndrome. Movement Disorders 11 (4): 431–3.

Seignot, M. J. N. (1961) Un cas de maladie des tics de Gilles de la Tourette gueri par le R-1625. Annales Medico-Psychologiques (Paris) 119: 578–9.

Shapiro, A. K., and Shapiro, E. S. (1968) Treatment of Gilles de la Tourette syndrome with haloperidol. British Journal of Psychiatry 114: 345.

Silver, A. A., Shytle, R. D., Philipp, M. K., Sanberg, P. R. (1996) Case study: Long-term potentiation of neuroleptics with transdermal nicotine in Tourette's syndrome. Journal of the American Academy of Child and Adolescent Psychiatry 35 (12): 1631–6.

Singer, H. S., Reiss, A. L., Brown, J. E., Aylward, E. H., Shih, B., Chee, E., Harris, E. L., Reader, M. J., Chase, G. A., Bryan, R. N., et al. (1993) Volumetric MRI changes in basal ganglia of children with Tourette's syndrome. Neurology 43 (5): 950–6.

Singer, H. S., Brown, J., Quaskey, S., Rosenberg, L. A., Mellits, E. D., Denckla, M. B. (1995a) The treatment of attention-deficit hyperactivity disorder in Tourette's syndrome: A double-blind placebo-controlled study with clonidine and desipramine. Pediatrics 95 (1): 74–81.

Singer, H. S., Schuerholz, L. J., Denckla, M. B. (1995b) Learning difficulties in children with Tourette syndrome. Journal of Child Neurology 10 (Suppl. 1): S58–61.

Spencer, T., Biederman, J., Wilens, T., Steingard, R., Geist, D. (1993) Nortriptyline treatment of children with attention-deficit hyperactivity disorder and tic disorder or Tourette's syndrome. Journal of the American Academy of Child and Adolescent Psychiatry 32 (1): 205–10.

Stein, D. J., Bouwer, C., Hawkridge, S., Emsley, R. A. (1997) Risperidone augmentation of serotonin reuptake inhibitors in obsessive-compulsive and related disorders. Journal of Clinical Psychiatry 58 (3): 119–22.

Steingard, R. J., Goldberg, M., Lee, D., DeMaso, D. R. (1994) Adjunctive clonazepam treatment of tic symptoms in children with comorbid tic disorders and ADHD. Journal of the American Academy of Child and Adolescent Psychiatry 33 (3): 394–9.

Stell, R., Thickbroom, G. W., Mastaglia, F. L. (1995) The audiogenic startle response in Tourette's syndrome. Movement Disorders 10 (6): 723–30.

Stern, J. S., and Robertson, M. M. (1997) Tics associated with autistic and pervasive developmental disorders. Neurologic Clinics 15 (2): 345–55.

Stokes, A., Bawden, H. N., Camfield, P. R., Backman, J. E., Dooley, J. M. (1991) Peer problems in Tourette's disorder. Pediatrics 87 (6): 936–42.

Swanson, J. M., Flockhart, D., Udrea, D., Cantwell, D., Connor, D., Williams, L. (1995) Clonidine and the treatment of ADHD: Questions about safety and efficacy. Journal of Child and Adolescent Psychopharmacology 5: 301–4.

Swedo, S. E., Leonard, H. L., Schapiro, M. B., Casey, B. J., Mannheim, G. B., Lenane, M. C., Rettew, D. C. (1993) Sydenham's chorea: Physical and psychological symptoms of St Vitus dance. Pediatrics 91 (4): 706–13.

Swedo, S. E., Leonard, H. L., Kiessling, L. S. (1994) Speculations on antineuronal antibody-mediated neuropsychiatric disorders of childhood. Pediatrics 93 (2): 323–6.

Swedo, S. E., Leonard, H. L., Mittleman, B. B., Allen, A. J., Rapoport, J. L., Dow, S. P., Kanter, M. E., Chapman, F., Zabriskie, J. (1997) Identification of children with pediatric autoimmune neuropsychiatric disorders associated with streptococcal infections by a marker associated with rheumatic fever. American Journal of Psychiatry 154 (1): 110–2.

Swerdlow, N. R., Magulac, M., Filion, D., Zinner, S. (1996) Visuospatial priming and latent inhibition in children and adults with Tourette's disorder. Neuropsychology, 10(4): 485–94.

Tanner, C. M., and Goldman, S. M. (1997) Epidemiology of Tourette syndrome. Neurologic Clinics 15 (2): 395–402.

Van der Linden, C., Bruggeman, R., Van Woerkom, T. (1994) Serotonin-dopamine antagonist and Gilles de la Tourette's syndrome: An open pilot dose-titration study with risperidone. Movement Disorders 9: 687–8.

Wagner, H. R., Reches, A., Fahn, S. (1985) Clonazepam-induced up-regulation of serotonin-1 binding sites in frontal cortex of rats. Neuropharmacology 24: 953–6.

Walkup, J. T., LaBuda, M. C., Singer, H. S., Brown, J., Riddle, M. A., Hurko, O. (1996) Family study and segregation analysis of Tourette syndrome: Evidence for a mixed model of inheritance. American Journal of Human Genetics 59 (3): 684–93.

Werry, J. S., Biederman, J., Thisted, R., Greenhill, L., Ryan, N. (1995) Resolved: Cardiac arrhythmias make desipramine an unacceptable choice in children. Journal of the American Academy of Child and Adolescent Psychiatry 34 (9): 1239–45.

Wolf, S. S., Jones, D. W., Knable, M. B., Gorey, J. G., Lee, K. S., Hyde, T. M., Coppola, R., Weinberger, D. R. (1996) Tourette syndrome: Prediction of phenotypic variation in monozygotic twins by caudate nucleus D2 receptor binding. Science 273 (5279): 1225–7.

Wolff, E. C. (1988) Psychotherapeutic interventions with Tourette's syndrome. In: Tourette's syndrome and tic disorders: Clinical understanding and treatment. Cohen, D. J., Bruun, R. D.,

Leckman, J. F. (eds.). Wiley, New York, pp. 207–22.

Ziemann, U., Paulus, W., Rothenberger, A. (1997) Decreased motor inhibition in Tourette's disorder: Evidence from transcranial magnetic stimulation. American Journal of Psychiatry 154 (9): 1277–84.

RESOURCES

National Organizations

Tourette Syndrome Association, Inc.
42–40 Bell Boulevard
Bayside, NY 11361-2820
telephone: (718) 224-2999;
(888) 4TOURET (toll free)
fax: (718) 279-9596
e-mail: tourette@ix.netcom.com

Contact the Tourette Syndrome Association, Inc., for a local Tourette Syndrome Association near you.

Example of a Local Organization

Tourette Syndrome Association
Rocky Mountain Region
1045 Lincoln
Suite 102
Denver, CO 80230
telephone: (303) 832-4166

Children who have Attention Deficit Disorder (Ch.ADD)
499 NW 70th Avenue, Suite 101
Plantation, FL 33317
telephone: (305) 587-3700;
(800) 233-4050
fax: (954) 587-4599

OC Foundation, Inc.
P.O. Box 70
Milford, CT 06460-0070
telephone: (203) 878-5669; Info line: (203) 874-3843
fax: (203) 874-2826

Newsletter

Medical Letter: A yearly summary of recent literature published by Tourette Syndrome Association, Inc.

General Reading for Adults

Bruun, R. D., and Bruun, B. (1994) A Mind of its own. Tourette's syndrome: A story and a guide. New York: Oxford University Press.

Comings, D. E. (1990) Tourette syndrome and human behavior. Duarte, CA: Hope Press.

Dornbush, M. P., and Pruitt, S. K. (1995) Teaching the tiger: A handbook for individuals involved in the education of students with attention deficit disorders, Tourette syndrome, or obsessive-compulsive disorder. Duarte, CA: Hope Press.

Du Paul, G., and Stoner, G. (1994) ADHD in the schools: Assessments and intervention strategies. New York: Guilford Press.

Haerle, T. (1992) Children with Tourette syndrome: A parents' guide. Rockville, Md.: Woodbine House.

Hughes, S. (1990) Ryan—A mother's story of her hyperactive/Tourette syndrome child. Duarte, CA: Hope Press.

Robertson, M. M., and Baron-Cohen, S. (1998) Tourette syndrome: The facts. 2nd ed. Oxford: Oxford University Press.

Sacks, O. (1986) The man who mistook his wife for a hat. London: Duckworth.

Sacks, O. (1995) An anthropologist on Mars. New York: Knopf.

Seligman, A. W. (1991) Echolalia: A novel. Duarte, CA: Hope Press.

Seligman, A. W., and Hilkevick, J. S. (1992) Don't think about monkeys: Extraordinary stories by people with Tourette syndrome. Duarte, CA: Hope Press.

Shapiro, A. K., et al. (1988) Gilles de la Tourette syndrome. 2nd ed. New York: Raven Press.

Shimberg, E. F. (1995) Living with Tourette syndrome. New York: Simon & Schuster.

General Reading for Young People

Buehrens, A. (1991) Hi, I'm Adam: A Child's Book about Tourette Syndrome. Duarte Calif.: Hope Press.

Internet Resources

Newsgroup/Unmoderated support groups on the Internet:
alt.support.tourette
alt.support.ocd.
alt.support.attn-deficit
k12.ed.special

Home Pages for Information on TS on the Internet

http://vh.radiology.uiowa.edu/Patients/IowaHealthBook/Tourette/

HomePage.html (home page for U. Iowa)
http://www.fairlite.com/ocd/ (information for patients and professionals)

Tourette Syndrome Association, Inc.
http://neuro-www2.mgh.harvard/edu/TSA/tsamain.nclk

Obsessive Compulsive Foundation, Inc.
http://pages.prodigy.com/alwillen/ocf.html

Children and Adults with Attention Deficit Disorders (Ch.ADD)
http://www.chadd.org

Southern California TSA Web Page
http://www.geocites.com/Hollywood/2219/

University of Iowa Virtual Hospital Page on TS
http://indy.radiology.uiowa.edu/Patients/IHB/Psych/Tourette/Home-Page.html

Yale's Home Page on TS and OCD
http://info.med.yale.edu/chldstdy/tsocd.htm

OCD Fairlite Home Page
http://www.fairlite.com/ocd/

4

Sex Chromosome
Aneuploidy in Males

Sex chromosome aneuploidy, an abnormal number of X or Y chromosomes, is the most common chromosomal abnormality that exists, having an overall incidence of 1 per 448 individuals (Linden et al., 1996; Nielsen and Wohlert, 1991). The incidence of these problems is even higher in utero; approximately 25% of all chromosome abnormalities detected by amniocentesis in women older than 35 years are sex chromosome abnormalities (Crandall et al., 1980). The majority of individuals with sex chromosome aneuploidies have normal intellectual abilities, although learning disabilities and mild emotional or behavioral problems are common. We are beginning to understand the behavioral and cognitive phenotype which is present in an unselected population of individuals with each disorder. The biases of earlier studies that screened institutional or prison populations (Jacobs et al., 1965; Price and Whatmore, 1967) have given way to the controlled findings of several longitudinal studies of sex chromosome aneuploidy (SCA) that identified patients at birth through unselected screenings (Nielsen and Wohlert, 1990; Ratcliffe et al., 1990; Robinson et al., 1986, 1990; Stewart et al., 1990; Walzer et al., 1990). Children with SCAs adapt less well to adversity than do their normal siblings, and the importance of a nurturing and supportive family in improving the outcome of children with SCAs has been documented (Bender et al., 1987). The outcome for fetuses of mostly professional parents that were diagnosed prenatally with SCAs has been excellent, probably because of a supportive environment and helpful background genes for cognitive and language abilities (Robinson et al., 1992).

This chapter focuses on the SCAs that occur in males, including 47,XXY, 47,XYY and 48,XXYY syndromes. Although the physical phenotype usually has

Neurodevelopmental Disorders: Diagnosis and Treatment, by Randi Jenssen Hagerman. New York: Oxford University Press, 1999. © Oxford University Press, Inc.

only minor abnormalities, the cognitive and behavioral phenotype is more remarkable and often requires the combined efforts of a treatment team that includes medical, psychological, and educational input.

47,XXY SYNDROME

Klinefelter and his colleagues (1942) first described this syndrome in males who presented with infertility, small testicles, gynecomastia (breast development), elevations in follicle stimulating hormone (FSH), and azoospermia in 1942. He did not know of the cytogenetic abnormality associated with this disorder until it was described by Bradbury and colleagues in 1956. Although mosaic patterns (46,XY/47,XXY) and variant patterns such as 48,XXXY can occur, the majority of people with Klinefelter syndrome (KS) have 47,XXY. KS occurs in approximately 1 per 600 individuals in the general population (Nielsen and Wohlert, 1991). The incidence increases with advanced maternal age; 33-year-old women have an incidence of 0.4 per 1,000 live births, but women of 49 years have an incidence of 14.6 per 1,000 live births (Hook et al., 1983). When diagnosis takes place at the time of amniocentesis, the survival rate is 92% in all pregnancies with 47,XXY and 99% in singleton pregnancies (Hook et al., 1983). KS is the most common cause of male hypogonadism, and it occurs in 8% of men presenting with infertility (Winter, 1990).

Patients with 47,XXY do not have consistent dysmorphic facial features (Figure 4.1), but their endocrine and learning problems key the clinician into considering the diagnosis.

Growth and Endocrine Changes

Infants with KS are normal at birth, but there is a tendency for a small head circumference, which usually remains within 1 SD below the mean throughout childhood (Stewart et al., 1990). The Toronto longitudinal study has followed 43 boys with 47,XXY throughout childhood and found a dramatic increase in the height percentiles between ages 5 and 8 years because of an increase in height velocity over that of normal boys (Stewart et al., 1990). The average height was at the 75th percentile by age 18, and the mean final adult height was 8 cm greater than the mean corrected midparental height. The height increase was mainly due to long legs; the sitting height was normal. The timing of puberty, that is, the onset of pubic hair, was found to be normal in patients with KS, compared with their siblings in the Denver longitudinal study (Salbenblatt et al., 1985), although the Toronto study found an occasional late maturer in the patients who were not treated with testosterone.

There is a primary Leydig cell deficiency in KS, and these are the cells that produce the majority of testosterone under control of leutenizing hormone (LH). Testicular biopsies in children with KS demonstrate spermatogonial depletion, but it is not until the onset of puberty that tubular fibrosis and hyalinization occur

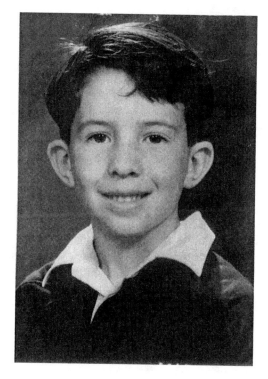

FIGURE 4.1: 7-year-old boy with 47,XXY syndrome. Although ears are mildy prominent, he does not have dysmorphic features.

because of the stimulation of LH and FSH (Winter, 1990). Infertility is the rule with rare exception (Laron et al., 1982). The enhanced levels of LH and FSH in puberty stimulate testicular estradiol secretion, leading to a high estradiol/testosterone ratio that may be significant for the development of gynecomastia (Winter, 1990). Although gynecomastia may be seen in early puberty in some normal males, it is more pronounced in boys with KS, and it is clinically significant in approximately 15%. In the Toronto study, males without gynecomastia in late adolescence had higher serum levels of testosterone than those with gynecomastia, and five of the males required bilateral mastectomies (Stewart et al., 1990). There is also enhanced conversion of testosterone to estradiol in KS, and this may contribute to the increased incidence of gynecomastia (Mandoki and Sumner, 1991).

The incidence of breast cancer is reported at 4% in males with KS, which is 20 times higher than in normal males, although it is similar to the breast cancer rate in females (Scheike et al., 1973). A subsequent study of cancer in 696 men with KS in Denmark did not find an increased rate of breast cancer, but instead found four cases of a rare cancer, primary mediastinal germ cell tumor, in adolescents and young adults (Hasle et al., 1995). The lifetime risk for this tumor is 1% for individuals with KS, but this represents a significantly increased risk over that of the general population. This risk is thought to relate to the incomplete migration of primordial germ cells from the endoderm of the yolk sac to the gonads, resulting in later malignant transformation. In KS there may be an increase in incomplete migration, or perhaps the elevation of gonadotropins (FSH and LH) in puberty causes a higher risk of malignant transformation (Hasle et al., 1995). There is no increased risk for other forms of cancer in KS.

Testosterone, FSH, and LH levels are normal prepubertally before 12 years of age in males with KS, but both FSH and LH increase to higher than normal levels by 14 years of age (Salbenblatt et al., 1985). The testicles increase in size as the testosterone levels rise in early puberty, but there is a subsequent decrease in size related to the fibrosis which occurs with high gonadrotropin levels (Salbenblatt et al., 1985). Most subjects with KS have a testicular volume between 3 and 6 ml in late puberty and adulthood, although an occasional patient may attain a volume of 10 ml (Stewart et al., 1990). The stretched penile length is usually within the normal range but can be slightly decreased (Stewart et al., 1990).

Although the timing of puberty is usually normal (Salbenblatt et al., 1985), 14 boys with KS and precocious puberty have been described in the literature (Bertelloni et al., 1996). In puberty the serum testosterone rises gradually, but 5 of the 43 Toronto patients did not reach the lower level of the normal range in adolescence, and the rest were in the low-normal to mid-normal range (Stewart et al., 1990). Testosterone therapy is indicated in males with KS; this is discussed further in the section on treatment.

Cognitive, Motor, and Language Development

Children with KS are described as quiet, shy, hypoactive, and language-delayed in early development (Mandoki and Sumner, 1991). Graham and colleagues (1988) found a primary language deficit in children with KS that includes auditory processing difficulties and auditory memory deficits with concomitant difficulties in expressive language. Problems with word retrieval, syntax, and narrative formulation were characteristic of the language phenotype. These problems lead to a lower Verbal IQ (VIQ) than Performance IQ (PIQ), although the Full-Scale IQ (FSIQ) on the WISC-R is usually within the normal range. In the Toronto study the mean VIQ was 84.6 (range 82–88) for the patients with KS and 104.2 for the controls, whereas the mean PIQ was 98.9 (range 93–103) for the patients with KS and 106.8 for the controls (Rovet et al., 1996). These data are similar to the scores of the Denver longitudinal study of 14 patients with 47,XXY who had a mean VIQ of 94.5, PIQ of 99, and FSIQ of 97 (Robinson et al., 1986) and the Boston longitudinal study of 13 patients with 47,XXY who had a mean VIQ of 95, PIQ of 111, and FSIQ of 103 (Walzer et al., 1990).

In KS, the VIQ and the PIQ do not correlate with each other as they do in normals (Netley et al., 1995). Perhaps they are more independent in KS because the VIQ is more significantly affected by the syndrome than the PIQ. In Toronto

18 males with KS had event-related potential (ERP) studies in the prepubertal period, during puberty, and in adulthood (Netley et al., 1995). Both an orthographic and a phonemic problem were present, and P3 peak latencies were studied in parietal and temporal regions. They found phonemic P3 latencies to be strongly associated with VIQ at all ages and unrelated to PIQ at any time. The P3 latency reflects neural processing times, and if the latency is long it provides a more substantial basis for learning and memory consolidation, which correlates positively with VIQ (Netley et al., 1995).

The Freedom from Distractibility factors from the Wechsler IQ subtest scores were also consistently lower at all ages in patients with KS than in controls (Rovet et al., 1996). This problem reflects difficulties with attention, although hyperactivity is not usually seen. Boys with KS are described as quiet and introverted, passive, and tending to withdraw from group activities (Rovet et al., 1996). Theilgaard (1984) studied young adult males with KS and found more problems with nervousness, passivity, less assertiveness, poor self-acceptance, decreased libido, and lower masculinity scores than in controls. On occasion more severe problems with attention deficit hyperactivity disorder (ADHD) may occur, as described in the following case history.

CASE HISTORY: JOHN (2)

John first presented to our Child Development Unit at age 6 years 10 months with a history of behavior and attention problems at school. He had been treated with methylphenidate (Ritalin) at a dose of 5 mg twice a day for a 2-month period, but his mother felt the medication was not helpful, so it was discontinued.

John's mother's pregnancy was normal. She delivered full-term vaginally, the birth weight was 8 lb. 5 oz., and John did well in the newborn period. His early motor milestones were normal, but his speech development was delayed, and he did not speak in sentences until 3 to 4 years of age. He has always had difficulty in following multiple directions, and he does better with just one direction at a time. In preschool he had some days when he would isolate himself from other children, and he was noted to have mild attentional problems. He also began to stutter in kindergarten. Because of his frustration with communication, he became aggressive at times with other kids. He would grab their arms or bite their hands, instead of verbally requesting them to do something. His aggression was mainly impulsive. In the first grade he had difficulty in staying on task with math, reading, and writing assignments, and his attention span was only 5 minutes.

Cognitive testing (WISC-III) carried out by the school demonstrated a Verbal IQ of 71, a Performance IQ of 108, and a Full-Scale IQ of 87. His highest subtest scores were 13 on Picture Completion and 15 on Picture Arrangement, with 12 on Block Design, but his subtest scores were only 2 on Vocabulary, 4 on Comprehension, 6 on Symbol Search, and 7 on Digit Span.

On examination, at 6 years 10 months, his height was 127.7 cm (90th percentile for age), weight was 23.3 kg (60th percentile for age), and head circumference was 53.1 cm (75th percentile for age). He had large prominent ears, with some cupping of the ear pinnae bilaterally, and a high arched palate. He also had a mild pectus excavatum and Tanner stage-1 prepubertal development, with a testicular volume of approximately 3 ml bilaterally. Palmar creases were normal; his finger joints demonstrated metacarpalphalangeal (MP) extension to 90°; and muscle tone and deep tendon reflexes were normal. On a computerized visual attention task, he scored in the abnormal range for number correct and in the borderline range for number of commissions.

John's overall diagnosis was of a language-based learning disability, in addition to a mild degree of ADHD. DNA *FMR1* testing was carried out because of his prominent cupped ears, in addition to his verbal deficit. The result showed two normal X chromosome alleles at 33 and 30 CGG repeats. A subsequent cytogenetics study documented his 47,XXY karyotype.

In a follow-up when John entered the second grade in school, he was having increasing problems with attention and concentration and disruptive behavior without his methylphenidate. Methylphenidate was restarted at a dose of 5 mg twice a day, and his attention span and disruptive behavior have significantly improved. The methylphenidate allows him to think about the results of his actions before acting impulsively. His desk in the classroom was previously separated from the other children because of his disruptive behavior, but now his desk is rejoined with the rest of the class. He received intensified special education support with an aide to help him in the regular classroom. He uses the computer daily at school, and computer software programs have improved his spelling, reading, and math.

Individualized special education remediation has been particularly helpful in reading. He continues to receive speech and language therapy in a small group setting in his classroom, and his stuttering is improving. The school social worker meets with him weekly, and a progress report is completed each day by his teachers with positive reinforcement. His self-image has also improved since he has participated in a gymnastics program that involves tumbling, in which he excels.

A rare patient has been described with more severe psychopathology, such as an acute paranoid disorder, autism, or psychosis (Stein and Siddiqui, 1986). This is most likely related to other background genes, although the mild cognitive and language deficits in KS may further predispose a patient to these problems. Most males with 47,XXY do not demonstrate significant behavior problems, and the patients who present to a developmental and behavior clinic represent a biased subgroup of patients with KS. Additional biased reports have described a few patients with KS who have fire-setting behavior; a study of 20 male arsonists detected one patient with KS (Miller and Sulkes, 1988; Virkkunen et al., 1987).

Significant motor deficits have been found in children with KS compared with controls. Children are usually described as motorically slow and awkward in early childhood, and school-aged children score lower on tasks of fine and gross motor coordination, speed dexterity, and strength than their siblings (Salbenblatt et al., 1987). In the Denver longitudinal study, 79% of the 14 males with 47,XXY had dysfunctional sensory-motor integration (Salbenblatt et al., 1987). In addition, hypotonia, hyperextensibility of finger joints, poor muscle strength, synkinetic or posturing movements, and tremor or dysmetria were seen. These problems interfered with handwriting tasks and impaired self-image and peer interactional abilities (Salbenblatt et al., 1987). In review of developmental milestones, the majority of boys with 47,XXY walked late, between 14 and 16 months (Salbenblatt et al., 1987). The combination of decreased muscle tone and poor joint proprioception led to diminished joint stability, resulting in an awkward gait pattern. These authors recommended periodic neuromuscular and sensory-motor integration evaluations with appropriate occupational therapy (OT) and physical therapy (PT) intervention (Salbenblatt et al., 1987).

Educational Problems

The cognitive, language, and attentional problems lead to poor school performance in boys with KS. Between 60 and 86% of the children receive some special education support, and many repeat at least one grade (Robinson et al., 1990; Rovet et al., 1996). Problems with reading and spelling are noted first and are related to the language deficits and phonological processing problems. Robinson and colleagues reported that 50% of the group followed in Denver had a specific dyslexia and that 11 of the 14 boys had some degree of reading-difficulty. Preschool language problems predicted the development of reading and comprehension problems in middle childhood (Graham et al., 1988). With increasing age, a greater number of patients with KS demonstrated academic difficulties. At age 20 years, 100% of patients in the Toronto study demonstrate a significant impairment in reading (Rovet et al., 1996). There is also a steady decline in math achievement scores throughout childhood, and by age 20, 100% of patients with KS have a significant impairment (Rovet et al., 1996). The problems in math are related to deficits in recall, working memory, and comprehension. The language deficits also interfere with solving word problems. By age 18, boys with KS were performing more than five grade levels below their expected placement (Rovet et al., 1996). The increasing academic difficulties are a reflection of their problems with comprehension and logical and conceptual thinking, which are more frequently demanded in higher grades. They are also restricted in their ability to obtain new information from print because of their reading disability, so they fall further behind (Rovet et al., 1996). Although the academic scores worsen with age, most patients graduate from high school, and some patients seek higher education. There is significant variability in the outcome of males with 47,XXY related to the environmental and family supports, background gene effects, and overall cognitive abilities.

The motor deficits in KS lead to problems in written language. The Toronto study found that by an average age of 14.5 years, the Test of Written Language mean score was at the 20.5 centile for boys with KS (Rovet et al., 1996). The motor deficits also interfere with participation in competitive sports, although boys can often excel in individual sports, such as biking, swimming, or hiking.

Psychopathology

The Denver longitudinal study has carried out a detailed psychiatric evaluation on 13 patients with 47,XXY and found that 54% received a psychiatric diagnosis compared with 14% of controls (Bender et al., 1995). These diagnoses included three patients with dysthymia, two with substance abuse, two with conduct disorder, and one with ADHD. These diagnoses are not surprising considering the high rate of academic and athletic failure in boys with KS. Most boys experienced a significant degree of frustration and low self-esteem even without a psychiatric diagnosis (Bender et al., 1995). In late adolescence, 5 of the 13 boys experienced great difficulty separating from family and living independently. Their separation was marked by anger, rebellion, and conflict, and four had problems with the law (Bender et al., 1995). Three of these individuals have problems in adult life with continuing anger and insecurity and have sought therapy. The most stable and supportive families had the children who had the least difficulty in transitioning into adult life (Bender et al., 1995).

A further study of environmental influences that affect the outcome of children with sex chromosome aneuploidy focused on the degree of dysfunction in families as measured by parenting skills, adverse stress events, and socioeconomic status (Bender et al., 1987). Children with SCA, including boys with 47,XXY, had a dramatic increase in school impairment and psychosocial impairment that was significantly different from the control siblings when they lived in a dysfunctional family compared to a nondysfunctional family (Bender et al., 1987). In contrast, language impairment increased in children with SCA in parallel to controls when they lived in a dysfunctional family. Therefore, children with SCA are more vulnerable to family dysfunction, and there is not simply an additive effect but a synergistic or mutually potentiating effect of a disturbed environment in school and psychosocial outcomes (Bender et al., 1987). Most children with SCA do not have the adaptive reserve to compensate for a dysfunctional environment. Family dysfunction and low socioeconomic status are not simply environmental measures but are also markers for other genetic factors that affect cognitive, language, and psychosocial development that can have an additive or synergistic effect on the outcome of a child with SCA.

Variant Patterns

The presence of mosaicism, meaning the existence of a normal cell line in addition to 47,XXY cells, will decrease the degree of deficits in all areas depending on the percentage of normal cells present. On the other hand, KS variants with a greater number of X chromosomes, such as 48,XXXY, and 49,XXXXY, will cause an increase in dysmorphic features and more severe language and cognitive impairment than in males with 47,XXY. Most boys with three or more X chromosomes will also have mental retardation. Polani first suggested that each extra X chromosome will reduce the IQ by 16 points (Polani, 1977). Borghgraef and colleagues pointed out that the Verbal IQ is consistently lower than the Performance IQ (on the WISC-R) in males with 49,XXXXY because of severe language impairment; in contrast, they show to a better performance on nonverbal tasks such as puzzles and sorting (Borghgraef et al., 1988). These individuals also have dysmorphic features, unlike males with 47,XXY, including a broad nasal bridge, epicanthal folds, short neck, hypogenitalism, a small thorax, and widely spaced nipples (Borghgraef et al., 1988; Linden et al., 1995). As a consequence of to the severe language deficit, they are often shy, quiet, and timid, although severe attentional problems, hyperactivity, and aggression have also been described (Borghgraef et al., 1988; Lomelino and Reiss, 1991).

An additional variant pattern in KS is 47,X,i(Xq)Y, where the second X chromosome is isodicentric with a missing Xp region and 2Xq regions are attached by a centromere. This has been reported in 19 cases to date, and it occurs in 0.3 to 0.9% of males with X chromosome polysomies (Arps et al., 1996). Males with this variant have normal intellectual abilities, elevations in LH and FSH, and low to normal testosterone after puberty; one-third evidence gynecomastia. These individuals do not have tall stature, a fact that suggests that the increased height in males with 47,XXY is due to the presence of additional Xp material. There are putative growth genes in the Xp region near the telemere (Arps et al., 1996). Therefore, the low testosterone levels and delayed closure of the epiphyses does not appear to be the sole cause of tall stature in KS.

Because KS is relatively common in the general population, it will co-occur on occasion with other disorders, and the clinical picture, including the cognitive outcome, is usually compounded for the worse. For instance, Butler and colleagues have described a boy with 47,XXY and Prader-Willi syndrome with significant developmental delays (Butler et al., 1997). The exception to this concept of compounding delays is the case in which KS co-occurs with fragile X syndrome. The extra X chromosome will be beneficial because it will produce significant levels of the FMR1 protein and thereby spare the patient with fragile X syndrome some degree of clinical involvement, depending on how much FMR1 protein is produced (see chapter 2). Approximately 1 in 155 males with fragile X syndrome will also have Klinefelter syndrome (Fryns and Van den Berghe, 1988).

Treatment

Patients with 47,XXY are normal at birth, and they are usually not diagnosed until the school-aged period when language and motor deficits become apparent or until adolescence or adulthood when small testicles or infertility are noticeable. With an increase in prenatal diagnosis, many of these children may also be identified before birth, and early intervention can occur when necessary. There is significant variability in this disorder, and not all boys with 47,XXY will require intervention. It is important for the family to be supportive of the child's needs whenever the diagnosis is made. A stable and nurturing family will make a difference in the outcome of the child (Bender et al., 1987). Often knowing the diagnosis will help to target appropriate interventions early.

> It was a relief to have a reason for his problems. We tell him he has an extra X chromosome that makes him extra special—A mother

Both motor and language intervention in the preschool period will improve development and perhaps lessen the need for therapy later in school. Appropriate intervention for a language-based learning disability includes vocabulary building, word retrieval work, and development of comprehension skills. The auditory processing deficits can also be addressed in therapy, although modifications in the classroom, such as repeating information, speaking in short sentences, giving auditory and visual information simultaneously, and decreasing ambient noise, can be helpful. These interventions are the same as what is recommended for children with ADHD, although children with KS usually do not have the hyperactivity. Newer computer technology targeted to improve auditory processing and language development, specifically the Fast Forward program (see Appendix 3), may be efficacious for this population (Tallal et al., 1996).

Because of the high incidence of dyslexia and milder reading problems, programs that target reading deficits early and that have been successful for dyslexia should be used as soon as possible. Examples are the Lindamood-Bell Learning Program or the Orton Gillingham program (Appendix 3). An intense phonological approach to reading should be initiated early. Computer programs such as the Edmark software for reading, which combines both visual and auditory feedback, should be utilized early in the child's education (see Appendix 2). Language therapy should focus not only on articulation problems but also on comprehension and higher linguistic concepts.

Math should also be targeted as a typical problem area early on, with intensive remediation and drills to demonstrate mastery (Rovet et al., 1996). The learning of new math concepts and word problems requires additional remediation, and when this is not available through the public schools, it should be obtained privately. Computer programs are also helpful for learning new math concepts, such as Millie's Math House or Math Blaster (see Appendix 2).

The motor problems, including fine and gross motor incoordination and sensory-motor integration deficits, often require early and continued intervention by an OT from the preschool period onward. Improvement in motor skills can help with a child's overall self-image and peer interactions, which are often problematic for these children. Individual sports, such as swimming, gymnastics, biking, and karate, should be emphasized instead of team sports.

> The more you wear him out with physical activity, the better he is—A mother

Although fine motor skills for handwriting will improve with occupational therapy, the use of a computer word processor should be initiated by third grade to facilitate written work. The Don Johnston Co:Writer is a word prediction program that will enhance the written language for the dyslexic speller (see Appendix 2). A spell checker on the word processor or a hand-held spelling computer may also be helpful.

Psychopharmacology and Counseling

Most children with KS do not require the use of medications to help with attention and concentration, although these problems should be assessed carefully because more significant problems in this area can occur and can be helped by stimulants (see the case history of John). Hyperactivity, ADHD, and aggression are more common in the variant patterns such as 49,XXXXY, as described previously. The stimulants are described in more detail in the next section, on males with 47,XYY, with whom they are used more commonly.

Depression and anxiety are occasionally seen in males with KS, and treatment should include the use of counseling on an individual basis. Group therapy to develop social skills with peers can also be helpful, and several programs exist to guide the development of these skills (Begum, 1996; Bloomquist, 1996; Frankel et al., 1997; Mundy, 1991). The speech and language pathologist can also use pragmatic language approaches to improve language skills in a group setting (see Appendix 3). Medications can also be used to improve anxiety or depression when counseling does not improve the problem.

The selective serotonin reuptake inhibitors (SSRIs) will enhance serotonin levels by blocking reuptake at the synapse; they are effective for treatment of depression and anxiety, in addition to obsessive-compulsive behavior in childhood and adulthood. These medications are used more frequently with other disorders such as Tourette syndrome and fragile X syndrome, but they are also occasionally used with patients with KS. For a more detailed discussion of SSRIs, see chapters 2 and 3.

Androgen Replacement Therapy

The replacement of testosterone in KS has several functions. It acts directly on muscle, where it stimulates an androgen receptor to stimulate transcription and build larger muscles, and it also closes the epiphyses of the bones. It prevents demineralization of the bones, thereby preventing development of osteoporosis. In reproductive tissues it is reduced to dihydrotestosterone, which has a greatly increased androgenic effect (Winter, 1990). In brain, fat cells, and Sertoli cells, testosterone is aromatized to estradiol, which then acts on estrogen receptors that can stimulate dendritic branching. A rise in testosterone will often decrease LH and FSH secretion and in some cases improve gynecomastia (Meikle et al., 1998; Winter, 1990).

Anecdotal evidence suggests that testosterone replacement therapy improves self-esteem, learning, attention, endurance, the development of secondary sexual characteristics, and interpersonal relations in individuals with KS (Winter, 1990). It is recommended that testosterone replacement begin at approximately 12 years of age, when the LH and FSH levels begin to increase and before significant gynecomastia develops (Winter, 1990).

One form of androgen replacement therapy used today is the intramuscular (IM) injection of testosterone esters, either testosterone enanthate or testosterone cypionate. With these agents, the testosterone levels rise sharply over 1 to 2 days and then gradually return to baseline levels over a 10-day period (Winter, 1990). Usually the injection is repeated every 2 to 3 weeks with a dose of 100 to 200 mg, and this continues throughout adolescence and adulthood.

Transdermal therapy with testosterone-impregnated skin patches provides a more even and physiological level of testosterone throughout replacement therapy. The first testosterone patches developed were worn on the scrotum and replaced daily. However, if the scrotum is small, they are hard to keep in place, and the scrotum on occasion must be shaved for adequate skin contact (Bagatell and Bremner, 1996). In a study of adolescent males treated with the scrotal patch, compliance was a problem (Linden and Robinson, 1991). A new nonscrotal permeation-enhanced testosterone transdermal (TTD) system has been developed and evaluated in 13 men with KS, aged 20 to 36 years (Meikle et al., 1998). Each patient used two TTD patches per day, which delivered 5 mg of testosterone daily. The patches were applied nightly to the back, thigh, abdomen, or upper arm on a rotating basis. After 6 months of therapy with the TTD system, the incidence, frequency, and severity of impotence and problems with libido, fatigue, and depression generally decreased, whereas the incidence of hot flashes increased from 11% of patients to 33%. Gynecomastia was a problem for five patients, and it resolved in three patients after treatment. Serum testosterone levels were boosted into the normal range, and LH and FSH levels decreased significantly, but only 46% and 38% of patients, respectively, decreased to the normal range. This study suggests that the nonscrotal TTD system is the most physiological and best tolerated replacement system for men with KS (Meikle et al., 1998).

Mandoki and Sumner describe a 16-year-old boy with 47,XXY who was originally referred because of temper outbursts and aggressive behavior, which were unusually severe for this diagnosis, but he responded well to a multimodal intervention (Mandoki and Sumner, 1991). He was born with a clubfoot and he experienced delays in his milestones. At 8 years old he had a Verbal IQ of 70, a Performance IQ of 80, and a Full-Scale IQ of 76 on the WISC-R. Prior to his diagnosis he experienced increasing academic failure and developed social withdrawal and increasingly disruptive and aggressive behavior. His treatment at diagnosis included individual counseling combined with propranolol, a beta blocker, at 80 mg four times a day to decrease aggression. He was subsequently treated with 200 mg of testosterone IM each month. The combination of propranolol, testosterone, and counseling dramatically improved his aggressive behavior and social interactions. He also requested and underwent surgery for suction lipectomy of both breasts, as well as bilateral orchiectomy, or removal of his testicles, with placement of testicle implants of normal size. His body image and self-esteem improved significantly with surgery. Finally, he received educational support and was placed in a vocational educational program where he was successful in school (Mandoki and Sumner, 1991). A multiprofessional approach can make a significant difference for these children, but early diagnosis and intervention can treat the early difficulties that lead to school failure and behavior problems.

47,XYY SYNDROME

The 47,XYY karyotype has been documented to occur in 1 per 894 live-born boys (Nielsen and Wohlert, 1991). Individuals with 47,XYY do not have dysmorphic facial features, and their IQ is usually within the normal range (Figure 4.2). They do not have the endocrine and fertility problems previously discussed for individuals with 47,XXY. However, they have tall stature, and they often have learning disabilities and significant emotional problems that are worthy of identification and treatment, as discussed later in this section. Early studies had identified a high incidence of 47,XYY males in prisons and hospitals related to a history of impulsivity and violence (Price and Whatmore, 1967), although controlled longitudinal studies of individuals identified at birth with 47,XYY have not found a significant incidence of incarceration (Nielsen and Wohlert, 1991). However, only a small number of males with 47,XYY have been followed longitudinally, so unbiased data is limited regarding outcome.

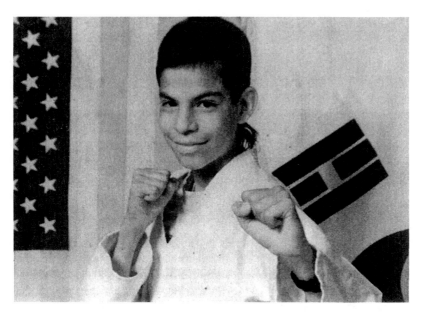

FIGURE 4.2:   Young man with 47,XYY syndrome. He does not have dysmorphic features.

Growth and Puberty

Growth through puberty has been followed in 14 boys with 47,XYY in the Edinburgh study, and their growth velocity increased throughout childhood compared with siblings (Ratcliffe et al., 1990). The onset of puberty and the development of pubic hair (mean age 13.8 years) was significantly later than that of their normal siblings (mean age 12.4 years) (Ratcliffe et al., 1990). Their testicular growth was normal and comparable to that of their siblings. Although their puberty was mildly delayed, their growth spurt was higher and of longer duration than that of controls. The mean height of 47,XYY boys at age 18 is 187.2 cm, and they exceeded the height of their fathers by at least 13 cm (Ratcliffe et al., 1990). Patients with 47,XYY are fertile.

Saliva or serum testosterone levels were studied in four males in the Denver longitudinal study and in seven males in the Edinburgh study. All values were within the normal range and not significantly different from controls (Ratcliffe et al., 1990; Robinson et al., 1986). One of four males with 47,XYY in the Denver study has had severe acne (Robinson et al., 1986). Although the prospective studies have not demonstrated differences in testosterone levels between males with 47,XYY and controls, other studies have demonstrated higher testosterone levels in males with 47,XYY than in controls (Schiavi et al., 1984).

In the Edinburgh study there was a death in infancy of a baby with 47,XYY and renal agenesis, and renal agenesis with hypoplastic lung also caused a death in an infant with 47,XYY in the Denmark study.

Cognitive, Academic, and Behavioral Development

The cognitive testing of 18 boys with 47,XYY in the Edinburgh study found a mean Verbal IQ of 101, Performance IQ of 105, and Full-Scale IQ (FSIQ) of 103 on the WISC-R, but all values were significantly lower than sibling controls (Ratcliffe et al., 1990). No male with 47,XYY had an IQ in the mentally retarded range, and four males had a PIQ greater than 120. There was a mild deficit in VIQ, but this was not as severe as was reported for the boys with 47,XXY. Four of the boys with 47,XYY experienced speech and language delays, and they received individual therapy (Ratcliffe et al., 1990).

In Denver, where four boys with 47,XYY have been followed longitudinally, only the VIQ was significantly lower than controls, and two boys had a PIQ that was 26 points higher than their VIQ (Robinson et al., 1986). Detailed speech and language testing demonstrated problems in processing linguistic information in all of the males, but language comprehension and speech production were good (Bender et al., 1983). A detailed neuromotor assessment demonstrated problems in all four, including hypotonia, motor planning problems, primitive reflex retention, poor bilateral coordination, and poor visual-perceptual-motor integration (Salbenblatt et al., 1987). Three of the four boys were late walkers, and three scored below the eighth percentile on the Bruininks-Oseretsky Test of Motor Proficiency (Salbenblatt et al., 1987).

In the Boston longitudinal study, 11 boys with 47,XYY have been progressively followed since identification at birth (Walzer et al., 1990). Cognitive testing demonstrated similar results to the Edinburgh study, that is, an IQ in the normal range, but three of the boys had a significantly lower VIQ than PIQ. Speech and language assessments were carried out routinely and demonstrated articulation deficits in three and speech dysfluency or stuttering in two patients. Nine of the 11 boys demonstrated a mild to moderate receptive and/or expressive language deficit, and six had auditory memory deficits (Walzer et al., 1990).

In the academic area, 42% of the 47,XYY group in Edinburgh required remedial reading, and one was identified with dyslexia which was significantly different from their sibling controls (18% required remediation) (Ratcliffe et al., 1990). Math scores were above the prediction for IQ.

In the Boston group, 5 of the 11 boys progressed adequately in their academics, but four of these five manifested problems with inattention, which led to problems in homework completion and distractibility that interfered periodically with academics (Walzer et al., 1990). Six of the 11 boys (55%) had significant learning disabilities which required resource room help over the years. Five of these six boys also manifested problems with inattention and impulsivity (Walzer et al., 1990). Therefore, a total of 9 of 11 boys (82%) had symptoms of ADHD that interfered with academics. The motor activity level was consistently higher in boys with 47,XYY than in controls during most of childhood. The teachers reported motor restlessness, fidgetiness, and excessive gross motor activity, including running or meandering about the room when they were expected to sit or stand quietly (Walzer et al., 1990). The distractibility in boys with 47,XYY usually began between 2 and 3 years of age, before their learning disabilities were diagnosed, whereas in boys with 47,XXY the distractibility began later, when they were struggling with comprehension or tasks they did not understand (Walzer et al., 1990). Although the learning and language deficits in boys with 47,XYY were less severe than in boys with 47,XXY, their disruptive and impulsive behavior more frequently was viewed as impairing teachability in boys with 47,XYY as compared with the shy and withdrawn behavior of boys with 47,XXY (Walzer et al., 1990).

In the Edinburgh study, questionnaires were utilized to study behavior, and a twofold increase was seen in tantrum behavior in 47,XYY boys compared with controls (86% versus 35%; Ratcliffe et al., 1990). Significant increases were also seen in solitary behavior in patients with 47,XYY (71%) compared with controls (28%) and in nonacceptance by peers (44% vs. 5%) (Ratcliffe et al., 1990). A personality questionnaire demonstrated a significantly increased factor score for "uncontrolled, follows own urges, careless of social rules" in boys with 47,XYY compared with sibling controls (Ratcliffe et al., 1990). Psychiatric referral took place in 50% of boys with 47,XYY compared with 9% of controls, and the reasons for referral included persistent tantrums in all cases and stealing in two cases, with police involvement (Ratcliffe et al., 1990).

Ratcliffe and Field (1982) have emphasized the tendency for reactive depression in males with 47,XYY when behavior problems are compounded by family dysfunction or other stressors in the environment. They recommend intensive treatment for depression, including individual and family psychotherapy combined with antidepressant medication and educational support as needed. They describe four patients who have done well with these interventions (Ratcliffe and Field, 1982).

In the Denmark longitudinal study of 20 boys with 47,XYY, one was involved in minor criminal activity and another was treated at a psychiatric day hospital, but both had experienced significant family dysfunction (Nielsen and Wohlert, 1991). Boys with 47,XYY syndrome are at increased risk for psychosocial problems when family dysfunction exists, similar to boys with 47,XXY, as previously discussed (Bender et al., 1987).

Although the longitudinal follow-up studies do not demonstrate that boys with 47,XYY consistently end up in jail, as clinic-referred case studies and early prison studies suggested, boys with 47,XYY often have problems with hyperactivity and impulse control that sometimes can lead to aggression. These problems were studied in a Danish population survey in which all men in Denmark who were in the top 15% of the height distribution (4,139) were studied cytogenetically, and 12 men with 47,XYY and 16 men with 47,XXY were identified (Schiavi et al., 1984). The authors found that 42% (5/12) of men with 47,XYY, 19% (3/16) of men with 47,XXY, and 9% of men with 46,XY had been convicted of one or more crimes, but they were usually minor offenses. In all three groups, those who had committed crimes had lower IQs than those who did not commit crimes. When IQ and socioeconomic status (SES) were controlled, the elevated crime rate compared with controls was reduced in the men with 47,XYY and disappeared in the men with 47,XXY (Schiavi et al., 1984).

The patients with sex chromosome anomalies and 46,XY controls matched on IQ and SES were studied with detailed psychological evaluations. The only interview measure that distinguished males with 47,XYY from controls was physical aggression, and the difference was mainly due to "aggression toward wife." All of the males with 47,XYY were described as occasionally aggressive, having emotional outbursts, and behaving impulsively when faced with frustration (Schiavi et al., 1984). These men typically used rigid and overcontrolled defenses to limit aggressive expression. Those patients with lower-than-average IQ seemed to have a lower tolerance for control of aggression in provocative situations (Schiavi et al., 1984). The large majority of the offenses committed by the men with 47,XYY was against property; there were only two offenses involving personal violence.

Males with 47,XXY were found to be more submissive and demonstrated antiaggressiveness on psychological testing than were controls and men with 47,XYY (Schiavi et al., 1984). This supports information from case histories that when aggression occurs in patients with 47,XXY it has a more disguised and defended form, whereas in males with 47,XYY it has a more direct and unpremeditated form (Schiavi et al., 1984). It is almost as if an abrupt mood change occurs more readily in males with 47,XYY than in males with 47,XXY. These problems can be addressed in treatment, as described in the next section.

There was a significant relationship between testosterone levels and criminal convictions among all of the study participants, including the 46,XY men (Schiavi et al., 1984). Men with 47,XYY had higher levels of testosterone, LH, and FSH than their controls, but the testosterone levels did not correlate with levels of aggression on the psychological testing (Schiavi et al., 1984). Elevations in hormonal levels have not been seen in the males with 47,XYY who were identified at birth and studied longitudinally.

Treatment

Males with 47,XYY do well in the newborn and infancy period, and they do not have dysmorphic features or medical problems. They are usually not diagnosed prenatally, and there is no maternal age effect for 47,XYY (Abramsky and Chapple, 1997). However, individuals with 47,XYY are more likely to be diagnosed between the ages of 1 and 10 years than are males with 47,XXY (Abramsky et al., 1997). This is probably because their motor and language milestones are often delayed, and they usually have more severe behavioral problems, including tantrums, than males with 47,XXY. In the preschool period, patients with 47,XYY should have a detailed motor and language evaluation to assess possible delays and outline their therapy needs. Many boys with 47,XYY could benefit from both OT therapy and speech and language therapy, but the outcome of such therapy has not been studied. Such intervention not only may make a difference in motor and language areas but also may be helpful for the child's self-image and emotional development, which appear to be most problematic in these patients. Severe tantrums may be related to the sensory integration problems reported by Salbenblatt et al. (1987) and may respond to sensory-integration occupational therapy.

Significant behavior problems require a psychological evaluation and counseling intervention, which can help with behavioral management and can also be directed to improving problems with anxiety and depression. Counseling can work synergistically with psychotropic medication. Two patients have been reported whose depression responded to tricyclic medication, imipramine, and desipramine, in addition to counseling. SSRI agents that boost the serotonin level are considered more effective and safer to use in childhood for treatment of depression and anxiety than tricyclics. SSRI agents do not prolong cardiac conduction, do not cause death or arrythmias in overdose, do not irritate the liver, and do not require the testing of serum levels, so they are easier to use in addition to being safer than tricyclics. We have seen a positive response to SSRIs in two patients with 47,XYY syndrome (see case history of Cory).

Impulsive behavior and mood swings may be related to the presence of ADHD. One patient with 47,XYY reported by Ratcliffe et al. (1990) responded well to methylphenidate for treatment of his hyperactivity or ADHD. Controlled studies have not been carried out regarding the efficacy of stimulant medication for the impulsivity or ADHD problems in males with 47,XYY. However, these medications are medically indicated for ADHD problems and can be utilized when a diagnosis of ADHD is made (AACAP, 1997). Stimulants also improve motor coordination, auditory processing, and social skills, so they may be beneficial in additional ways in this population (Barkley, 1990). Stimulants can be combined with an SSRI agent, such as fluoxetine (Prozac), sertraline (Zoloft), or fluvoxamine (Luvox), which may be added to improve depression, anxiety, obsessive compulsive behavior, irritability/aggression, or disruptive behavior disorder (Zubieta and Alessi, 1993).

Clonidine is an alpha-adrenergic presynaptic agonist which lowers norepinephrine levels both centrally and peripherally. It has been used as an antihypertensive agent, and it has an overall calming effect for children with severe hyperactivity (Hagerman et al., 1998; Hunt et al., 1990). Clonidine may also be helpful for aggression in combination with ADHD, but the side effects include sedation. Clonidine is available in both a pill and a patch form (Catapres TTS patch), although the patch can be irritating to the skin in approximately 40% of patients (Hagerman et al., 1998). For more information about clonidine, see chapters 2 and 3 of this book.

When mood lability or aggression do not respond to stimulants, clonidine, or SSRI agents, then mood stabilizers, such as carbamazepine (Tegretol), valproic acid, gabapentin, and lithium should be considered. Ratcliffe et al. (1990) described one boy with 48,XXYY and severe tantrum behavior who was treated with carbamazepine when his EEG demonstrated a posterior spike wave discharge, although clinical seizures were not present. Carbamazepine, valproic acid, and gabapentin are anticonvulsants, as well as mood stabilizers, but they can improve mood instability even when the EEG is normal. This patient did well on carbamazepine, but it may have been because of carbamazepine's psychotropic effect.

When aggression is severe and does not respond to the stimulants, SSRIs, or mood stabilizers, or when thinking becomes distorted with psychotic elements, an antipsychotic agent may be necessary. Risperidone is a relatively new atypical antipsychotic which has a lower risk of long-term motor side effects such as tardive dyskinesias and extrapyramidal symptoms because of a combined serotonergic and dopaminergic blockade (Kapur and Remington, 1996). It is not only helpful in psychosis but also has been beneficial in patients with aggression or disruptive behavior and ADHD and in patients with pervasive developmental disorders and cognitive deficits (Fisman and Steel, 1991; Simeon et al., 1995). It is particularly helpful in treating paranoid ideation, aggressive and impulsive behavior, and mood swings (Simeon et al., 1995). A rare patient with 47,XYY has been described as having schizophrenia (Rajogopalan et al., 1998).

CASE HISTORY: CORY

Cory is now an 18-year-old young man with 47,XYY syndrome who has had a long history of behavioral problems, including ADHD.

His biological mother was a Cherokee Indian, but he was given up at birth by his biological mother and was in a foster home until he was adopted at 20 months of age. His developmental milestones were mildly delayed, with walking at 15 to 16 months, words at 2 years, and sentences at 3 years of age. In early childhood, he developed problems with distractibility, a short attention span, and hyperactivity. More significant problems developed in preschool, including frequent aggression and fighting. He had an explosive and unpredictable temper, which caused significant difficulties both at home and at school because of physical aggression toward himself and teachers. At 5 years of age he began speech and language therapy, which continued for 3 years. He did not qualify for special education help until he was in the sixth grade and having problems academically and behaviorally. At 7 years of age the WISC-R demonstrated a Verbal IQ of 97, a Performance IQ of 133, and a Full-Scale IQ of 116.

At 12 years of age, Cory was referred to our Child Development Unit because his aggressive behavior raised concern for possible fetal alcohol syndrome, although there was no known history of alcohol intake by his biological mother. He did not have physical features of fetal alcohol syndrome, and his height was greater than the 95th percentile for his age, his weight was at the 60th percentile for his age, and his head circumference was at the 70th percentile for his age. A genital exam demonstrated normal testicular volume, with a Tanner stage-2 pubertal development. His extremities were normal, deep tendon reflexes were 2+ and symmetrical, and his neurological examination was normal. Because of his tall stature and severe behavioral problems, cytogenetic testing was carried out and demonstrated a 47,XYY karyotype.

A methylphenidate (Ritalin) trial was recommended beginning at 5 mg twice a day to three times a day, but he became more aggressive on methylphenidate, so it was discontinued. He was enrolled in a day treatment program, which decreased his aggression and helped him to become more productive academically.

On reevaluation at age 16, Cory was in a high school setting where he was failing most of his subjects. Achievement testing Woodcock Johnson-Revised Achievement test at age 16 demonstrated a math score of 69, a reading score of 82, and a spelling score of 100. An overall psychological assessment included WISC-III testing, which demonstrated a Verbal IQ of 78, a Performance IQ of 100, and a Full-Scale IQ of 87. His lowest subtest scores were 2 on Comprehension, 4 on Arithmetic, 5 on Digit Span, 6 on Symbol Search, and 6 on Coding. His highest scores included 12 on Object Assembly and 12 on Picture Arrangement. At one point during the testing he suddenly became angry, abruptly left his seat, and walked out of the room. He also became more agitated when he was frustrated by the cognitive testing. His subtest scores demonstrated significant weaknesses, particularly in mathematical reasoning, which may affect his ability to develop the functional skills he will need to maintain a job. He also had a striking weakness on tasks measuring common sense reasoning and social judgment, which is reflective of his significant difficulty in making sound social decisions. He had severe problems with attention and concentration which appeared to interfere with his testing and may be part of the reason for his significant IQ drop from his test scores when he was 7 years of age.

His social-emotional evaluation was characterized by grandiose ideas, paranoid thinking, and loosely connected ideas. On projective testing he demonstrated avoidance of feelings, with boredom, confusion, or sleep substituting for most emotions; recurring images of death, suicide, or violent behavior; and disconnection between parents and children. He appeared to be depressed, although he was unable to label his feelings of sadness. He had feelings of worthlessness and loss, and his feelings of hurt and rejection appeared to be translated into extreme anger regarding his mother's remarriage. His loose thinking and somewhat paranoid and suspicious ideation were of great concern to the examiners. His overall diagnosis included depression, ADHD, and conduct disorder, in addition to a learning disorder with a deficit in verbal intellectual abilities. He was treated with paroxetine because of a previous negative response to fluoxetine and sertraline. One month later risperidone was started at a dose of 1 mg at bedtime. His paroxetine, which was increased to 20 mg a day, has improved his mood, and depression, and his risperidone has decreased his aggression, stabilized his mood, and improved his attentional problems and agitation.

Intensive counseling was also recommended for him, either privately or through the county mental health center. Although his medication and limited counseling have helped, he continues to have ongoing difficulties in school with academics, and he continues to be severely handicapped socially and emotionally. His volatile temper has interfered with his school progress and has also led to frequent job dismissals.

48,XXYY SYNDROME

Muldal and Ockey (1960) first described the 48,XXYY karyotype as the "double male." Since this description, over 100 patients have been documented in the medical literature, and these individuals are considered a variant of Klinefelter syndrome (Borgaonkar et al., 1970; Hasle et al., 1995; Meschede et al., 1995; Sorensen et al., 1978). Boys with 48,XXYY represent 2.3% of patients with KS (Hasle et al., 1995). There are important differences, however, between boys with 47,XXY and 48,XXYY, and some authors have questioned whether 48,XXYY males should be included under the umbrella of KS (Grammatico et al., 1990). Although males with 48,XXYY have the endocrine features of KS, they have more severe cognitive deficits, behavioral problems, and dysmorphic features than males with 47,XXY, as described in this section.

The incidence of 48,XXYY syndrome was originally estimated at 1 out of 50,000 (Sorensen et al., 1978), but a recent report found the 48,XXYY karyotype in 1 out of 17,000 males in a newborn screening (Nielsen and Wohlert, 1991). Because of the rarity of this disorder, longitudinal and unbiased data of a large group of patients identified through newborn screening are not available. Because most of the clinical information is based on a clinic-referred population who presented with cognitive or behavioral problems, there is likely a skewing of the information presented here toward more significant problems.

Physical and Endocrine Features

Males with 48,XXYY have the endocrine features of KS, including small testes, elevations of FSH and LH from puberty onward, and tall stature. In a survey of 53 cases, 62% of those older than 12 years had gynecomastia, 18% had a small penis, 54% had a female pubic hair distribution, and 6 out of 53 or 11%, had cryptorchidism (Borgaonkar et al., 1970). Children with 48,XXYY were generally tall, and 31% were above the 90th percentile (Borgaonkar et al., 1970). Of those patients older than 16 years, 80% were over 71 inches tall (Borgaonkar et al., 1970). In a review of 16 cases of 48,XXYY syndrome, the adult height was found to exceed the height of males with 47,XXY by about 3 inches (Ferguson-Smith, 1966). The testicular biopsies are similar to males with 47,XXY, including hyalinization of seminiferous tubules and fibrosis during puberty and adulthood and little or no spermatogenesis (Bloomgarden et al., 1980; Borgaonkar et al., 1970).

Minor skeletal abnormalities are more frequent in males with 48,XXYY than in males with 47,XXY, but there is no consistent finding that is helpful diagnostically (Figure 4.3). The skeletal problems may include digital abnormalities, such as shortened fingers or clinodactyly, cubitus valgus or varus, radioulnar synostosis, clubfoot, flat feet, kyphoscoliosis, lordosis, and hip abnormalities (Borgaonkar et al., 1970; Borghgraef et al., 1991; Linden et al., 1995). Dermatoglyphic findings have been unusual, including a reduced total ridge count, a frequent distally placed palmar triradius, simian crease in 21%, and an increased number of arches on the fingertips (Borgaonkar et al., 1970). Vascular problems are more frequent than what has been reported in males with 47,XXY and 47,XYY. Varicose veins and ulcers on the extremities were reported in 5 of 53 cases (Borgaonkar et al., 1970). The etiology of the vascular and ulcer problems has been debated, and there is evidence for arteriole involvement in the lower extremities, increased edema of the lower extremities, increased platelet aggregation, a deficit of fibrinolysis related to androgen deficiency, and enhanced thromboembolism (Grammatico et al., 1990).

Congenital heart disease is more common in 48,XXYY males than in 47,XXY or 47,XYY males, and it occurs in 8% (Meschede et al., 1995). Tetrology of Fallot, atrial septal defect, and pulmonic stenosis has been reported in males with 48,XXYY (reviewed by Meschede et al., 1995).

Neurological, Cognitive, and Behavioral Features

Epilepsy is more frequently seen in males with 48,XXYY than in males with 47,XXY or 47,XYY. Seizures or an abnormal EEG were reported in 23% of the 53 males with 48,XXYY surveyed by Borgaonkar et al. (1970). More recently seizures were found in three of four patients reported by Borghgraef et al. (1991), but seizures are often not mentioned in case reports (Linden et al., 1995).

A review of cognitive testing in 33 males with 48,XXYY demonstrated that

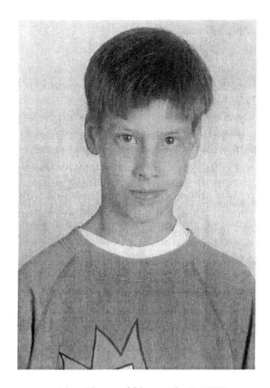

FIGURE 4.3: 12-year-old boy with 48,XXYY syndrome. He has a broad nasal bridge and mild epicanthal folds.

60% had an IQ less than 70, 30% had an IQ between 71 and 80, and 9% were
above 80, specifically 84, 87, and 90 (Borgaonkar et al., 1970). Speech and
language development is delayed, and the Verbal IQ is usually lower than the
Performance IQ, which is also typical of the 47,XXY males described previously.
Consistent motor testing has not been reported, but several patients have been
described as clumsy or having psychomotor delays.

Only 17% of 53 patients reviewed by Borgaonkar and colleagues (1970) are
described as having good social judgment; the other 83% are described as having
deviant behavior including aggression and delinquency. However, 66% of this
sample were karyotyped because of behavior problems or cognitive deficits (Borgaonkar et al., 1970). Subsequent clinical reports have emphasized shy and timid
behavior combined with sudden outbursts of anger leading to aggression or obstinate behavior. There seems to be a mood instability problem in many patients
not unlike what has been described for 47,XYY patients, although the shyness
and timidity of 47,XXY patients is also seen.

CASE HISTORY: DAVID (2)

David is now a 12-year-old boy who was diagnosed with 48,XXYY syndrome at 6 years of age after presenting with significant developmental delays and cognitive testing, demonstrating a Verbal IQ of 69, a Performance IQ of 78, and a Full-Scale IQ of 71 on the WISC-R. His mother had a normal pregnancy with him, and his birth weight was normal. He did well in the newborn period. He was described as an easy baby who rarely cried, and he slept most of the time. His developmental milestones were mildly delayed, with walking between 16 and 17 months, words at 2½ years of age, and short sentences at 3½ years of age. He was described as stiff and uncoordinated, and he was frequently frustrated with both language and motor tasks. He became more emotionally labile at 2 years of age, and tantrums were a frequent problem. He would become anxious or fearful in new situations, and in general he was fidgety and distractible but not overtly hyperactive. He has had difficulties with appropriate peer interactions because of his anxiety. He perseverates in language, frequently chews his nails, and has poor eye contact.

His medical history included recurrent otitis media infections in early childhood and a prophylactic 6-month course of antibiotics. Mitral valve prolapse was diagnosed after a cardiology evaluation that was precipitated by a history of fatigue and low energy. At 2 years of age he had a bilateral orchiopexy for undescended testicles.

In school David was placed in a self-contained special education program for children with significant limitations in intellectual capacity. He received speech and language therapy and occupational therapy through his special education program.

On examination at age 6, his height was at the 80th percentile, his weight was at the 50th percentile, and his head circumference was at the 60th percentile. He was shy and somewhat anxious during the exam, and he would verbalize in only single words or very short phrases. His ear pinnae were not prominent, but they were somewhat compressed superiorly. He had epicanthal folds bilaterally, with a mildly broad nasal bridge. He had a grade 1/6 systolic murmur, which was consistent with his mitral valve prolapse diagnosis. His genitalia demonstrated normal prepubertal development with testicles measuring 3 ml bilaterally. He had double-jointed thumbs and clinodactyly of the fifth finger bilaterally. Palmar creases were normal, and he had thin, long fingers. He had motor coordination problems on examination, including difficulty with alternating movements at fast rates. Tandem walking was mildly unstable, and he was only able to balance on either foot for 10 seconds and to hop on either foot for less than 10 hops. Visual motor coordination problems were seen in his design copying and handwriting.

David's treatment program included intensifying his speech and language therapy and adding sensory integration occupational therapy. He was tried on methylphenidate (Ritalin) at a dose of 5 mg twice a day, but it was not helpful for improving his attention span. At 9 years of age, sertraline (Zoloft) at a dose of one-half of a 50-mg tablet was tried to decrease his anxiety, mood lability, and tantrum behavior. Sertraline helped these problems, but it was subsequently discontinued after he improved in these areas.

In follow-up at age 11, he was having increasing problems with moodiness and outburst behavior occurring once per day in an abrupt fashion, although in general he was described as shy and quiet. He would yell, scream, cry, or even punch people who were near him when he became upset. Over the past 2 months, his mother felt that he experienced frequent anger and perhaps sadness. On one occasion he angrily cut his hair in an irregular fashion. It was recommended that he be placed back on sertraline at a dose of 50 mg in the morning and also have ongoing counseling. These interventions have dramatically decreased his outburst behavior, and his mood has improved. In school his attention and concentration problems persist, and he is quite distractible, particularly to noises outside of the classroom. When he is integrated into the regular classroom, he puts his head down on his desk and cries, so he has spent most of his time in a self-contained special education program. Academic testing at age 12 years 2 months, when he was in the sixth grade, demonstrated composite scores for reading and math at the 2.6 grade level on the Wechsler Individual Achievement Test. On the Woodcock-Johnson-Revised tests of cognitive ability, his Processing Speed Cluster Score was at the 2.6 grade level, and his Comprehension-Knowledge Cluster Score was at the 1.7 grade level. His age-equivalent score was 7 years 6 months on the Developmental Test of Visual Motor Integration, which is a standard score of 79.

He has not had problems with ulcers or leg aches, but his mother has noted that perfusion to his feet is sometimes poor, with a blue hue in his feet.

When violent or aggressive behavior is seen, it usually occurs impulsively and may be part of a generalized picture of ADHD as is seen in males with 47,XYY, as described previously. More significant cognitive deficits occur in the male with 48,XXYY than in the male with 47,XYY, and these cognitive problems can lead to an increase in frustration with many of the demands placed on the child both at home and at school. The cognitive deficits are also a marker for more severe CNS dysfunction, which in this patient population is often associated with poor self-control and mood instability. One male has been described with 48,XXYY and late-onset psychosis beginning at age 36 after a childhood marked by aggression, impulsivity and cognitive deficits (Verbal IQ of 54 and Performance IQ of 74; Lee, 1996). Having an additional X chromosome has been suggested to predispose an individual to schizophrenia, although this may be simply related to the cognitive and language deficits seen in individuals with an extra X (Crow, 1988).

Treatment

Usually individuals are now diagnosed with 48,XXYY syndrome because of language and motor delays noted within the first 4 years of life or because of behavior problems in early childhood including hyperactivity, impulsivity, or aggression. The work-up for individuals with 48,XXYY includes detailed language, motor, and psychological evaluations so that the severity of these problems can be documented to guide a treatment plan. Most of these individuals require OT and speech and language therapy to improve their motor and language development beginning in the preschool period.

The degree of impulsivity, inattentiveness, and hyperactivity should be carefully assessed because stimulant medication might be helpful for the child who has ADHD. Methylphenidate (Ritalin), dextroamphetamine (Dexedrine), Adderall (a mixture of four dextro- and levo-amphetamine salts), or pemoline (Cylert) may be helpful in controlling the impulsivity and aggression. Pemoline has been associated in rare instances with hepatic failure, so the other stimulants should be tried first (Adcock et al., 1998). Stimulants may also be helpful for controlling the abrupt outbursts of anger that have been described in childhood. Clonidine, described previously, may also be helpful for calming severe hyperactivity or improving aggression (Hagerman et al., 1998). If the clonidine causes significant sedation, then guanfacine (Tenex), a more selective alpha$_{2A}$-adrenergic presynaptic agonist, can be used.

Moodiness, irritability, and even aggression have been known to respond to SSRI agents in other disorders (see chapters 2 and 3 for a more complete discussion of serotonin agents), but there is a lack of even anecdotal evidence regarding the efficacy of serotonin agents in 48,XXYY syndrome. In our experience SSRIs can be helpful, as described in the previous case history, particularly for children with significant anxiety, depression, or a poor self-image. They will improve mood and decrease anxiety, which can be a precipitant of aggression.

More severe aggression or mood instability may require the use of mood-stabilizing agents, including valproic acid, carbamazepine, gabapentin, or lithium, but again there is a lack of even anecdotal evidence regarding the efficacy of these agents in the treatment of mood instability or aggression in patients with 48,XXYY syndrome. Risperidone, a new atypical antipsychotic agent that blocks both dopamine and serotonin receptors, has been shown to be helpful in the treatment of aggression in combination with ADHD or PDD, as described previously (Fisman and Steel, 1991; Simeon et al., 1995). We have seen a benefit of this medication in one boy with 48,XXYY syndrome (Figure 4.4).

CASE HISTORY: JACK

Jack is a 6½-year-old boy who was referred for evaluation to our Child Development Unit because of behavioral difficulties. His birth weight was normal, 7 lbs. 13 oz., but he had mild difficulties with sucking and feeding during the first few days of life. He subsequently had gastroesophageal reflux and esophagitis in the first few weeks of life, which gradually resolved. Recurrent ear infections in the first year required PE tube placement at 10 months of age. He had pneumonia at 2 years of age and subsequently had chronic respiratory problems with reactive airway disease.

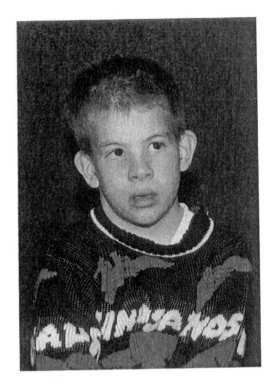

FIGURE 4.4: 6½-year-old boy with 48,XXYY syndrome. Note broad nasal bridge, epicanthal folds, and prominent ears.

His developmental milestones were delayed, with sitting at approximately 8 months, crawling at 12 months, and walking at 18 months. He began to use single words at 3 years of age and two-word phrases at 4 years of age. Because of his severe language delays and mildly dysmorphic features, cytogenetic testing was done and revealed a karyotype of 48,XXYY.

At approximately 3 years of age, Jack developed significant hyperactivity combined with aggression, which became a problem for his developmental preschool program. Because of these difficulties, he was placed on clonidine, with one-half of a 0.1 mg tablet three times a day. The clonidine had a calming effect, but it also caused sedation. On one occasion, he climbed up into the cupboard and overdosed on clonidine, which required hospitalization, so this medication was discontinued. Methylphenidate (Ritalin) was also tried at approximately 3½ years of age, but it caused side effects, including irritability and hyperactivity, and it was discontinued. Dextroamphetamine (Dexedrine) was subsequently started in treatment of his ADHD, beginning at 2.5 mg in the morning and 2.5 mg in the afternoon. This medication helped his concentration and overactivity, but it has not improved his aggressive or oppositional behavior. He seems to become aggressive with very minimal provocation, and oppositional behavior also occurs subsequently. He has smeared feces on the walls and windows at home, and he has a history of being cruel to the family's new puppy. On one occasion he attempted to set fire to his room after obtaining a lighter. His mother feels that he knows that he is different, and that this is causing a great difficulty with his self-esteem. He also stuffs cotton balls up his nose, and these have been removed several times by the parents, although on one occasion it required a surgical intervention.

Psychological testing at age 5½ using the Kaufman Assessment Battery for children demonstrated a Mental Processing Composite of 79, with Sequential Processing at 83 and Simultaneous Processing at 80. On the Vineland he had a Communication score of 53, Daily Living of 45, Socialization of 55, Motor of 46, and an overall Adaptive Behavior Composite of 46.

On examination at age 6½, Jack's height is at the 75th percentile, weight is at the 80th percentile, and head circumference is at the 75th percentile. He has a broad nasal bridge with epicanthal folds and slightly prominent ears. His palate is somewhat high-arched, his hair is coarse, and he has a double whorl centrally. His posterior hairline is low, and he has a short broad neck, with a hint of neck webbing. Blood pressure and heart rate were normal, and heart exam was normal. Testes are descended (3 ml bilaterally), and he has a normal phallus. His finger joints are mildly hyperextensible, and he has a bridged palmar crease bilaterally. His extremities show mild hypotonia, with upper and lower extremity deep tendon reflexes at 1+ bilaterally.

Because of the severity of his aggression, even with dextroamphetamine at a dose of 10 mg three times per day, risperidone was started beginning at 0.5 mg at bedtime, and intensive counseling was recommended. So far the risperidone has helped to decrease his aggression, but outbursts still occur, so the dose was increased to 1 mg at bedtime. This dose has been more effective for him without significant side effects, and counseling has been initiated.

Males with 48,XXYY have the endocrine problems associated with KS and should be treated with testosterone therapy as described previously. One 31-year-old male with 48,XXYY was successfully treated with 200 mg of IM depotestosterone once a month (Sourial and Fenton, 1988). He experienced an improvement in self-image after the development of appropriate secondary sexual characteristics. On testosterone, he also experience a decrease in his sexual fantasies, which were associated with impulsivity and aggression. He was also successfully treated with propranolol (10 mg three times a day) for a coarse tremor in his hands.

Another patient with 48,XXYY syndrome diagnosed at age 27 subsequently underwent a trial of methyltestosterone but experienced "touchy, grumpy, changeable" behavior and exacerbation of aggression with treatment, so methyltestosterone was discontinued (Lee, 1996). This patient was subsequently diagnosed with psychosis after he developed auditory hallucinations, delusions of control, thought insertion, and thought broadcasting (Lee, 1996). The psychotic process may have interfered with his androgen therapy, making this an unusual case. In general, testosterone therapy is recommended at 12 years of age before the LH and FSH levels rise as described previously in 47,XXY syndrome (Meikle et al., 1998; Winter, 1990).

CONCLUSIONS AND FUTURE DIRECTIONS

Males with SCA may experience a variety of learning and behavior problems that may not be diagnosed until adulthood. Lifelong struggles with these difficulties, combined with family dysfunction, can lead to a poor outcome in our society. Clinicians must consider SCAs in tall males who have language and motor problems combined with mood fluctuations or outburst behavior. Early and intensive intervention that combines motor and language therapy with special education support and counseling will lead to the best outcome. Psychopharmacology can also be helpful for attentional problems and mood fluctuations, but we are only in the early stages of documenting benefit. A focus on the mood instability problem is important, particularly for the subgroup with intermittent aggression. Future work needs to include controlled studies which have neuropsychological and emotional measures to document the benefits of psychopharmacological intervention. Innovative educational programs, such as Fast Forward and other computer technology, should be studied in a controlled fashion to document their efficacy in improving auditory processing and other language deficits for children with SCAs. Further studies of the environmental factors and the background genetic factors that put a subgroup of individuals with SCAs at high risk for a poor prognosis will allow clinicians to target this group for the most intensive and efficacious intervention available.

ACKNOWLEDGMENTS   I thank Mary Linden, Bruce Bender, James Salbenblatt, Arthur Robinson, Sheila Tunnel, Mrs. Parent, Mrs. Capps, Mr. Corbett, and Mrs. Gamboa and Mrs. Renee Rupe for critically reviewing this manuscript and giving me cogent comments to improve the quality of this work. The MCH training grant no. MCJ-089413 and the Children's Hospital Research Foundation partially supported this work.

REFERENCES

AACAP (1997) Practice parameters for the assessment and treatment of children, adolescents, and adults with attention deficit hyperactivity disorder. Journal of American Academy of Child and Adolescent Psychiatry 36 (Suppl. 10): 085S–121S.

Abramsky, L., and Chapple, J. (1997)

47,XXY (Klinefelter syndrome) and 47,XYY: Estimated rates of and indication for postnatal diagnosis with implications for prenatal counselling. Prenatal Diagnosis 17 (4): 363–8.

Adcock, K. G., MacElroy, D. E., Wolford, E. T., Farrington, E. A. (1998) Pemoline therapy resulting in liver transplantation. Annals of Pharmacotherapy 32: 422–4.

Arps, S., Koske-Westphal, T., Meinecke, P., Meschede, D., Nieschlag, E., Harprecht, W., Steuber, E., Back, E., Wolff, G., Kerber, S., Held, K. (1996) Isochromosome Xq in Klinefelter syndrome: Report of 7 new cases. American Journal of Medical Genetics 64 (4): 580–2.

Bagatell, C. J., and Bremner, W. J. (1996) Androgens in men — uses and abuses. New England Journal of Medicine 334 (11): 707–14.

Barkley, R. A. (1990) Attention deficit hyperactivity disorder: A handbook for diagnosis and treatment. Guilford, New York.

Begum, R. W. (1996) Social skills lessons and activities. Center for Applied Research in Education, West Nyack, New York.

Bender, B. G., Fry, E., Pennington, B., Puck, M., Salbenblatt, J., Robinson, A. (1983) Speech and language development in 41 children with sex chromosome anomalies. Pediatrics 71 (2): 262–7.

Bender, B. G., Linden, M. G., Robinson, A. (1987) Environment and developmental risk in children with sex chromosome abnormalities. Journal of the American Academy of Child and Adolescent Psychiatry 26: 499–503.

Bender, B. G., Harmon, R. J., Linden, M. G., Robinson, A. (1995) Psychosocial adaptation of 39 adolescents with sex chromosome abnormalities. Pediatrics 96 (2, Pt. 1): 302–8.

Bertelloni, S., Baroncelli, G., Battini, R., Saggese, G. (1996) Central precocious puberty in Klinefelter syndrome: A case report with longitudinal follow-up of growth pattern. American Journal of Medical Genetics 65 (1): 52–5.

Bloomgarden, Z. T., Delozier, C. D., Cohen, M. P., Kasselberg, A. G., Engel, Rabin, D. (1980) Genetic and endocrine findings in a 48, XXYY male. Journal of Clinical Endocrinology and Metabolism 50 (4): 740–3.

Bloomquist, M. L. (1996) Skills training for children with behavior disorders: A parent and therapist guide book. Guilford, New York.

Borgaonkar, D. S., Mules, E., Char, F. (1970) Do the 48, XXYY males have a characteristic phenotype? Clinical Genetics 1: 272–93.

Borghgraef, M., Fryns, J. P., Smeets, E., Marien, J., van den Berghe, H. (1988) The 49,XXXXY syndrome. Clinical and psychological follow-up data. Clinical Genetics 33: 429–34.

Borghgraef, M., Fryns, J. P., Van Den Berghe, H. (1991) The 48,XXYY syndrome: Follow-up data on clinical characteristics and psychological findings in 4 patients. Genetic Counseling 2 (2): 103–8.

Bradbury, J. T., Bunge, R. G., Boccabella, R. A. (1956) Chromatin test in Klinefelter's syndrome. Journal of Clinical Endocrine Metabolism 16: 689.

Butler, M. G., Hedges, L. K., Rogan, P. K., Seip, J. R., Cassidy, S. B., Moeschler, J. B. (1997) Klinefelter and trisomy X syndromes in patients with Prader-Willi syndrome and uniparental maternal disomy of chromosome 15 — a coincidence? [Letter to the editor]. American Journal of Medical Genetics 72 (1): 111–4.

Crandall, B. F., Lebherz, T. B., Rubinstein, L., Robertson, R. D., Sample, W. F., Sarti, D., Howard, J. (1980) Chromosome findings in 2,500 second trimester amniocenteses. American Journal of Medical Genetics 5 (4): 345–56.

Crow, T. J. (1988) Sex chromosomes and psychosis. British Journal of Psychiatry 153: 675–83.

Ferguson-Smith, M. A. (1966) Sex chromatin, Klinefelter's syndrome and mental deficiency. In: The sex chromatin. Moore, K. L. (ed.). Saunders, Philadelphia, pp. 277–315.

Fisman, S., and Steele, M. (1991) Use of risperidone in pervasive developmental disorders: A case series. Journal of Child and Adolescent Psychopharmacology 6 (3): 177–190.

Frankel, F., Myatt, R., Cantwell, D. P., Feinberg, D. T. (1997) Parent-assisted transfer of children's social skills training: Effects on children with and without attention-deficit hyperactivity disorder. Journal of the American Academy of Child and Adolescent Psychiatry 36 (8): 1056–64.

Fryns, J. P., and Van den Berghe, H. (1988) The concurrence of Klinefelter syndrome and fragile X syndrome. American Journal of Medical Genetics 30: 109–13.

Graham, J. M., Bashir, A. S., Stark, R. E., Silbert, A., Walzer, S. (1988) Oral and written language abilities of XXY boys: Implications for anticipatory guidance. Pediatrics 81: 795–806.

Grammatico, P., Bottoni, U., De Sanctis, S., Sulli, N., Tonanzi, T., Onorio, A. C., Del Porto, G. (1990) A male patient with 48,XXYY syndrome: Importance of distinction from Klinefelter's syndrome. Clinical Genetics 38: 74–8.

Hagerman, R. J., Bregman, J. D., Tirosh, E. (1998) Clonidine. In Psychotropic medication and developmental disabilities: The international consensus handbook. Reiss, S., and Aman, M. G. (eds.). Ohio State University Nisonger Center, Columbus, Ohio, pp. 259–69.

Hasle, H., Mellemgaard, A., Nielsen, J., Hansen, J. (1995) Cancer incidence in men with Klinefelter syndrome. British Journal of Cancer 71 (2): 416–20.

Hook, E. B., Cross, P. K., Schreinemachers, D. M. (1983) Chromosomal abnormalitiy rates at amniocentesis and in live-born infants. Journal of the American Medical Association 249 (15): 2034–8.

Hunt, R. D., Capper, L., O'Connell, P. (1990) Clonidine in child and adolescent psychiatry. Journal of Child and Adolescent Psychopharmacology 1: 87–102.

Jacobs, P. A., Brunton, M., Melville, M. M., Brittain, R. P., McClemont, W. F. (1965) Aggressive behavior, mental sub-normality and the XYY male. Nature 208 (17): 1351–2.

Kapur, S., and Remington, G. (1996) Serotonin-dopamine interaction and its relevance to schizophrenia. American Journal of Psychiatry 153: 466–76.

Klinefelter, H. F., Reifenstein, E. C., Albright, F. (1942) Syndrome characterized by gynecomastia aspermatogenes without A-leydigism and increased excretion of follicle stimulating hormone. Journal of Clinical Endocrine Metabolism 2: 615–27.

Laron, Z., Dickerman, Z., Zamir, R., Galatzer, A. (1982) Paternity in Klinefelter's syndrome: A case report. Archives of Andrology 8: 149–51.

Lee, J. W. (1996) An XXYY male with schizophrenia. Australian and New Zealand Journal of Psychiatry 30 (4): 553–6.

Linden, M. G., and Robinson, A. (1991) Transdermal testosterone supplementation in adolescent males with Klinefelter syndrome. Clinical Research 39: 97.

Linden, M. G., Bender, B. G., Robinson, A. (1995) Sex chromosome tetrasomy and pentasomy. Pediatrics 96 (4, Pt. 1): 672–82.

Linden, M. G., Bender, B. G., Robinson, A. (1996) Intrauterine diagnosis of sex chromosome aneuploidy. Obstetrics and Gynecology 87 (3): 468–75.

Lomelino, C. A., and Reiss, A. L. (1991) 49, XXXXY syndrome: Behavioural and developmental profiles. Journal of Medical Genetics 28: 609–12.

Mandoki, M. W., and Sumner, G. S. (1991) Klinefelter syndrome: The need for early identification and treatment. Clinical Pediatrics 30 (3): 161–4.

Meikle, A. W., Dobs, A. S., Arver, S., Caramelli, K. E., Sanders, S. W., Mazer, N. A. (1998) Androgen replacement in the treatment of Klinefelter's syndrome: Efficacy and safety of a non-scrotal permeation-enhanced testosterone transdermal system. Endocrine Practice 4 (1): 17–22.

Meschede, D., Nekarda, T., Kececioglu, D., Loser, H., Vogt, J., Miny, P., Horst, J. (1995) Congenital heart disease in the 48,XXYY syndrome. Clinical Genetics 48 (2): 100–2.

Miller, M. E., and Sulkes, S. (1988) Firesetting behavior in individuals with Klinefelter syndrome. Pediatrics 82: 115–7.

Muldal, S., and Ockey, C. H. (1960) Double male: New chromosome constitution in Klinefelter's syndrome. Lancet 2: 492–3.

Mundy, J. (1991) Let's talk. Western Psychological Services, Los Angeles.

Netley, C., Taylor, M. J., Molan, M. (1995) Event-related potentials (ERPs) and intelligence in neonatally identified 47,XXY males. Clinical Genetics 47 (3): 150–4.

Nielsen, J., and Wohlert, M. (1990) Sex chromosome abnormalities found among 34,910 newborn children: Results from a 13-year study in Arhus, Denmark. In: Children and young adults with sex chromosomes aneuploidy. Evans, J. A., Hamerton, J. L., Robinson, A. (eds.). Wiley Liss for the National Foundation, March of Dimes, New York. Birth Defects: Original Article Sseries 26 (4): 209–23.

Polani, P. E. (1977) Abnormal sex chromosomes, behaviour mental disorders. In Developments in psychiatric research. Tanner, J. M. (ed.). Hodder and Stoughton, London, pp. 89–128.

Price, W. H., and Whatmore, P. B. (1967) Behavior disorders and pattern of crime among XYY males identified at a maximum security hospital. British Medical Journal 1: 533–6.

Rajogopalan, M., MacBeth, R., Varma, S. L. (1998) XYY chromosome anomaly and schizophrenia. American Journal of Medical Genetics (Neuropsychiatric Genetics) 81: 64–5.

Ratcliffe, S. G., and Field, M. A. S. (1982) Emotional disorders in XYY children: Four case reports. Journal of Child Psychology and Psychiatry 23 (4): 401–6.

Ratcliffe, S. G., Butler, G. E., Jones, M. (1990) Edinburgh study of growth and development of children with sex chromosome abnormalities. In: Children and young adults with sex chromosomes aneuploidy. Evans, J. A., Hamerton, J. L., Robinson, A. (eds.). Wiley Liss for the National Foundation, March of Dimes, New York. Birth Defects: Original Article Series 26 (4): 1–44.

Robinson, A., Bender, B., Borelli, J., Winter, J. S. (1986) Sex chromosome aneuploidy, prospective and longitudinal studies. In Ratcliffe, S. G., and Paul, N. (eds.). Vol. 22. Liss, New York, pp. 23–71.

Robinson, A., Bender, B. G., Linden, M. G., Salbenblatt, J. A. (1990) Sex chromosome aneuploidy: The Denver Prospective Study. In: Children and young adults with sex chromosomes aneuploidy. Evans, J. A., Hamerton, J. L., Robinson, A. (eds.). Wiley Liss for the National Foundation, March of

Dimes, New York. Birth Defects: Original Article Series 26 (4): 59–115.

Robinson, A., Bender, B. G., Linden, M. G. (1992) Prognosis of prenatally diagnosed children with sex chromosome aneuploidy. American Journal of Medical Genetics 44 (3): 365–8.

Rovet, J., Netley, C., Keenan, M., Bailey, J., Stewart, D. (1996) The psychoeducational profile of boys with Klinefelter syndrome. Journal of Learning Disabilities 29 (2): 180–96.

Salbenblatt, J. A., Bender, B. G., Puck, M. H., Robinson, A., Faiman, C., Winter, J. S. D. (1985) Pituitary-gonadal function in Klinefelter syndrome before and during puberty. Pediatric Research 19 (1): 82–6.

Salbenblatt, J. A., Meyers, D. C., Bender, B. G., Linden, M. G., Robinson, A. (1987) Gross and fine motor development in 47,XXY and 47,XYY males. Pediatrics 80 (2): 240–4.

Scheike, O., Visfeldt, J., Petersen, B. (1973) Breast carcinoma in association with the Klinefelter's syndrome. Acta Pathological Microbiologica Scandinavica 81: 352–8.

Schiavi, R. C., Theilgaard, A., Owen, D. R., White, D. (1984) Sex chromosome anomalies, hormones, and aggressivity. Archives of General Psychiatry 41: 93–9.

Simeon, J. G., Carrey, N. J., Wiggens, D. M., Milin, R. P., Hosenbocus, S. N. (1995) Risperidone effects in treatment-resistent adolescents: Preliminary case reports. Journal of Child and Adolescent Psychopharmacology 5 (1): 69–79.

Sorensen, K., Nielsen, J., Jacobsen, P., Rolle, T. (1978) The 48,XXYY syndrome. Journal of Mental Deficiency Research 22: 197–205.

Sourial, N., and Fenton, F. (1988) Testosterone treatment of an XXYY male presenting with aggression: A case report. Canadian Journal of Psychiatry 33: 846–50.

Stein, M. B., and Siddiqui, A. R. (1986) Acute paranoid disorder and Klinefelter's syndrome. Canadian Journal of Psychiatry 31: 434–5.

Stewart, D. A., Bailey, J. D., Netley, C. T., Park, E. (1990) Growth, development, and behavioral outcome from mid-adolescence to adulthood in subjects with chromosome aneuploidy: The Toronto study. In: Children and young adults with sex chromosomes aneuploidy. Evans, J. A., Hamerton, J. L., Robinson, A. (eds.). Wiley Liss for the National Foundation, March of Dimes, New York. Birth Defects: Original Article Series 26 (4): 131–88.

Tallal, P., Miller, S. L., Bedi, G., Byma, G., Wang, X., Nagarajan, S. S., Schreiner, C., Jenkins, W. M., Merzenich, M. M. (1996) Language comprehension in language-learning impaired children improved with acoustically modified speech [see comments]. Science 271 (5245): 81–4.

Theilgaard, A. (1984) A psychological study of the personalities of XYY and XXY men. Acta Psychiatrica Scandinavia 315: 1–133.

Virkkunen, M., Nutila, A., Goodwin, F. K., et al. (1987) Cerebralspinal fluid monoamine metabolite levels in male arsonists. Archives of General Psychiatry 44: 241–7.

Walzer, S., Bashir, A. S., Silbert, A. R. (1990) Cognitive and behavioral factors in the learning disabilities of 47,XXY and 47,XYY boys. In: Children and young adults with sex chromosomes aneuploidy. Evans, J. A., Hamerton, J. L., Robinson, A. (eds.). Wiley Liss for the National Foundation, March of Dimes, New York. Birth Defects: Original Article Series 26 (4): 45–58.

Winter, J. S. D. (1990) Androgen therapy in Klinefelter syndrome during adolescence. In: Children and young adults with sex chromosomes aneuploidy.

Evans, J. A., Hamerton, J. L., Robinson, A. (eds.). Wiley Liss for the National Foundation, March of Dimes, New York. Birth Defects: Original Article Series 26 (4): 235–45.

Zubieta, J. K., and Alessi, N. E. (1993) Is there a role of serotonin in the disruptive behavior disorders? A literature review. Journal of Child and Adolescent Psychopharmacology 3 (1): 11–35.

RESOURCES

Klinefelter Syndrome and Associates, Inc. (KS & Associates)
P.O. Box 119
Roseville, CA 95678-0119
Contact: Melissa Aylstock, Executive Director
telephone: (916) 773-1449
fax: (916) 773-1449
http://www.genetic.org
e-mail: ks47xxy@ix.netcom.com

XXY Network
Contact: Robert Grace
telephone: 209-533-2679
e-mail: xxynetwork@mlode.com

Support for XXY adults and parents of boys with XXY syndrome

Contact: Renee Rupe
4336 S. Kalispell Circle
Aurora, CO 80015
telephone: (303) 766-2050
e-mail: amazonb@worldnet.att.net

Support for parents of boys and adults with XXYY syndrome

Children's Kluge Center (Klinefelter Clinic University of Virginia)
Contact: Shirley Berry
telephone: (800) 627-8596

Contact: Allan D. Rogol, MD, PhD
telephone: (804) 924-5895
e-mail: ADR2hscmail.mcc.virginia.edu

Alliance of Genetic Support Groups
35 Wisconsin Circle, Suite 440
Chevy Chase, MD 20815

telephone: (301) 336-GENE
http://www.medhelp.org/www/agsg.htm

National Organization for Rare Disorders, Inc. (NORD)
Fairwood Professional Bldg.
100 Route 37
New Fairfield, CT 06812
(203) 746-6518
http://www.nord-rdb.com/~orphan

Klinefelter Syndrome Brochures

Understanding Klinefelter Syndrome
National Institutes of Child Health and Development (NICHD).
P.O. Box 29111
Washington, DC 20040

There is no charge for this booklet.

Klinefelter Syndrome
Klinefelter Syndrome and Associates.
P.O. Box 119
Roseville, CA 95678-0119

There is no charge for this pamphlet.

Klinefelter's Syndrome, The X-tra Special Boy and For Boys Only, A Supplement
Diane Plumridge, Christene Barkost, and Stephen LaFranchi.

You can order the above informative Klinefelter Syndrome pamphlets for $3.50 for the main pamphlet and $1.25 for the supplement from the Oregon Health Sciences University at the following

address. (Make checks payable to Child Development and Rehabilitation Center.)
Attn: CDRC Publications
Oregon Health Sciences University, CDRC
P.O. Box 574
Portland, Oregon 97207
telephone: (503) 279-8342

Klinefelter's Syndrome—An Orientation
Johannes Neilson.
Turner Center
Cytogenetic Laboratory
Skovagervej 2
DK-8240 Risskov, Denmark

There is no charge for this booklet.

Books

The student with a genetic disorder.
Plumridge, D., Bennett, R., Dinno, N., Branson, C.
Springfield, IL: Thomas.

Describes the educational implications for special education teachers and for physical therapists, occupational therapists, and speech pathologists. Available from Charles C. Thomas, 2600 South First St., Springfiled, IL 62794-9265. ISBN 0-398-05839-3. $75.95 hardback, $39.95 softback

Web Sites

http://www.genetic.org/ks/index.shtml
Klinefelter Syndrome and Associates is a nonprofit support organization for the genetic condition Klinefelter Syndrome and its variants.

http://www.genetic.org
This site is sponsored by Klinefelter Syndrome and Associates and is designed to provide support and education for families and professionals dealing with genetic conditions.

http://www.tmoon.com/ks/ks.htm
A mother of a Klinefelter syndrome boy tells her story.

http://www.medhelp.org/www/agsg.htm
The Alliance of Genetic Support Groups is a nonprofit organization dedicated tohelping individuals and families who have genetic disorders.

http://ajoupath.ajou.ac.Kr/bulletin/bulletin.html
An XYY discussion board

http://home.att.net/~amazonb
For information regarding XXYY syndrome

5

Sex Chromosome Aneuploidy in Females

This chapter will focus on the most common sex chromosomal aneuploidies (SCAs) that occur in females: Turner syndrome, which involves loss of all or part of the second X chromosome, and 47,XXX syndrome, in addition to tetrasomy, 48,XXXX, and pentasomy, 49,XXXXX. Approximately 1 of 2,500 newborn females has Turner syndrome, but the majority (99%) of all 45,X pregnancies are aborted spontaneously in early pregnancy, usually before amniocentesis is performed (Hook and Warburton, 1983). It is likely that over 1% of conceptions involve X chromosome loss and that 10% of spontaneously aborted fetuses have a 45,X karyotype (Neely and Rosenfeld, 1994; Rosenfeld et al., 1994). The incidence of 47,XXX syndrome is 1 per 1,000, making it the most common SCA in females (Nielsen and Wohlert, 1990).

TURNER SYNDROME

Although Otto Ullrich in 1930 described a case that was later defined as X monosomy in the German literature, it is Henry Turner who is credited with describing this syndrome when he reported seven patients with short stature, congenital webbed neck, sexual infantilism, and cubitus valgus in 1938 (Turner, 1938). Gonadal dysgenesis or streak ovaries were identified in 1944 as the cause of sexual infantilism in this syndrome, and Ullrich subsequently described lymphadema and excessive neck folds in infancy in 1949 (Ullrich, 1949). It was not until 1959 that the phenotype in Turner syndrome (TS) was found to be associated with X chromosome monosomy (45,X) (Ford et al., 1959). Several large series of

Neurodevelopmental Disorders: Diagnosis and Treatment, by Randi Jenssen Hagerman. New York: Oxford University Press, 1999. © Oxford University Press, Inc.

cytogenetic abnormalities associated with TS have been reported; these are reviewed by Neely and Rosenfeld (1994). Over 50% of patients with TS have 45,X, approximately 6% of patients have 46,X,iso(Xq), and 30% of patients have mosaicism, usually with 45,X/46,XX or 45,X/46,X,iso(Xq), although rarer types of mosaicism such as 45,X/46,XY and 45,X/47,XXX have also been reported (Neely and Rosenfeld, 1994). Occult mosaicism may be more common, and it is postulated that mosaicism with a normal cell line in the fetal membranes may be necessary for adequate placental function and fetal survival (Saenger, 1996). In general, individuals with mosaicism have fewer physical and cognitive features than individuals with the 45,X karyotype, as described in the following sections.

Physical Phenotype

Facial Features

The typical facial features of TS, including neck webbing (pterygium colli) and a low posterior hairline, are related to fetal lymphatic obstruction. This problem also causes downward slanting of the eyes, epicanthal folds, and posterior rotation of the ears (Figure 5.1). Other physical features associated with the lymphatic

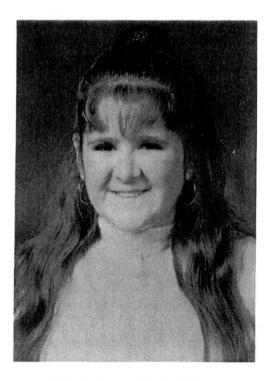

FIGURE 5.1:   A 15-year-old girl with Turner syndrome.

drainage problem include edema of the hands and feet noted at birth, characteristic dermatoglyphics, and nail dysplasia. The nails may be hypoplastic (underdeveloped), hyperconvex, or even upturned. The skeletal dysplasia associated with TS causes a small jaw (micrognanthia) and a high arched palate. Typical physical features associated with TS are outlined in Table 5.1.

Bone and Growth Abnormalities

Short stature and growth failure are the hallmarks of the TS phenotype, and the cause appears to be a combination of skeletal dysplasia, growth hormone secretion dysfunction, and estrogen deficiency (Neely and Rosenfeld, 1994). Intrauterine growth is mildly retarded, with a mean reduction of birth weight of 540 grams and 2.8 cm in birth length compared to normals (Neely and Rosenfeld, 1994). Growth velocity in the first 3 years of life is normal, but a progressive decline in growth velocity for the rest of childhood is present, and there is no pubertal growth spurt in adolescence (Neely and Rosenfeld, 1994). By 10½ years of age the whole growth curve for TS is below the 5th percentile of the normal growth curve. Standards for growth have been published for TS, and they are helpful to judge the effectiveness of growth hormone therapy in TS (Naeraa and Nielsen, 1990).

Patients with TS appear to be stocky, having short legs and a square-shaped torso and shield-like chest with the appearance of a wide internipple distance. Hypoplasia of the cervical vertebrae contributes to the short neck and short stature (Rosenfeld, 1989). The bone dysplasia includes a number of abnormalities, including a short fourth metacarpal, a wide carrying angle of the lower arms (cubitus valgus, which is caused by a developmental abnormality of the trochlear head); genu valgum, or bowing out of the lower legs; tufting of the distal phalanges; and a bayonet deformity of the wrists, resulting in lateral and dorsal bowing of the radius and occasional subluxation of the distal ulna (Rosenfeld, 1989). There is limited evidence of osteopenia with coarse trabecular pattern of the vertebrae or carpal bone seen on X-ray, but this may be secondary to the estrogen deficiency in TS (Neely and Rosenfeld, 1994).

Sexual Development

Although the ovaries of fetuses with TS are normal in the first trimester, there is a degeneration process of the oogonia and oocytes that leads to fibrosis of the ovary, usually by the time of birth (Rosenfeld, 1989). The fibrosis leads to streak ovaries, and the uterus is usually hypoplastic. The high frequency of mosaicism may allow for some functional ovarian tissue in a limited number of patients so that early breast development may occasionally be seen and a rare patient may menstruate in early puberty. The loss of the short arm only of the X is associated with a higher prevalence of retained ovarian function, including nonstreak ovaries and early breast development (Neely and Rosenfeld 1994). Testosterone production from the adrenals may allow for pubic or axillary hair. The ovarian failure leads to elevations of gonadotropins, follicle stimulating hormone (FSH), and

TABLE 5.1: Phenotypic Features of
Turner Syndrome

Phenotypic feature	Percentage with problem
Growth	
short stature	100
short neck	40
cubitus valgus	47
short metacarpals	37
genu valgum	35
micrognathia	60
high arched palate	38
nail dysplasia	13
Head and Neck	
webbed neck	25
low posterior hairline	42
strabismus	18
ptosis	11
Cardiac	
coarctation of aorta	20
bicuspid aortic valve	34–50
aortic root dilation	10
Renal	
double collecting systems	8
horseshoe kidney	7
renal abnormalities	6
obstruction	6
absent kidney	3
Reproductive	
gonadal failure	96
infertility	99
Miscellaneous	
multiple pigmented nevi	26
Hashimoto's thyroiditis	34
hypothyroidism	10
hypertension	7

Adapted from Lippe (1990), Neely and Rosenfeld (1994),
and Rosenfield (1989).

luteinizing hormone (LH) after age 10 years (Rosenfeld, 1989); and, when sensitive assays are employed, these elevations may be seen in early to mid-childhood.

Only a few successful pregnancies have occurred naturally in women with TS, and most of these individuals have mosaicism. It is important to explain to the families that gonadal failure is most probable but that 10 to 20% of patients may initiate puberty, 2% to 8% may menstruate, and fewer than 1% will have a successful pregnancy naturally (Rosenfeld, 1989; Saenger, 1996).

Cardiovascular and Renal Abnormalities

There is some evidence that the edema present in utero is the cause of the cardiovascular problems associated with TS (Neely and Rosenfeld, 1994). The two most common problems are coarctation of the aorta (narrow or stenotic area of the aorta) seen in 20% and bicuspid aortic valve seen in 34 to 50% (Saenger, 1996) (see also Table 5.1). Dilation of the aortic root may also occur. These defects predispose patients to aortic stenosis, bacterial endocarditis, hypertension, and on rare occasion aortic dissection or aneurysm (dilation of the vessel wall). In a mail survey, 15 of 237 respondents (6.3%) had aortic dilation and two of these patients had a dissection, which can be catastrophic (Lin et al. 1998). Pregnancy is a high-risk time for aortic dissection, and two patients with TS have died suddenly in pregnancy with this complication (Lin et al., 1998).

Approximately one-third of patients with TS have renal abnormalities, as noted in Table 5.1, but these problems are more common in individuals with the 45,X karyotype (45%) than in all of the other karyotypes combined (18%) (Neely and Rosenfeld, 1994). Approximately 6% of individuals with TS have an obstruction of the collecting system, and they require urological referral because surgery may be necessary. Abnormalities of the renal vascular system may lead to hypertension.

Molecular Clinical Correlations

Early cytogenetic studies suggested that deletions of the short arm of the X more frequently resulted in short stature, whereas deletions of the long arm more frequently lead to ovarian dysgenesis. Ovarian dysgenesis occurred in 93% of patients with Xq- but in only 65% of patients with Xp-, whereas short stature occurred in 43% of patients with Xq- but in 88% of patients with Xp- (Neely and Rosenfeld, 1994). Cytogenetic studies of various deletion patients suggest that a locus controlling stature occurs at Xp22. Deletion studies of the long arm, however, have shown the presence of ovarian dysfunction at almost all sites, so multiple genes are involved in ovarian function. Further studies have shown that proximal genes are associated with ovarian failure, whereas distal genes are associated with preserving ovarian function (Zinn et al., 1998). A recent study by Zinn et al. (1998) found that traits for high-arched palate, autoimmune thyroid disease, short stature, and ovarian failure mapped to Xp11.2–p22.1 in a series of deletion patients with TS. One candidate gene for ovarian failure within this region is

ZFX at Xp21.2. It encodes a transcription factor of unknown function (Zinn et al., 1998).

Approximately 5% of patients with TS have mosaicism such as 45,X/46,XY, which includes a Y chromosome line. Some of these individuals demonstrate ambiguous genitalia and mixed gonadal dysgenesis with a combination of streak ovaries and dysgenetic testicular elements. However, when fetuses are identified prenatally with 45,X/46,XY, 85 to 90% are normal phenotypic males and only 10% demonstrate mixed gonadal dysgenesis (Hsu, 1989). The presence of the Y chromosome increases the incidence of gonadal malignancy, specifically gonadoblastoma or dysgerminoma, and the risk is thought to be 15 to 20% in patients with dysgenetic gonads (reviewed by Neely and Rosenfeld, 1994). In these cases a prophylactic gonadectomy is usually recommended. With the use of molecular markers for a Y line in individuals with TS, up to 15% have evidence of previously undetected Y material. It is unclear if these individuals with occult Y material are also at the same risk for gonadal malignancy (Neely and Rosenfeld, 1994).

The phenotype in TS is hypothesized to be caused by the halved expression of those genes on the X chromosome which are not X-inactivated. The pericentromeric regions on the long and short arm and the distal portion of the short arm have regions which are not inactivated and involve multiple genes (reviewed by Neely and Rosenfeld, 1994). In males, the Y chromosome supplies the second dose of critical TS genes; therefore, TS genes are predicted to be X-Y homologues and to escape X-inactivation, and there are presently 18 candidate genes (Zinn et al., 1998).

Recent studies suggesting a differential effect in the phenotype depending on which parent the single X came from are consistent with an imprint effect on the X chromosome. Studies with DNA testing have documented that the X is of maternal origin approximately 80% of the time in females with TS (Neely and Rosenfeld, 1994). There is no difference in the rate of fetal demise depending on the source of the X, but limited data suggest an absence of renal and cardiac abnormalities when the X comes from the father (reviewed by Neely and Rosenfeld, 1994).

A recent report by Skuse et al. (1997) demonstrated a possible imprint effect in the cognitive and behavioral phenotype in TS. They studied 80 females with TS, of whom 55 had a maternally derived X and 25 had a paternally derived X. The females with a paternally derived X had a higher Verbal IQ, better results on an executive function task measuring behavioral inhibition, and better scores on a social cognition behavior checklist than females with a maternally derived X chromosome. They concluded that there may be a genetic locus for social cognition and language abilities that is imprinted and is not expressed from the maternally derived X chromosome (Skuse et al., 1997). The social cognition checklist included several questions which reflect attention deficit hyperactivity disorder (ADHD) symptoms, such as "behavior often disrupts normal family life" or "interrupts conversation" or "has difficulty following commands unless they are carefully worded." This suggests that what is termed social cognition in this study is strongly reflective of ADHD symptoms, which may also have an imprint effect that deserves further study. Both subgroups were equally impaired on nonverbal or visual-spatial tasks. Three females with TS were found to have autism, and all three were found to have a maternally derived X chromosome (Skuse et al., 1997).

Neurocognitive and Neuroanatomical Findings

Cognitive studies have traditionally documented visual-spatial perceptual problems in girls with TS that lead to a lowered Performance IQ of approximately 12 points compared with Verbal IQ on the WISC-III (Rovet, 1995b). The mean IQ of over 200 girls with TS was 94.6 compared with 103.9 in controls (Rovet, 1995b). Deficits in visual memory, spatial reasoning, design copying, mental rotations, visual discrimination, visual sequencing, and visual-motor coordination have been documented. Girls with TS are considered to have a nonverbal learning disability (NVLD), although their profile is somewhat atypical, because their visual perceptual problems are not global (Rovet, 1995b). Deficits in math appear to be related to visual-spatial deficits, because stepwise procedures are difficult (Rovet, 1995b). The math problems are also consistent with a NVLD. Mazzocco (1998) found evidence that math deficits in TS correlated with elements of executive function, and this problem may underlie both the math and some of the visual-spatial deficits.

There is considerable variability in the cognitive phenotype, and 10 to 20% of women with TS exhibited higher nonverbal than verbal abilities (Pennington et al., 1985). Detailed neuropsychological testing also demonstrated verbal deficits compared with controls in women with TS, which suggests global brain dysfunction and not just right-hemisphere problems consistent with NVLD (Pennington et al., 1985; Rovet, 1995b).

There also appears to be a developmental progression in the cognitive deficits of TS. The verbal-performance IQ discrepancy may be more dramatic in the preadolescent than in the adolescent, suggesting that the verbal abilities may be vulnerable to the lack of estrogen or pubertal changes in adolescence (Rovet and Buchanan, 1999). Studies of evoked potential responses have demonstrated that females with TS who were given estrogen replacement therapy in early adolescence and had normal estrogen levels had a comparable waveform profile to normal females, whereas the females who received their estrogen therapy late failed to show a normal response (Johnson and Ross, 1994).

Achievement Testing

Although the majority of girls with TS are excellent readers with adequate spelling and written language skills, they have difficulty in completing tasks and in their written work, and the majority have moderate to severe problems in mathematics (Rovet, 1995a; Rovet and Buchanan, 1999). The fact-recall problem in math improved as the children with TS aged, but the procedural deficits, which included confusion about component steps in problems, reflect core deficits (Rovet et al.,

1994). Mazzocco (1998) compared the types of math difficulties in girls with TS, fragile X syndrome, and controls and found that a higher percentage of girls with TS made operation and alignment errors on math calculations than did the other groups. The math scores of girls with TS also correlated significantly with a line-orientation task and with the WISC-R third-factor scores, which reflect attention and memory problems in addition to visual-perceptual problems (Mazzocco, 1998). In a study of young girls aged 5 to 6 years with TS compared with controls, deficits were already present in math reasoning relative to vocabulary development (M. M. M. Mazzocco, personal communication 1998).

Girls with TS attain reading levels that are higher than what is predicted based on their IQs and compared with age-matched controls (Temple and Carney, 1996). They have strengths in both phonological reading skills and lexical reading skills. In TS there is genuine hyperdevelopment of reading skills.

Motor Abilities

Mild delays in early motor milestones are common in girls with TS. In the Denver longitudinal follow-up study, four of nine nonmosaic girls with TS were delayed in walking (14.3 months or later), but all were walking by 17 months, whereas none of the mosaic girls were delayed (Bender et al., 1984). In a more detailed motor assessment utilizing the Bruininks-Oseretsky Test of Motor Proficiency, four of five nonmosaic girls scored below the first percentile in the battery composite with neurological signs of hypotonia, retension of primitive asymmetric and symmetric tonic neck reflexes, and dysfunctional sensory-motor integration (Salbenblatt et al., 1989). Four girls with a mosaic status had motor percentiles between 8 and 72 and were not significantly different from controls. Ross and colleagues have found continued motor problems throughout childhood in a group of 78 girls with TS compared with controls (Ross et al., 1996a). These girls had a decreased sense of athletic ability and a poor physical self-image. They performed worst on motor tasks that also had spatial demands. These studies suggest the need for early motor intervention with sensory-integration therapy. Further studies regarding the effect of estrogen replacement on motor function are needed to guide treatment.

Neuroanatomical Studies

In a magnetic resonance imaging (MRI) study of 30 age-matched girls with TS and controls, no significant differences were seen in overall brain volume, but there was a smaller proportion of tissue, both grey and white matter, within the right and left parietal regions in girls with TS than in controls (Reiss et al., 1995). In addition, a larger proportion of brain tissue volume was seen in the right inferior parietal-occipital region in girls with TS than in controls. However, these gross neuroanatomical findings did not correlate with the neurocognitive testing which was carried out on the subjects (Reiss et al., 1995). In an MRI study of adults with TS (mean age 30 years 7 months) compared with controls a significant decrease in overall cerebral volume, in addition to decreased region-to-brain ratios of the parietal-occipital cortex, hippocampus, and lenticular and thalamic nuclei, were seen in women with TS (Murphy et al., 1993). The neuroanatomical abnormalities were less severe in women who had a mosaic pattern than in those with full X monosomy (Murphy et al., 1993). These results point out the deleterious effect of X monosomy on brain development, but the more dramatic effect of age on brain changes suggest that the estrogen deficiency problem may compound brain problems in TS. It is difficult to assess brain neuroanatomy on and off estrogen because estrogen replacement is generally recommended in TS, as described later in this chapter. It is known that estrogen has significant effects on verbal fluency, performance on spatial tasks, verbal memory tests, and fine motor skills (McEwen et al., 1997). Ovarian steroids have effects throughout the brain, including the catecholaminergic neurons in the brainstem and midbrain, serotonergic systems in the midbrain, and the cholinergic system of the basal forebrain; estrogens also regulate and induce synaptogenesis, particularly in the hippocampus (McEwen et al., 1997). The replacement of estrogen is important not only for sexual development but also, and perhaps most important, for optimal brain function.

A recent positron emission tomography (PET) study demonstrated significant global hypermetabolism in most brain areas except the association areas of the neocortex, including the right superior parietal area, the right and left superior temporal, insula, and occipital association areas, and the left inferior and midtemporal regions, all of which demonstrated hypometabolism in women with TS compared with controls (Murphy et al., 1997). The authors found a significant correlation between the right–left differences on cognitive testing and the metabolic differences on PET. The hypometabolism findings in the temporal and parietal lobes continued to be significant even after correction for size differences between brain regions in patients with TS and controls. The hypometabolism likely reflects differences in the structure and function of brain neural networks. The social deficits in TS may also be related to the hypometabolism. The insula emphasizes the behavioral relevance of a stimulus, and lesions of the insula result in social isolation (Murphy et al., 1997). The right parietotemporal regions are important in producing and understanding affective components of speech, so hypometabolism in both of these areas may lead to the social difficulties seen in TS (Murphy et al., 1997).

Only four autopsy descriptions of patients with TS have been reported (reviewed by Rovet and Buchanan 1999; Pennington et al., 1985). One case had no brain pathology, another demonstrated a neuronal migration defect, another had mild cortical dysplasia in the centrum semiovale, another had diffuse atrophy, and another had arteriosclerotic abnormalities that were most pronounced in the right temporal-parietal region (Reske-Nielsen et al., 1982). These cases were published before 1985, and there is a need for further studies to see if any consistency is present in the neuroanatomical findings.

Behavioral Features

Although severe psychopathology is usually not seen in girls with TS, several reports have documented problems with immaturity, inattention, social competence, self-esteem, and school performance compared with controls (McCauley et al., 1995; Romans et al., 1997; Rovet and Ireland, 1994). In a study of 97 girls with TS aged 7 to 14 years, 51% had an elevated T score on the Achenbach Child Behavior Checklist (CBCL) hyperactivity scale compared with 14% of controls (McCauley et al., 1995). The girls with TS also rated themselves lower on popularity, school competence, social competence, and physical appearance than controls. A decline in self-concept was also documented in girls with TS as they grew into early adolescence. Most interestingly, socioeconomic status did not correlate with any of the behavioral measures in girls with TS, whereas in controls the higher the socioeconomic status, the higher the self-esteem and social competence and the fewer behavioral concerns. In contrast also to controls, the Verbal IQ did not correlate with the behavioral or self-concept measures in girls with TS, although the it did correlate with school competence. It appears that the presence of TS has an overriding effect on the usually strong predictive factors of socioeconomic status and IQ on psychosocial functioning (McCauley et al., 1995).

The degree of physical involvement from TS, including height and number of dysmorphic features, also did not correlate with psychosocial functioning (McCauley et al., 1995). In a similar study of 103 girls with TS which utilized the CBCL, patients with TS and karyotypes that included deletions, rearrangements, and Y chromosome material were more likely to have elevated behavior problem scores than those with X-monosomy, mosaicism, or an isochromosome (Rovet and Ireland, 1994). This study demonstrated that height was associated with social competence (in contrast to the McCauley study) but not with behavior problems (Rovet and Ireland, 1994). The etiology for the social and behavior problems in TS is complex and not simply related to growth issues. The executive function deficits, in addition to other neuropsychological problems perhaps exacerbated by estrogen deficiency, take a toll on self-image and social/behavioral abilities.

A follow-up to the McCauley et al. (1995) study utilized estrogen replacement in 31 girls between the ages of 12 and 14 years with TS (Ross et al., 1996b). Significant increases were subsequently documented in their self-reported self-esteem and psychological well-being; parents also reported significant improvements in problem behaviors on the CBCL, including the social problems and the aggressive scales. Such improvements were not seen in a subgroup of 16 adolescents with TS who were not treated with estrogen. This effect of estrogen may be secondary to the physical effects of estrogen on sexual maturation or it may be secondary to a direct effect on brain function, perhaps related to estrogen's effect on the serotonin system. There was no correlation between the stages of breast development and the self-esteem or behavioral measures in this study, so it is likely that estrogen's central effect made a difference. This study suggests that estrogen replacement should begin between 12 and 14 years instead of the traditional recommendation of waiting until after 14 years so that height growth will not be compromised (Ross et al., 1996b).

An important point of the behavioral studies is that a significant percentage of girls with TS is unaffected by social problems (24%) or by behavioral problems (71%; Rovet and Ireland, 1994). In a detailed psychiatric evaluation of nine females with TS and six females with a mosaic karyotype, none demonstrated a psychiatric diagnosis of psychopathology (Bender et al., 1995). Learning disabilities were common, and four of the nine females with X-monosomy were in special education. Most were described as socially reticent, having only one or two friends instead of a wide social network, and many had concerns about their physical self-image. In contrast, the mosaic girls were more outgoing, socially well adjusted, and basically indistinguishable from controls (Bender et al., 1995).

Hyperactivity and/or attentional problems, often consistent with a diagnosis of ADHD, have been reported for a subgroup of girls with TS, although it appears to be less of a problem for individuals identified through newborn screening than in clinic populations (Bender et al., 1995). Cognitive testing usually demonstrates a lower score on the Freedom from Distractibility factor of the Weschler Intelligence Scales in girls with TS than in controls, but other tests of attention and concentration are usually deficient also (Stefanatos et al., 1995). The attentional problems appear to be related to executive function deficits, including working memory problems (Romans et al., 1997). One investigator feels that the working memory problems are a core deficit in TS that also underlies the poor visual-spatial processing (Berch, 1996).

Treatment

Sometimes the diagnosis of TS occurs prenatally by chance, since maternal age is not associated with an increased incidence of TS. Counseling at this time should emphasize that girls with TS usually have normal intellectual abilities, combined with short stature, infertility, and other congenital abnormalities (Table 5.1). Additional learning problems related to visual-spatial deficits and visual-motor coordination problems should also be addressed. The variability in the clinical phenotype and the fact that mosaicism also adds to this variability should be discussed (Committee on Genetics/AAP, 1995). Guidelines have been established for appropriate follow-up of all individuals diagnosed with TS. These are outlined in the subsequent sections (Committee on Genetics/AAP, 1995; Rosenfeld et al., 1994; Saenger, 1996).

Infants and Toddlers

The diagnosis of TS often occurs in the newborn period because of congenital lymphedema that causes a webbed neck, a low hairline, and swelling of the hands and feet. The diagnosis is made by cytogenetic studies, but use of fluorescent in situ hybridization (FISH) studies for detection of cells with both Xs increases the detection of mosaicism to 60%, in contrast to 34% with conventional techniques (Saenger, 1996).

Once the diagnosis is made, a cardiology consultation and evaluation that includes ultrasonography or MRI should be carried out because the incidence of bicuspid aortic valve is as high as 50%, and the incidence of coarctation of the aorta is approximately 20% (Saenger, 1996). Approximately 9% may also have aortic root dilation, and these individuals are at risk for aortic dissection (Committee on Genetics/AAP, 1995). If a significant cardiac abnormality is detected, prophylactic antibiotics are recommended during surgical or dental procedures associated with bacteremia (bacteria in the blood) to prevent subacute bacterial endocarditis (heart infection). Cardiac disease or complications are the single source of early mortality in TS; therefore, these problems must be addressed once the diagnosis is made. Careful cardiology follow-up at least on a yearly basis is necessary (Saenger, 1996).

Renal disease is also commonly seen (Table 5.1), so renal ultrasonography is also recommended at the time of diagnosis (Rosenfeld et al., 1994). Structural abnormalities require urological consultation and a workup to rule out infection. Hydronephrosis and pylonephritis are common in abnormalities that cause obstruction (Saenger, 1996). Hypertension is also common in TS even without cardiac or renal problems, so the blood pressure should be assessed at each examination (Committee on Genetics/AAP, 1995).

Feeding problems are occasionally seen in infants with TS because of hypotonia of the cheeks and lips, dysfunctional tongue movements, poor chewing skills, and a general oral motor dyspraxia (Mathisen et al., 1992). A high arched palate and a small jaw may also contribute to feeding problems. If problems with sucking, swallowing, or chewing occur, then referral to an occupational therapy (OT) for therapy to improve feeding is helpful. The OT can also provide therapy to improve overall motor coordination and facilitate attainment of motor milestones. As the child becomes a toddler, sensory-motor integration (SI) therapy can help with hyperarousal to sensory stimuli, motor planning, and both fine and gross motor coordination. For a more detailed discussion of SI therapy, see chapter 2.

In the newborn period, the parents should be told that the edema may last for months and may recur at a later time. For significantly dysmorphic features, plastic surgery is available and occasionally utilized, although keloid formation is commonly seen in TS. Gargan has recently reported a surgical procedure to release the dense fibrous band that extends from the mastoid process to the acromion and is associated with the webbing of the neck (Gargan, 1997). Their large V-Y plasty releases the band, removes the web and most of the abnormal hairline, and corrects the vertical deficiency of skin in the neck.

Orthopedic problems such as congenital hip dislocation occasionally occur, so the hips should be examined carefully in the newborn period (Rosenfeld et al., 1994). Scoliosis is also seen in approximately 10% but is more commonly diagnosed in adolescence; it requires orthopedic consultation (Saenger, 1996).

Recurrent otitis media occurs in up to 60% of infants and toddlers with TS (Saenger, 1996). The cause probably relates to the facial structural changes, although hypotonia may also facilitate collapse of the eustachian tube. Aggressive treatment of recurrent otitis media includes the use of prophylatic antibiotics or insertion of PE tubes to eliminate a conductive hearing loss and facilitate normal language development. Adenoidectomy is not routinely recommended because the high arched palate, small jaw, and small lower face appear to predispose the patients to velopharyngeal incompetence when the adenoids are removed (Saenger, 1996). Sensorineural hearing loss also occurs in TS, but it is more common in adulthood and is thought to be related to premature aging of the hearing system (Hultcrantz and Sylven, 1997).

Early ophthalmological problems such as strabismus and ptosis are not un-common (Table 5.1) and require ophthalmological consultation when noted to avoid amblyopia. Stool guaiac testing is also recommended periodically because abnormal mesenteric vascular development can cause gastrointestinal bleeding, and an increased incidence of Crohn's disease and ulcerative colitis have been reported in TS (Saenger, 1996). Another autoimmune process, Hashimoto's thy-roiditis, causes hypothyroidism in 10 to 30% of girls with TS (Saenger, 1996). This may increase to 50% in adulthood, and screening for hypothyroidism is recommended every 1 to 2 years throughout life (Committee on Genetics/AAP, 1995).

Short stature is a universal problem in children with TS, unless significant mosaicism is present. Growth should be plotted on the growth chart developed for TS (Committee on Genetics/AAP, 1995). Growth hormone (GH) therapy should be initiated as soon as the height drops below the 5th percentile of the normal female growth curve, which usually occurs between 2 and 9 years of age (Saenger, 1996). However, the optimal time for initiation of GH therapy is controversial, although such therapy is often started between 4 and 5 years of age beginning with a dose of 0.05 mg/kg/day of GH (Rosenfeld et al., 1994). GH therapy should be carried out by a pediatric endocrinologist, and growth should be monitored at 3- to 6-month intervals. When GH therapy is started after 9 years, or if growth is far below the fifth percentile, then consideration should be given to adding an anabolic steroid, such as oxandrolone, at a dose of 0.0625 mg/kg/day to GH (Joss et al., 1997; Rosenfeld et al., 1994).

One of the most extensive studies reported so far involved 70 patients who started therapy at a mean age of 9.3 years (range 4.7–12.4 years) (Rosenfeld et al., 1998). These patients were treated with either GH alone or GH with oxandrolone (0.0625 to 0.125 mg/kg/day). Patients were initially treated with three weekly injections of GH at a dose of 0.125 mg/kg. After 2 years they were switched to 0.375 mg/kg/wk divided into seven daily injections. Patients treated with GH alone reached a mean height of 150.4 cm, which was 8.4 cm taller than their mean projected adult height, and patients treated with GH plus oxandrolone attained a mean height of 152.1 cm, which was 10.3 cm taller than their mean projected adult height. Both regimens were beneficial in stimulating growth to a reasonable goal of 150 cm, which is about 5 feet, in girls with TS. Oxandrolone with GH was somewhat superior to GH alone, and significant side effects were not seen. Oxandrolone at a dose of 0.0625 mg/kg/day did not excessively stimulate bone maturation and was well tolerated. This study also included estrogen treatment at a minimum age of 14 years. Conjugated estrogens were initiated at 0.3 mg/day and increased to 0.625 mg/day after 6 months. At 1 year estrogen replacement was given cyclically, and progesterone was added (Rosenfeld et al., 1998).

Some recent protocols have used an escalation of the dose of GH. For instance, Van Teunenbroek and colleagues carried out a stepwise increase in dose from 28 to 42 to 56 IU/M^2/week with an average of 6.4 years at initiation of therapy (van Teunenbroek et al., 1996). There were significant gains in growth at the highest dose without an acceleration in bone maturation, but dividing the injection to twice a day compared to once a day made no difference in height growth (van Teunenbroek et al., 1997).

GH therapy should be continued until a satisfactory height has been obtained or until the bone age exceeds 15 years and growth slows to less than 2 cm per year (Saenger, 1996). Early introduction of estrogen replacement accelerates bone maturation and stimulates epiphyseal fusion, which decreases the final height prediction, as discussed later in this chapter. GH therapy does not cause cardiac problems, nor does it influence the cognitive abilities of patients with TS (Ross et al., 1997; Silverman and Friedlander, 1997).

School-Aged Children

GH therapy, as described previously, usually continues through the school-aged period, and attention to learning problems becomes of optimal importance during this time. The cognitive profile discussed previously is associated with learning disabilities involving visual-spatial perception, visual-motor coordination, attentional problems, and memory difficulties (Bender et al., 1984; Pennington et al., 1985; Rovet, 1995b; Rovet et al., 1994; Salbenblatt et al., 1989; Williams et al., 1991). Although these problems are significant compared with controls in groups of patients with TS, there are some individuals who may not have these difficulties and may not require remediation. For those who do have these problems, special education support can help with the visual-perceptual problems as they relate to academic difficulties, which are most typical in math. Williams et al. (1992) have shown that verbal mediation techniques can improve the visual-spatial perceptual problems in TS. This type of tutoring support usually takes place in a pull out situation, but it can also be incorporated into the regular class time and carried out in a small group or individually within the class. Tutoring can also be obtained privately outside of school, particularly if the student does not qualify for special education support. Many students with learning disabilities struggle academically but do not qualify for special education programs in the school. These children often do well with private tutoring.

The fine and gross motor difficulties combined with visual-motor coordination problems seen in the majority of girls with TS may benefit from occupational therapy (OT). If sensory processing problems are also present, then a sensory-integration OT approach is often helpful. However, controlled studies to evaluate the efficacy of OT therapy in TS have not been carried out. To facilitate the children's written work, which is often laborious because of visual-motor coordination and ADHD problems, girls with TS can be taught keyboard skills and the use of a computer word processor early on in elementary school. The special education teacher can facilitate the use of computers on a daily basis.

A variety of computer software can be helpful for visual-spatial deficits, such as Kid Pixs, which utilizes drawing and graphics; Blocks in Motion, which helps visual spatial processing; and Trudy's Time and Place House, which helps map and directional skills. More advanced games that improve visual perceptual skills include Tetris and Shanghai (see Appendix 2). Software for improving math difficulties includes Math Blaster and Millie's Math House (see Appendix 2). Some girls may need additional work in the language area, particularly concept formation and verbal memory. These students may qualify for language therapy through the school, and computer software can also be utilized to improve these skills.

The attentional problems are often mild and may respond well to structure and behavioral programming (see case history of Sally). Cognitive approaches that help the child guide her behavior by using reauditorization, in which the child repeats the instructions or information, or self-talk can be helpful for the child with inattention or impulsivity problems. Programs that require the child to think out loud to review her options and strategies for problem solving can help with defining the task, focusing attention, and decreasing impulsivity (Kosiewicz et al., 1982).

On occasion the ADHD symptoms do not respond optimally to structure and cognitive programming, and further treatment is needed. ADHD symptoms respond usually to stimulant medication, specifically methylphenidate (Ritalin), dextroamphetamine (Dexedrine), a mixture of dextro- and levoamphetamine salts (Adderall), or pemoline (Cylert) (AACAP, 1997; Arnold et al., 1998). Pemoline is not a drug of choice because of the recent rare reports of liver failure associated with pemoline's use (Berkovitch et al., 1995; Hochman et al., 1998). The other stimulants do not cause these difficulties, although side effects usually include appetite suppression and cardiovascular stimulation. Stimulants can be used in individuals with cardiac disease, but the cardiologist should be consulted first. Careful monitoring of blood pressure is needed because stimulants may exacerbate hypertension. Follow-up medication checks should occur every 3 to 6 months to follow growth percentiles, heart rate, and blood pressure and to discuss the response to medication so that the dosage can be adjusted. A typical starting dose is 5 mg of methylphenidate twice or three times a day. If a long-acting preparation is needed to avoid the midday dosing, Adderall, a Dexedrine spansule, or a slow-release methylphenidate can be given in the morning only.

Tricyclic antidepressants such as imipramine or desipramine can also be used to treat ADHD, but these medications prolong cardiac conduction, which is a problem in individuals with heart disease.

If significant dysthymia or depression occur, particularly in adolescence when the self-image may be poor, counseling should be initiated. The additional use of an antidepressant can be beneficial, and the safest and most effective are the selective serotonin reuptake inhibitors (SSRIs). Examples of these medications include fluoxetine (Prozac), sertraline (Zoloft), and fluvoxamine (Luvox). These medications not only improve mood and depression but also help with anxiety and obsessive-compulsive behavior (Alderman et al., 1998). These difficulties are rarely a problem in TS, so the reader is referred to chapters 2 and 3 for further information on these medications.

Adolescence and Adulthood

The most important issue in adolescence is estrogen replacement. The timing of estrogen use is somewhat controversial. Early estrogen replacement may compromise final height growth, so most clinicians suggest delaying estrogen replacement until 14 to 15 years of age (Saenger 1996), although earlier treatment may help both cognitive and emotional development. Treatment should begin with a low daily dosage, for example, 0.3 mg of conjugated estrogens (Premarin). This dose can be gradually increased to 1.25 mg so that feminization progresses gradually. Some patients feel that breast development is inadequate even with appropriate estrogen doses, but this may be secondary to limited breast anlage or the shield chest deformity (Saenger, 1996). In the second year of therapy, a progestin agent can be added, medroxyprogesterone acetate (Provera), for 12 days each month.

Adults with TS require long-term estrogen and progestin replacement. Breakthrough bleeding is often a problem if the dose is too low, but higher doses of estrogen may cause excessive breast tenderness. Some women prefer the transdermal estradiol patch (Estraderm 50 to 100 micrograms), which is applied twice weekly. The new transdermal estradiol matrix patch, Climara, is applied once a week and often causes less skin irritation than Estraderm (Saenger, 1996). The progestin agent is usually medroxyprogesterone acetate (5 to 10 mg/day), or norethindrone (1 to 2 mg/day), and it is given for 10 to 12 days each month. It can also be prescribed continuously with estrogen for women who do not wish to menstruate (Saenger, 1996).

Most women with TS are infertile, although an occasional patient, about 2 to 8%, may have spontaneous menses, and a smaller percentage may be fertile. Just over 20 pregnancies have been reported in the literature, and in some cases occult mosaicism was detected in ovarian tissue (Magee et al., 1998). For those women who become pregnant, there is a high rate of reproductive failure, including 29% having spontaneous abortion, 10% having stillbirth, and 20% having congenital anomalies, including chromosomal problems (Magee et al., 1998). Women with TS who are pregnant must be counseled regarding these high rates of fetal wastage and congenital problems, and they should be offered prenatal diagnosis. Pregnant women with TS should also be followed closely for cardiovascular complications, such as aortic dissection, as discussed previously.

New reproductive options, including in vitro fertilization (IVF), allow women with TS to become pregnant and not have the high rates of fetal wastage or congenital abnormalities that are seen in the rare spontaneous pregnancies. IVF techniques involve an egg donor who may be a relative or an anonymous donor and fertilization of the donor eggs in the laboratory, with subsequent implantation of two fertilized eggs in the uterus of the women with TS. Before this procedure, women with TS must undergo a medical evaluation to detect cardiac or renal problems which could interfere with the pregnancy. Pregnancy rates from IVF vary from 25 to 58%, and they typically do not differ between patients with TS and other oocyte recipients (Vockrodt and Williams, 1994). Although the IVF procedure is expensive, approximately $8,000 per cycle, it allows a woman with TS to have a pregnancy; this option was not available previously.

The medical follow-up for the adolescent with TS includes assessment of thyroid function every 1 to 2 years; comprehensive physical examinations at least once a year that include a blood pressure check and an assessment for scoliosis, lordosis, and kyphosis; and periodic cardiology follow-up as prescribed by the consulting cardiologist (Committee on Genetics/AAP, 1995; Roge et al., 1997). Renal anomalies require more careful follow-up for urinary tract infections, and orthodontics should be considered for malocclusion problems related to a small jaw. Pigmented nevi tend to increase in adolescence, and they should be removed if they are consistently rubbed by clothing (Committee on Genetics/AAP, 1995). Melanoma occurs only rarely in TS (Gare et al., 1993).

Many adolescents with TS are well adjusted, but some girls experience social difficulties related to ADHD symptoms, including impulsivity, or related to a poor self-image, leading to social withdrawal. These individuals may require individual or group counseling to improve their social skills. In a study comparing girls with TS, girls with fragile X syndrome, and controls, the girls with TS were found to have poorer ability in identifying social cues for peer conflict situations but not for scenarios that did not involve conflict (Freund et al., 1999). This problem correlated with attention/concentration deficits and with nonverbal perceptual skills. In addition, a decreased ability to generate social responses was associated with decreased interpersonal skills. Overall, the girls with TS generated more immature social strategies (Freund et al., 1999). Individual or group therapy can target these problems with a treatment program that includes role-playing and practice in learning of specific strategies to improve these problems (Begum, 1996; Bloomquist, 1996).

In adulthood, a key concern is prevention of osteoporosis. Women should continue on estrogen replacement therapy throughout adulthood. Women should also be given adequate calcium intake (1.2 g/day) and participate in regular weight-bearing exercise (Saenger, 1996). If lymphedema becomes a problem, support hose are helpful, and a diuretic can be used, but surgery is rarely helpful (Rosenfeld et al., 1994). Patients should also be watched for anorexia nervosa and inflammatory bowel disease (Saenger, 1996). Monitoring for hypothyroidism, urinary tract infections, and hypertension should also continue, and a yearly comprehensive medical evaluation is recommended (Rosenfeld et al., 1994). Glucose intolerance is common, and insulin resistance may worsen with obesity; cholesterol levels are often increased in TS, so this should be monitored with appropriate dietary recommendations as needed (Saenger, 1996).

Sensorineural hearing loss and middle-ear infections are common in adulthood and affect approximately 15% of patients (Saenger, 1996). In mid-adulthood a mid-frequency hearing loss with a dip at 2 kHz was common and usually progressed with age in a study of 40 women with TS (Hultcrantz and Sylven, 1997). This problem usually led to social hearing problems and the need for hearing aids. Periodic audiometric evaluations are recommended to detect and treat these problems early.

Most adult women with TS adapt well to adult life without significant psychopathology (Bender et al., 1995). They tend to move into sexual relationships at a later age than peers, and they are less likely to marry than their peers, but this may be secondary to inadequate estrogen replacement in adulthood. Sex education and sexual therapy can be helpful for women who are experiencing difficulty with sexuality issues (Rovet, 1996).

CASE HISTORY: SALLY

Sally is now a 15-year-old girl with Turner syndrome, 45,X karyotype, who was diagnosed at 7 years of age.

Her mother had a normal pregnancy and vaginal delivery, and Sally had a birth weight of 6 pounds 2½ ounces. Her mother noticed that her fingers were somewhat puffy after birth, but a diagnosis of Turner syndrome was not made until she was 7. Her early development included hypotonia, and she did not sit independently until 12 months of age. She walked at 18 months and rode a tricycle at 3 years of age. She is somewhat cautious with gross motor activities, and even now she does not ride a bicycle because of balance problems, awkwardness, and cautiousness in attempting difficult motor tasks. She said words at 2 years of age and sentences just subsequently, but she had difficulty with articulation until she was 4 years of age. Speech and language therapy was started in kindergarten and continued through the 6th grade in school.

She has difficulty in following multiple directions, and she has had ongoing problems with inattentiveness, distractibility, and impulsive behavior in school. The teachers felt that she was hearing only about 70% of what was presented in school, and she also would frequently forget to do things, such as turning in her papers. She has never had hyperactivity, but she was diagnosed with attention deficit disorder without hyperactivity when she went through a detailed medical work-up at 7 years of age. She was started on methylphenidate (Ritalin) in the fifth grade, and the teachers felt it was a lifesaver for her. She began with a dose of 5 mg twice a day, and her current dose is 10 mg in the morning, 10 mg after lunch, and sometimes a 5-mg dose in the late afternoon to help with homework. The teachers saw a great improvement in her concentration and in her organizational abilities on methylphenidate.

Sally has received her speech and language therapy in school, but she has not received tutoring or special education support for her visual-perceptual problems. Math is one of her most difficult subjects. She reads well, but sometimes it is hard for her to settle down to read, and she does better reading on a subject in which she is interested. She has poor self-esteem and is often unsure of herself. She is somewhat bothered by being short; her present height is 4′ 9″.

Because she was felt to be growing fairly well in childhood, she was not given growth hormone, but she began estrogen replacement at 12 years of age. She was started on Premarin then, and later Provera was added for cycling. She takes 5 mg of Provera for the last 10 days of her cycle, and then she stops for a week during menstruation. She was found to be hypothyroid at 7 years of age, and she was started on Synthroid at that time.

With her estrogen replacement, her mother felt that she matured quite significantly with calmer behavior, fewer mood fluctuations, and less crying behavior, and she also became more outgoing. She is comfortable in talking with adults and younger children, but she still has difficulty with peer interactions at school. She is described as a loner who does not have close friends, but she also does not reach out for friendships. She does not appear to be depressed, but she could use some help with facilitating peer interactions, perhaps through a social-skills-building group.

After her diagnosis of Turner syndrome was made, Sally underwent a detailed cardiology evaluation, which was normal, and her kidney assessment was also normal. She had a bout of high blood pressure, 157/115, at age 13, which stayed consistently elevated. She was taken off methylphenidate for a 6-week period, but this made no difference in her blood pressure, which remained elevated. When off methylphenidate, her concentration skills deteriorated, so the methylphenidate was restarted. She was treated with losartan (Cozaar), an angiotensin II receptor antagonist antihypertensive medication, and she had a good response to this.

The family history is significant for short stature; there are several individuals in the family who are 5′: her mother is 5′4″, and her father is 5′9½″. There is no family history of significant attentional problems or hyperactivity.

Cognitive testing demonstrates a Verbal IQ of 91, a Performance IQ of 83, and a Full-Scale IQ of 86 on the WISC-III. Sally is now going into the 11th grade; she has plans to go to college, study journalism, and become a sports reporter. She says that she doesn't play sports, but she enjoys watching sports and she is looking forward to reporting on sports.

47,XXX SYNDROME

The first report of the 47,XXX karyotype was in a woman with normal intellectual abilities who presented with secondary amenorrhea (lack of menstrual periods) in 1959 (Jacobs et al., 1959). Since that time several hundred females have been reported with this karyotype, and the incidence of 47,XXX, or triple X, is 1 per 1,000 (Nielsen and Wohlert, 1990). The incidence of this disorder also varies with the age of the mother; for instance, the incidence is 0.4 per 1,000 for a 33-year-old mother, but it gradually rises to 6.5 per 1,000 for a 49-year-old mother

(Hook et al., 1983). For fetuses diagnosed at the time of amniocentesis with 47,XXX, the fetal survival rate is good, with 99% surviving to term (Hook et al., 1983).

Women with 47,XXX syndrome usually have normal physical features, with tall stature and normal fertility, but they also may have significant cognitive deficits leading to learning disabilities and significant emotional problems. Early reports reviewed by Barr and colleagues found a four- to fivefold increased prevalence of XXX syndrome in mental institutions which included people with mental retardation or psychosis compared with the general population (Barr et al., 1969). Subsequent multicenter longitudinal studies of unbiased populations identified at birth have shown a better outcome than earlier biased case reports, but significant learning and emotional problems are a difficulty for many girls who are identified at birth with 47,XXX (Netley, 1986). They have the most significant intellectual deficits of the common SCAs identified in the longitudinal follow-up studies (Bender et al., 1986; Robinson et al., 1990) (Figure 5.2). The information on 47,XXX is based on the experience of seven research groups who followed 46 females from birth through adolescence. An additional study of individuals with SCAs diagnosed prenatally and followed long term demonstrates development comparable to siblings and better than the postnatal longitudinal follow-up studies (Robinson et al., 1992). However, this study involved a high SES cohort, with 85% of parents who were college graduates and often professionals. The overall IQ and outcome is improved for this group, most likely because the background genes and the environment are optimal for better performance.

Physical Features

The majority of girls with 47,XXX have a normal physical phenotype, although some minor anomalies, including epicanthal folds and clinodactaly, are seen

Estimated Full Scale IQ Distributions For SCA and Control Children

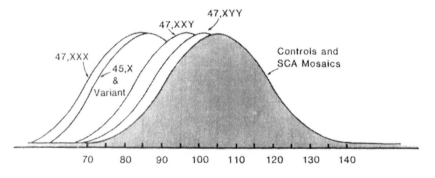

FIGURE 5.2:   Estimated Full-Scale IQ distributions for children with SCA and controls. Reprinted with permission from Bender et al. 1986.

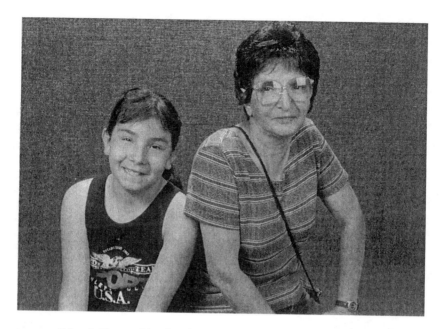

FIGURE 5.3:   A 13-year-old girl with XXX syndrome and her mother, who also has XXX syndrome.

occasionally (Barr et al., 1969; Linden et al., 1988) (Figure 5.3). The majority have a height above the 75th percentile (Linden et al., 1988), although one follow-up study identified a subgroup with a height growth below the 50th percentile (Ratcliffe et al., 1990). Another report described two case studies of intrauterine growth retardation (IGR) associated with 47,XXX, and a review of the literature found other cases with IGR and persistent short stature during development (Chudley et al., 1990).

Overall puberty and reproductive competence are normal for girls with 47,XXX. The onset of puberty, defined as the appearance of breast budding, occurred slightly later (mean age 11.2 years) in girls with 47,XXX than in controls (mean age 10.4; Ratcliffe et al., 1990). Menarche was also delayed about 1 year compared with controls; it occurred at a mean age of 13.6 years. In the Edinburgh study, 1 of 16 girls with 47,XXX followed longitudinally developed secondary amenorrhea and was found to have persistently raised gonadotrophins (LH and FSH) (Ratcliffe et al., 1990). On further investigation with laparoscopy, one ovary was found to be a streak gonad and the other contained very few follicles. One wonders if there was mosaicism and if two of the three Xs were lost in the ovarian tissue. In the Denver follow-up study of 11 girls with 47,XXX, two developed precocious puberty, but the rest had normal hormonal levels except that FSH was occasionally in the upper normal range or slightly greater (Linden et al., 1988). Fertility is normal for the majority of girls with 47,XXX, and 8 of the 11 girls followed in Denver have become pregnant. Of 13 offspring, one child died of sudden infant death at 4 months, another had craniosynostosis surgery, but the remaining 11 children are normal (M. Linden, personal communication 1998). Women with 47,XXX are at a slightly increased risk to have children with chromosomal abnormalities, so prenatal counseling is recommended.

Development

Early motor milestones are delayed in some girls with 47,XXX, and the mean age for walking was 16.2 months with a range of 11 to 22 months in the Denver follow-up study (Linden et al., 1988). By age 2, delays were seen in language development; single words were used at a mean of 18.5 months, and phrases were spoken at 31.8 months. Nine of 11 had documented problems with articulation, and one girl was diagnosed with selective mutism and did not speak until 40 months of age (Linden et al., 1988). Girls with 47,XXX syndrome had the most severe problems with speech and language abilities of all of the major groups of SCAs studied in follow-up (Bender et al., 1983).

Detailed motor testing was carried out in 10 girls with 47,XXX in the Denver follow-up study, and 9 demonstrated sensory-motor integration dysfunction (Salbenblatt et al., 1989). In addition, low tone was seen in 6, and it was associated with poor strength, poor joint stability, and gait abnormalities. Seven had difficulties with balance, rapid alternating movements, motor planning, and bilateral coordination. These problems were seen in both fine and gross motor skills, and the authors recommended early motor intervention with periodic assessments of neuromuscular and sensory-motor integration by an occupational therapist (Salbenblatt et al., 1989). Poor coordination persisted into adolescence, and individual sports were more satisfying than team sports (M. Linden, personal communication 1998).

Cognitive, Behavioral, and Academic Features

Typically, the Verbal IQ (VIQ) is lower than the Performance IQ (PIQ), which is the opposite of what is seen in girls with Turner syndrome. In a pooled cohort of 32 international patients with 47,XXX, the mean VIQ was 87, which was 19 points below the control group's VIQ, and the PIQ was 95 (Netley, 1986). Two of the highest subtest scores were Coding and Digit Span, which suggests a lack of significant attentional problems (Ratcliffe et al., 1990). In Edinburgh the girls were assessed with the Matching Familiar Figures test, and they did not demonstrate deficits in impulsivity (Ratcliffe et al., 1990). These results and clinical impressions suggest that ADHD is not typically seen in patients with 47,XXX. However, immature behavior and a preference for playing with younger children was usually reported by parents (Linden et al., 1988). Shy and quiet behavior was most commonly seen, and perhaps the verbal deficit predisposed the girls to this behavior.

In the international cohort of 32 girls, 71.4% received educational interventions in school (Netley, 1986). In the Denver sample of 11 girls, 9 required special education support and 3 were in full-time special education classes (Bender et al., 1991). The Edinburgh cohort was studied with the British Ability Scales; the reading centile for the group of girls with 47,XXX was at 11.8, whereas the math centile was slightly better at 18.6, although both scores were far lower than controls (Ratcliffe et al., 1990).

In the Denver cohort a detailed psychosocial evaluation, including a psychiatric interview, took place between 12 and 19 years of age; 6 of the 11 girls had a diagnosis of dysthymia, 1 had a diagnosis of conduct disorder, and 3 had a diagnosis of adjustment disorder (Bender et al., 1995). Four of the girls were hospitalized in psychiatric settings during adolescence, two because of suicide attempts, one for alcohol and drug abuse, and one because of overtly psychotic symptoms. The girls with 47,XXX syndrome demonstrated the greatest degree of difficulty cognitively and behaviorally compared with the main SCA groups (Bender et al., 1995). High school was a very frustrating experience for almost all of these girls, and less than half finished their high school degree. They typically did not participate in extracurricular activities such as sports, music, or clubs, and 4 of the 11 girls became pregnant in high school (Bender et al., 1995). Three of this cohort have successfully moved into adulthood, but only one successfully completed college and is free of psychosocial problems; the other two have experienced significant depression. Family strength and SES status has played less of a role in predicting successful outcome in girls with 47,XXX than in the other SCA groups (Bender et al., 1995).

A recent follow-up psychiatric evaluation in young adulthood of 11 women in the Denver cohort demonstrated 11 psychiatric diagnoses, with affective disorder (dysthymia and depression) and substance abuse/dependence disorder being the most prevalent (Harmon et al., 1998). Two of the women have been married twice, compared with none of the controls, and relationship difficulties were a common concern for these women. There was a significant correlation between lower IQ and poorer psychological adaptation (Harmon et al., 1998). Although significant psychosocial problems were common, the variability in this syndrome is great, and most adults are self-sufficient, have married, are raising children, and are competitively employed (Harmon et al., 1998). Another longitudinal study of girls with 47,XXX demonstrated a better psychosocial outcome, but the SES status and the IQ scores were higher than in the Denver study (Rovet et al., 1995).

Treatment

Infancy and Toddlers

Babies with 47,XXX syndrome usually do well in the newborn period and do not typically require treatment. They usually do not have more physical problems, such as ear infections, than controls. Mild developmental delays in motor milestones and more significant delays in language skills may precipitate testing in the toddler period. Children with delays should be placed in a developmental preschool setting where they can receive both motor and language therapy. Individualized and group motor and language therapy should continue through the school-aged period for the children who have language and motor deficits.

School-Aged Children

The most significant problems for girls with 47,XXX syndrome involve learning disabilities and emotional difficulties, which can lead to a high rate of school failure. Therefore, girls with this diagnosis should be thoroughly evaluated in cognitive, educational, motor, language, and emotional areas at the beginning of school and periodically as needed. Many of these girls need ongoing motor and language therapy, in addition to special education support. Because of the high rate of dysthymia or depression, early intervention to boost self-image and positive behavior reinforcement to make sure these individuals feel successful in school should be helpful. Because shyness and social interactional deficits are common, a social-skills-building group can be organized at school to improve these difficulties (Begum, 1996; Bloomquist, 1996).

If dysthymia or depression develop, individual counseling and antidepressant medication can be helpful. SSRIs are most commonly used to treat depression, and fluoxetine (Prozac) has the widest experience in pediatric populations (Sovner et al., 1998). Since these girls typically do not have ADHD, the mild activation effect of fluoxetine will not exacerbate hyperactivity and may help shyness or social withdrawal. If selective mutism is present, as was seen in one patient in the Denver cohort, then fluoxetine is the drug of choice for this problem. The side effects of the SSRIs are typically minimal and include mild stomachache, loose stools, insomnia, or mania. The SSRI agents are usually well tolerated, and blood testing for liver function or blood count is not necessary. The SSRIs do not have the cardiac toxicity that is seen with tricyclic antidepressants, so EKGs are not needed in follow-up (Sovner et al., 1998).

Rustagi and Fine (1987) reported a 12-year-old girl with XXX who presented with emotional immaturity, trichotillomania (recurrent pulling out of one's hair), enuresis, and chronic skin picking. Individual and family therapy with a focus on cognitive and behavioral approaches and a detailed explanation of the diagnosis improved her self-esteem, socialization, and affect remarkably. This patient also had an unusual red blood cell morphology, including schistocytes and ovalocytes, which have been previously reported in girls with 47,XXX and may be an associated finding (reviewed by Rustagi and Fine, 1987).

Adolescence and Adulthood

The high dropout rate and the high pregnancy rate in high school demonstrate the need for vocational training and alternative educational programming in some girls with 47,XXX. Such programming should involve a community work component to make the high school experience more practical for future vocational needs. Other girls with 47,XXX may successfully complete their education with little or no assistance, and each patient should be individually assessed to clarify her needs educationally and psychosocially. Problems with dysthymia or depression may continue into adulthood and can be treated with an SSRI, as discussed here, and counseling.

CASE HISTORY: JULIA

Julia is a 13-year-old girl with 47,XXX syndrome that was diagnosed at the time of amniocentesis. Her mother also has 47,XXX syndrome, and was 40 years old at the time of her pregnancy with Julia. Her mother was ill with a viral infection 6 weeks before her due date, and she went into premature labor and delivered by a repeat C-section. The birth weight was 5 pounds, and Julia was hospitalized for a month after birth because of a ventricular septal defect (VSD) and pulmonic stenosis diagnosed in the first few days of life. The VSD gradually closed spontaneously, and she did not require surgery.

Her developmental milestones included walking at 11 months, riding a tricycle at 3½ years, words at 3 years, and phrases at 4 years of age. She underwent a speech and language evaluation at 3½ years, and was found to be 6 months delayed in receptive language and 12 months delayed in expressive language with moderate to severe articulation problems. She was treated with speech and language therapy twice a week in the preschool period and then entered special education in kindergarten. She is mainstreamed into the regular classroom but receives pull out special education support for academic subjects, including math, reading, and written language, and ongoing speech and language therapy. She will be going into the sixth grade at middle school in the fall.

Julia has never been hyperactive, but attention and auditory processing problems have been a difficulty for her and relate to her moderate-to-severe speech and language delays. School testing has demonstrated a Verbal IQ of 60 and a Performance IQ of 87 on the WISC-III.

Her past medical history includes multiple otitis media infections in the first several years of life, and she also has reactive airway disease, for which she uses a nebulizer as needed. Although her VSD has closed, she is followed at 2-year intervals by a cardiologist because her pulmonic valve is minimally dysplastic, causing a mild pulmonic stenosis and mild pulmonic regurgitation. She also has moderate poststenotic dilation of her main pulmonary artery.

On examination at age 11, Julia was quiet, and it was difficult for her to speak in complete sentences. Her height was at the 15th percentile, weight at the 50th percentile, and head circumference at the 60th percentile. Her facial features included mildly prominent ears, with a skin tag in front of her right ear. She has small palpebral fissures and a broad nasal bridge with a mild degree of synophrys (hairiness connecting the two eyebrows). A chest exam was normal, and her heart exam demonstrated a grade-2/6 short, early peaking, medium-pitched systolic ejection murmur best heard at the left sternal border. This murmur radiated into the left anterior lung field. She also had a systolic ejection click. A genitalia exam demonstrated normal prepubertal development. Deep tendon reflexes were 2+ and symmetrical. Palmar creases were normal, and there was no hyperextensibility of the finger joints, but there was a mild degree of tapering at the tips of her fingers. She had difficulty with fast or alternating rates in finger movements. She had problems in following multiple directions, and it was difficult for her to talk in full sentences because of problems in formulating and organizing information. She made multiple visual errors in reading at the third-grade level, but her comprehension was approximately 80% for what she read. She demonstrated visual motor coordination problems in her design copying and in her writing.

Juila was briefly tried on stimulant medication, but this caused an increase in outburst behavior and did not help her attention in school, so it was discontinued. She continues to receive special education support through school for reading, written language, and math, and she continues in speech and language therapy through school twice a week.

TETRASOMY AND PENTASOMY

Carr and colleagues described the first case of tetrasomy, 48, XXXX, in 1961 (Carr et al., 1961). These women are usually tall, but minor facial and orthopedic anomalies are more common in them than what is seen in 47,XXX girls, including epicanthal folds, hypertelorism (widely spaced eyes), nystagmus, clinodactaly, and radioulnar synostosis (Figure 5.4) (Linden et al., 1995). Fewer than 50 cases have been described. One-half of these had normal menarche, and the other half had menstrual dysfunction (Linden et al., 1995).

Mental retardation is seen in tetrasomy. The VIQ is usually lower than the PIQ, similar to what has been reported in males with tetrasomy and pentasomy (see chapter 4) (Borghgraef et al., 1988). Polani (1977) suggested that each extra X chromosome will reduce the IQ by 16 points.

There is no consistent behavioral phenotype, and descriptions have included shy, pleasant, friendly, cooperative, aggressive, and emotionally labile personalities (Linden et al., 1995). Approximately half of the reports have described periodic outbursts of unstable behavior described as angry and disruptive (Linden et al., 1995).

Pentasomy, 49,XXXXX, is extremely rare and has even more severe features than tetrasomy, including mental retardation, short stature, coarse facial features, microcephaly, congenital heart defects including VSD and patent ductus arteriosis, generalized joint laxity with multiple dislocations, talipes equinovarus (clubfoot), single palmar creases, small uterus, and reduced fertility (Linden et al., 1995).

The treatment for tetrasomy and pentasomy involves a combination of special education, counseling as needed, and medical intervention as previously described. The following case of a girl with 48,XXXX illustrates treatment issues.

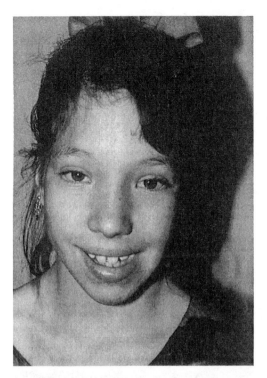

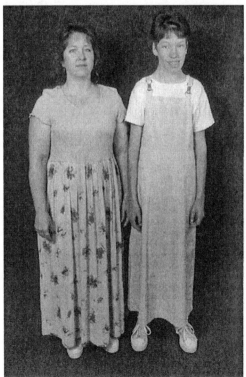

FIGURE 5.4: (a) A girl with XXXX syndrome at 11 years of age Note the broad nasal bridge and mild jaw deviation to the left. (b) Same girl at 15 years of age after a growth spurt, which places her above the 98th percentile for age (178 cm); she is significantly taller than her mother.

CASE HISTORY: JODY

Jody is a 15-year-old girl with 48,XXXX syndrome. Her mother's pregnancy had minimal spotting in the second and third months, which disappeared. Her mother delivered full-term vaginally, the birth weight was 6 pounds 9½ ounces, and the Apgar scores were 7 and 8. In the newborn period she had mild difficulties in coordinating a suck, and she was described as hypotonic. She was unable to sit independently until 9 months of age, although she walked at 15 months. She was significantly delayed in language milestones, and she did not say words until approximately 3 years of age. She had physical therapy, occupational therapy, and speech and language therapy during the preschool period. In school she has had difficulties in fine motor coordination, which have affected her handwriting, although she enjoys drawing. She also has mild difficulty in chewing meat, related to oral motor coordination problems. She received OT therapy until the fourth grade and speech and language therapy and special education support throughout her schooling.

Jody's past medical history includes just a few otitis media infections and one hospitalization for pneumonia at 3 years of age. Her baby teeth have been slow to come out, and the dentist has had to pull several teeth to encourage her adult teeth to emerge. She has soft enamel, and cavities are frequent for her.

She has never been hyperactive, but she has had problems with inattention and impulsivity throughout her school experience. In early childhood she was described as withdrawn, shy, and socially anxious, but her social interactions have improved with age, and she became more outgoing by the fifth grade. In the fifth grade she was mainstreamed into the regular classroom for about 30% of the time, in addition to special education classes and speech and language therapy.

At 11 years of age, cognitive testing using the WISC-III demonstrated a Verbal IQ of 63, a Performance IQ of 73, and a Full-Scale IQ of 64, with a Freedom from Distractibility score of 50.

Her family history is significant for ADHD problems in her father and in her brother, who responded well to methylphenidate.

On examination at age 11½, her weight was at the 30th percentile, her height was at the 70th percentile, and head circumference was at the 90th percentile. Jody was shy at first during the examination, and at one point when she was frustrated with a writing task, she became more emotional, almost to the point of tears. Her head was normocephalic, her ear pinnae were not prominent—although the top of the ears were somewhat compressed—and her ear canal was quite narrow. She had a broad nasal bridge with epicanthal folds bilaterally. Her filtrum was flat but not elongated, and her dentition demonstrated enamel dysplasia. Her palate was narrow, and braces were in place. Her voice was hoarse. Her chest exam was normal, as was her heart exam, and her spine was straight. Her torso was somewhat long and narrow, and her legs were long. Genitalia demonstrated normal prepubertal development, and she did not have palpable breast buds. Her extremities demonstrated mild tapering of her fingers, and clinodactyly (turning in of the fifth finger) bilaterally. Her finger joints were not hyperextensible, and palmar creases were normal. Her second through fifth toes were short bilaterally. Deep tendon reflexes were 1+ and symmetrical in all four extremities. She demonstrated fine motor coordination problems and difficulties in coordinating a skip. She had problems in processing multiple directions, and also with right and left directionality, which required repetition. She was a slow auditory processor and would sometimes get confused with too much information. She demonstrated visual motor coordination problems, and she had difficulty with design copying at the 6-year age level. She was able to read adequately at the third-grade level, and her comprehension was 70% for what she read, but when a third-grade story was read to her, her comprehension dropped to 30%.

Jody's treatment plan included a trial of methylphenidate (Ritalin), a stimulant medication to improve her auditory processing and attentional problems in school. This did not have a significant benefit to her at age 11, so it was discontinued. The stimulant medication, however, was re-tried at age 15 because her mother felt that, with the initiation of puberty, she had more difficulty in staying focused at school. She was described by her teachers as very spacy and unfocused. She had started menstruating at age 14. Methylphenidate was retried at a dose of 10 mg twice a day, and this made a remarkable difference for her in school. The teachers feel that her attention and concentration are dramatically improved, and it is "a night and day difference when she is on medication." She continues to receive special education support for academic subjects and also for speech and language therapy.

Her growth in follow-up at age 15 has increased remarkably, and she is well above the 98th percentile for her age at 178 cm. She continues in braces, and she has a significant deviation of her jaw to the left. She enjoys school, she reads at the fifth-grade level, and she is accepted by her peers, although she is shy. She has not had significant emotional problems, and her self-image is good. She uses a computer word processor to enhance her written work, and she has initiated vocational training in school.

CONCLUSION

With optimal intervention, which includes medical, educational, and psychological support as needed, girls with SCA can lead relatively normal lives. However, the clinician and the educator must be aggressive in their intervention, so that these girl's vulnerabilities do not lead to school failure and a poor self-image. The knowledge about what is expected in each disorder can help to guide treatment, but it must be individualized for each child. Our goal of a happy, healthy, and successful childhood will lead to the best outcome in adulthood.

ACKNOWLEDGMENTS   This work reported in chapter 5 was supported in part by MCH grant no. MCJ089413. I am indebted to Mary Linden, Ron Rosenfeld, and Michele Mazzocco for their careful review and cogent comments and to Mrs. Calkins and Mrs. Pellegrini for helpful information. I also thank Tracy Kovach for helpful information regarding computer technology.

REFERENCES

AACAP (1997) Practice parameters for the assessment and treatment of children, adolescents, and adults with attention deficit hyperactivity disorder. Journal of American Academy of Child and Adolescent Psychiatry 36 (Suppl. 10): 085S–121S.

Alderman, J., Wolkow, R., Chung, M., Johnston, H. F. (1998) Sertraline treatment of children and adolescents with obsessive-compulsive disorder or depression: Pharmacokinetics, tolerability, and efficacy. Journal of American Academy of Child and Adolecent Psychiatry 37 (4): 386–94.

Arnold, L. E., Gadow, K., Pearson, D. A., Varley, C. K. (1998) Stimulants. In: Psychotropic medication in developmental disabilities: The international consensus handbook. Reiss, S., and Aman, M. G. (eds.). Ohio State University Nisonger Center, Columbus, pp. 224–43.

Barr, M. L., Sergovich, F. R., Carr, D. H., et al. (1969) The triplo-X female: An appraisal based on a study of 12 cases and a review of the literature. Canadian Medical Association Journal 101: 247–58.

Begum, R. W. (1996) Social skills lessons and activities. Center for Applied Research in Education, West Nyack, New York.

Bender, B., Fry, E., Pennington, B., Puck, M. H., Salbenblatt, J., Robinson, A. (1983) Speech and language development in 41 children with sex chromosome anomalies. Pediatrics 71 (2): 262–7.

Bender, B., Puck, M., Salbenblatt, J., Robinson, A. (1984) Cognitive development of unselected girls with complete and partial X monosomy. Pediatrics 73 (2): 175–82.

Bender, B. G., Puck, M. H., Salbenblatt, J. A., Robinson, A. (1986) Cognitive development of children with sex chromosome abnormalities. In: Cognitive development of children with sex chromosome abnormalities. Smith, S. (ed.). College Hill Press, San Diego, pp. 175–201.

Bender, B. G., Linden, M., Robinson, A. (1991) Cognitive and academic skills in children with sex chromosome abnormalities. Reading and writing: An interdisciplinary journal 3: 315–7.

Bender, B. G., Harmon, R. J., Linden, M. G., Robinson, A. (1995) Psychosocial adaptation of 39 adolescents with sex chromosome abnormalities. Pediatrics 96: 302–8.

Berch, D. B. (1996) Memory. In Turner syndrome across the lifespan. Rovet, J. (ed.). Klein Graphics, Toronto.

Berkovitch, M., Pope, E., Phillips, J., Koren, G. (1995) Pemoline-associated fulminant liver failure: Testing the evidence for causation. Clinical Pharmacology and Therapeutics 57 (6): 696–8.

Bloomquist, M. L. (1996) Skills training for children with behavior disorders: A parent and therapist guide book. Guilford, New York.

Borghgraef, M., Fryns, J. P., Smeets, E., Marien, J., van den Berghe, H. (1988) The 49,XXXXY syndrome. Clinical and psychological follow-up data. Clinical Genetics 33: 429–34.

Carr, D. H., Barr, M. L., Plunkett, E. R. (1961) An XXXX sex chromosome complex in two mentally defective females. Canadian Medical Association Journal 84: 131–7.

Chudley, A. E., Stoeber, G. P., Greenberg, C. R. (1990) Intrauterine growth retardation and minor anomalies in 47,XXX children. In: Children and young adults with sex chromosomes aneuploidy. Evans, J. A., Hamerton, J. L., Robinson, A. (eds.). Wiley Liss for the National Foundation, March of Dimes, New York. Birth Defects: Original Article Series 26 (4): 267–72.

Committee on Genetics/American Academy of Pediatrics (1995) Health supervision for children with Turner syndrome. Pediatrics 96 (6): 1166–72.

Ford, C. E., Miller, O. J., Polani, P. E., de Almeida, J. C., Briggs, J. H. (1959) A sex chromosome anomaly in a case of gonadal dysgenesis (Turner's syndrome). Lancet 1: 711–3.

Freund, L. S., Reiss, A. L., Baumgardner, T., Denckla, M. B. (1999) Social information processing in girls with fragile X or Turner syndrome. Manuscript submitted for publication.

Gare, M., Ilan, Y., Sherman, Y., Ben-Chetrit, E. (1993) Malignant melanoma in Turner's syndrome. International Journal of Dermatology 32: 743–4.

Gargan, T. J. (1997) Web neck deformity in Turner syndrome. Plastic and Reconstructive Surgery 99 (3): 871–4.

Harmon, R. J., Bender, B. G., Linden, M. G., Robinson, A. (1998) Transition from adolescence to early adulthood: Adaptation and psychiatric status of women with 47,XXX. Journal of American Academy of Child and Adolecent Psychiatry 37 (3): 286–91.

Hochman, J. A., Woodard, S. A., Cohen, M. B. (1998) Exacerbation of autoimmune hepatitis: Another hepatotoxic effect of pemoline therapy. Pediatrics 101 (1): 106–8.

Hook, E. B., and Warburton, D. (1983) The distribution of chromosomal genotypes associated with Turner's syndrome: Live birth prevalence rates and

evidence for diminished fetal mortality and severity in genotypes associated with structural X abnormalities or mosaicism. Human Genetics 64: 24–7.

Hook, E. B., Cross, P. K., Schreinemachers, D. M. (1983) Chromosomal abnormalitiy rates at amniocentesis and in live-born infants. Journal of the American Medical Association 249 (15): 2034–8.

Hsu, L. Y. F. (1989) Prenatal diagnosis of 45,X/46,XY mosaicism—A review and update. Prenatal Diagnosis 9: 31–48.

Hultcrantz, M., and Sylven, L. (1997) Turner's syndrome and hearing disorders in women aged 16–34. Hearing Research 103 (1–2): 69–74.

Jacobs, P. A., Baikie, A. G., Brown, C. W. M., et al. (1959) Evidence for the existence of the human "super female." Lancet 2: 423–5.

Johnson, R., and Ross, J. (1994) Event-related potential indications of altered brain development in Turner syndrome. In: Atypical cognitive deficits in developmental disorders: Implications for brain function. Broman, S., and Grafman, J. (eds.). Erlbaum, Hillsdale, N.J.

Joss, E. E., Mullis, P. E., Werder, E. A., Partsch, C. J., Sippell, W. G. (1997) Growth promotion and Turner-specific bone age after therapy with growth hormone and in combination with oxandrolone: When should therapy be started in Turner syndrome? Hormone Research 47 (3): 102–9.

Kosiewicz, M. M., Hallahan, D. P., Lloyd, J., Graves, A. W. (1982) Effects of self-instruction and self-correction procedures on handwriting performance. Learning Disabilities Quarterly 5: 71–8.

Lin, A., Lippe, B., Rosenfeld, R. G. (1998) Further delineation of aortic-dilation, dissection and rupture in patients with Turner syndrome. Pediatrics 102 (1): 134. http://www.pediatrics.org/cgi/content/full/102/1/el2.

Linden, M. G., Bender, B. G., Harmon, R. J., Mrazek, D. A., Robinson, A. (1988) 47,XXX: What is the prognosis? Pediatrics 82 (4): 619–30.

Linden, M. G., Bender, B. G., Robinson, A. (1995) Sex chromosome tetrasomy and pentasomy. Pediatrics 96 (4, Pt. 1): 672–82.

Lippe, B. M. (1990) Primary ovarian failure. In: Clinical Pediatric Endocrinology. S. A. Kaplan (ed.). Saunders, Philadelphia, pp. 325–66.

Magee, A. C., Nevin, N. C., Armstrong, M. J., McGibbon, D., Nevin, J. (1998) Ullrich-Turner syndrome: Seven pregnancies in an apparent 45,X woman. American Journal of Medical Genetics 75: 1–3.

Mathisen, B., Reilly, S., Skuse, D. (1992) Oral-motor dysfunction and feeding disorders of infants with Turner syndrome. Development of Child Neurology 34: 141–9.

Mazzocco, M. M. M. (1998) A process approach to describing mathematics difficulties in girls with Turner syndrome. Pediatrics 102:492–6.

McCauley, E., Ross, J. L., Kushner, H., Cutler, G., Jr. (1995) Self-esteem and behavior in girls with Turner syndrome. Journal of Developmental Behavior in Pediatrics 16 (2): 82–8.

McEwen, B. S., Alves, S. E., Bulloch, K., Weiland, N. G. (1997) Ovarian steroids and the brain: Implications for cognition and aging. Neurology 48 (suppl. 7): S8–S15.

Murphy, D. G., De Carli, C., Daly, E., et al. (1993) X-chromosome effects on female brain: A magnetic resonance imaging study of Turner's syndrome. Lancet 342: 1197–1200.

Murphy, D. G., Mentis, M. J., Pietrini, P., Grady, C., Daly, E., Haxby, J. V., De La Granja, M., Allen, G., Largay, K., White, B. J., Powell, C. M., Horwitz, B., Rapoport, S. I., Schapiro, M. B. (1997) A PET study of Turner's syndrome: Effects of sex steroids and the X chromosome on brain. Biological Psychiatry 41 (3): 285–98.

Naeraa, R. W., and Nielsen, J. (1990) Standards for growth and final height in Turner's syndrome. Acta Paediatrica Scandinavia 79: 182–90.

Neely, E. K., and Rosenfeld, R. G. (1994) Phenotypic correlations of X-chromosome loss. In: Molecular genetics of sex determination. Wachtel, S. S. (ed.). Academic Press, San Diego, pp. 311–39.

Netley, C. (1986) Summary overview of behavioral development in individuals with neonatally identified X and Y aneuploidy. In: Children and young adults with sex chromosomes aneuploidy. Evans, J. A., Hamerton, J. L., Robinson, A. (eds.). Wiley Liss for the National Foundation, March of Dimes, New York. Birth Defects: Original Article Series 22: 293–306.

Nielsen, J., and Wohlert, M. (1990) Sex chromosome abnormalities found among 34,910 newborn children: Results from a 13-year study in Arhus, Denmark. In: Children and young adults with sex chromosomes aneuploidy. Evans, J. A., Hamerton, J. L., Robinson, A. (eds.). Wiley Liss for the National Foundation, March of Dimes, New York. Birth Defects: Original Article Series 26 (4): 209–23.

Page, D. C. (1995) Mapping and targeting Turner genes. In: Turner syndrome in a life span perspective: Research and clinical aspects. Albertsson-Wikland, K. A., and Ranke, M. B. (eds.). Elsevier Press, Amsterdam, pp. 297–308.

Pennington, B. F., Heaton, R. K., Karzmark, P., Pendleton, M. G., Lehman, R., Shucard, D. W. (1985) The neuropsychological phenotype in Turner syndrome. Cortex 21: 391–404.

Polani, P. E. (1977) Abnormal sex chromosomes, behaviour mental disorders. In: Developments in psychiatric research. Tanner, J. M. (ed.). Hodder and Stoughton, London, pp. 89–128.

Ratcliffe, S. G., Butler, G. E., Jones, M. (1990) Edinburgh study of growth and development of children with sex chromosome abnormalities. In: Children and young adults with sex chromosomes aneuploidy. Evans, J. A., Hamerton, J. L., Robinson, A. (eds.). Wiley Liss for the National Foundation, March of Dimes, New York. Birth Defects: Original Article Series 26 (4): 1–44.

Reiss, A. L., Mazzocco, M. M. M., Greenlaw, R., Freund, L. S., Ross, J. L. (1995) Neurodevelopmental effects of X monosomy: A volumetric imaging study. Annals of Neurology 38: 731–8.

Reske-Nielsen, E., Christensen, A., Nielsen, J. (1982) A neuropathological and neuropsychological study of Turner's syndrome. Cortex 18: 181–91.

Robinson, A., Bender, B. G., Linden, M. G., Salbenblatt, J. A. (1990) Sex chromosome aneuploidy: The Denver Prospective Study. In: Children and young adults with sex chromosomes aneuploidy. Evans, J. A., Hamerton, J. L., Robinson, A. (eds.). Wiley Liss for the National Foundation, March of Dimes, New York. Birth Defects: Original Article Series 26 (4): 59–115.

Robinson, A., Bender, B. G., Linden, M. G. (1992) Prognosis of prenatally diagnosed children with sex chromosome aneuploidy. American Journal of Medical Genetics 44 (3): 365–8.

Roge, C., Cooper, M., Tarnoff, H. (1997) Health supervision for children with Turner syndrome [Letter to the editor; Comment]. Pediatrics 99 (1): 145–6; 147 [discussion].

Romans, S., Roeltgen, D., Kushner, H., Ross, J. (1997) Executive function in girls with Turner syndrome. Developmental Neuropsychology 13: 24–40.

Rosenfeld, R. G. (1989) Turner syndrome: A guide for physicians. Turner's Syndrome Society, Stanford, Cal., pp. 23.

Rosenfeld, R. G., Tesch, L., Rodriguez-Rigau, L. J., McCauley, E., Albertsson-Wikland, K., Asch, R., Cara, J., Conte, F., Hall, J. G., Lippe, B., Nagel, T. C., Neely, E. K., Page, D. C., Ranke, M., Saenger, P., Watkins, J. M., Wilson, D. M. (1994) Recommendations for diagnosis, treatment, and management of individuals with Turner syndrome. Endocrinologist 4 (5): 351–8.

Rosenfeld, R. G., Attie, K. M., Frane, J., Brasel, J. A., Burstein, S., Cara, J. F., Charnausek, S., Gotlin, R. W., Kuntze, G., Lippe, B. M., Mahoney, P. C., Moore, W. V., Saenger, P., Johanson, A. J. (1998) Growth hormone therapy of Turner's syndrome: Beneficial effect on adult height. Journal of Pediatrics 132: 319–24.

Ross, J. L., Kushner, H., Roeltgen, D. P. (1996a) Developmental changes in motor function in girls with Turner syndrome. Pediatric Neurology 15 (4): 317–22.

Ross, J. L., McCauley, E., Roeltgen, D., Long, L., Kushner, H., Feuillan, P., Cutler, G. B., Jr. (1996b) Self-concept and behavior in adolescent girls with Turner syndrome: Potential estrogen effects. Journal of Clinical Endocrinology and Metabolism 81 (3): 926–31.

Ross, J. L., Feuillan, P., Kushner, H., Roeltgen, D., Cutler, G. B., Jr. (1997) Absence of growth hormone effects on cognitive function in girls with Turner syndrome. Journal of Clinical Endocrinology and Metabolism 82 (6): 1814–7.

Rovet, J. (1995a) Behavioral manifestations of Turner syndrome in children: A unique phenotype. In: Turner syndrome in a life span perspective: Research and clinical aspects. Albertsson-Wikland, K. A., and Ranke, M. B. (eds.). Elsevier Press, Amsterdam, pp. 297–308.

Rovet, J. (1995b) Turner syndrome. In:

Syndrome of nonverbal learning disabilities: Neurodevelopmental manifestations. Rourke, B. P. (ed.). Guilford, New York, pp. 351–71.

Rovet, J. (1996) Turner syndrome across the lifespan. Klein Graphics, Toronto.

Rovet, J., and Buchanan, L. (1999) Turner syndrome: A cognitive neuroscience approach. In: Neurodevelopmental disorders: Contributions to a new framework from the cognitive neurosciences. Tager-Flusberg, H. (ed.). MIT Press, Cambridge, Mass.

Rovet, J., and Ireland, L. (1994) Behavioral phenotype in children with Turner syndrome. Journal of Pediatric Psychology 19 (6): 779–90.

Rovet, J., Szekely, C., Hockenberry, M. (1994) Specific arithmetic deficits in children with Turner syndrome. Journal of Clinical and Experimental Neuropsychology 16: 820–39.

Rovet, J., Netley, C., Bailey, J., Keenan, M., Stewart, D. (1995) Intelligence and achievement in children with extra X aneuploidy: A longitudinal perspective. American Journal of Medical Genetics 60 (5): 356–63.

Rustagi, P. K., and Fine, P. M. (1987) Diagnosis and treatment of a child with X-polysomy. Journal of the American Academy of Child and Adolescent Psychiatry 26 (4): 593–4.

Saenger, P. (1996) Turner's syndrome. New England Journal of Medicine 335 (23): 1749–54.

Salbenblatt, J. A., Meyers, D. C., Bender, B. G., Linden, M. G., Robinson, A. (1989) Gross and fine motor development in 45,X and 47,XXX girls. Pediatrics 84 (4): 678–82.

Silverman, B. L., and Friedlander, J. R. (1997) Is growth hormone good for the heart? Journal of Pediatrics 131: S70–S74.

Skuse, D. H., James, R. S., Bishop, D. V., Coppin, B., Dalton, P., Aamodt-Leeper, G., Bacarese-Hamilton, M.,

Creswell, C., McGurk, R., Jacobs, P. A. (1997) Evidence from Turner's syndrome of an imprinted X-linked locus affecting cognitive function [see comments]. Nature 387 (6634): 705–8.

Sovner, R., Pary, R.J., Dosen, A., Geyde, A., Barrera, F. J., Cantwell, D. P., Huessy, H. R. (1998) Antidepressants. In: Psychotropic medication in developmental disabilities: The international consensus handbook. Reiss, S., and Aman, M. G. (eds.). Ohio State University Nisonger Center, Columbus, pp. 179–200.

Stefanatos, G., Roeltgen, D., Kushner, H., Cutler, J., Gordon, B. (1995) Turner syndrome: Neurodevelopment from childhood through adolescence. American Journal of Medical Genetics 58: 74–82.

Temple, C. M., and Carney, R. (1996) Reading skills in children with Turner's syndrome: An analysis of hyperplexia. Cortex 32 (2): 335–45.

Turner, H. (1938) A syndrome of infantilism, congenital webbed neck, and cubitus valgus. Endocrinology 23: 566–74.

Ullrich, P. (1949) Turner's syndrome and status Bonnevie-Ullrich. American Journal of Human Genetics 1: 179–202.

van Teunenbroek, A., de Muinck Keizer-Schrama, S. M., Stijnen, T., Jansen, M., Otten, B. J., Delemarre-van de Waal, H. A., Vulsma, T., Wit, J. M., Rouwe, C. W., Reeser, H. M., Gosen, J. J., Rongen-Westerlaken, C., Drop, S. L. (1996) Yearly stepwise increments of the growth hormone dose results in a better growth response after four years in girls with Turner syndrome. Journal of Clinical Endocrinology and Metabolism 81 (11): 4013–21.

van Teunenbroek, A., de Muinck Keizer-Schrama, S., Stijnen, T., Waelkens, J., Wit, J. M., Vulsma, T., Gerver, W. J., Reeser, H., Delemarre-van de Waal, H., Jansen, M., Drop, S. (1997) Growth response and levels of growth factors after two years growth hormone treatment are similar for a once and twice daily injection regimen in girls with Turner syndrome. Clinical Endocrinology 46 (4): 451–9.

Vockrodt, L., and Williams, J. K. (1994) A reproductive option for women with Turner's syndrome. Journal of Pediatric Nursing 9 (5): 321–5.

Williams, J. K., Richman, L. C., Yarbrough, D. B. (1991) A comparison of memory and attention in Turner syndrome and learning disability. Journal of Pediatric Psychology 16 (5): 585–93.

Williams, J. K., Richman, L. C., Yarbrough, D. B. (1992) Comparison of visual-spatial performance strategy training in children with Turner syndrome and learning disabilities. Journal of Learning Disabilities 25 (10): 658–64.

Zinn, A. R., Tonk, V. S., Chen, Z., Flejter, W. L., Gardner, H. A., Guerra, R., Kushner, H., Schwartz, S., Sybert, V. P., Van Dyke, D. L., Ross, J. (1998) Evidence for a Turner syndrome locus or loci at Xp11.2–p22.1. American Journal of Human Genetics 63: 1757–66.

RESOURCES

The Turner's Syndrome Society of the United States
1313 Southeast 5th Street, Suite 327
Minneapolis, Minnesota 55414
telephone: (800) 365-9944
fax: (612) 379-3619
http://www.turner-syndrome-us.org

Turner Syndrome Society of Canada
7777 Keele St, Fl 2
Concord, Ontario, Canada L4K 1Y7
telephone: (416) 660-7766   Contact: Sandi Hofbauer
fax: (416) 660-7450

Turner Center For Information, Counseling, and Research
The Psychiatric Hospital in Aarhus
Skovagervej 2
DK-8240 Risskov, Denmark
telephone: +45 86 17 77 77
fax: +45 86 17 59 77
e-mail: mpr@cybernet.dk
http://www.aaa.dk/turner/index.htm

English versions of Danish booklets by Johannes Nielsen are available.

Triple X Support Group and Newsletter
Contact: Rita Kuhn, (908) 232-2773

Newsgroup

alt.support.turner-syndrom

General Readings

Rosenfeld, R. G. (1992) Turner syndrome: A guide for physicians, 2nd ed. Minneapolis, Minn.: The Turner's Syndrome Society.

Rosenfeld, R. G., and Grumbach, M. M. (eds.). (1990) Turner syndrome. New York: Marcel Dekker.

Plumridge, D. (1987) Good things come in small packages: The whys and hows of Turner syndrome. Portland, Ore.: University of Oregon Health Sciences Center.

Reiser, P. A., and Underwood, L. E. Turner syndrome: A guide for families. Minneapolis, Minn.: The Turner's Syndrome Society.

Albertsson-Wikland, K. A., and Ranke, M. B. (eds.). (1995) Turner syndrome in a life span perspective. Elsevier Press. New York.

Rovet, J. (ed.). (1996) Turner syndrome across the lifespan. Toronto. Klein Graphics.

6

Angelman Syndrome and Prader-Willi Syndrome

Angelman syndrome (AS) and Prader-Willi syndrome (PWS) are two distinct neurodevelopmental disorders that are linked genetically because they both are caused by a deletion in the 15q11–q13 region. In AS, the distinguishing clinical features are severe mental retardation, microcephaly, lack of language, ataxia, and seizures. In PWS, the clinical features are different, including severe hypotonia in infancy, subsequent hyperphagia (overeating with a lack of normal satiation) and rapid weight gain after the first year, obsessive compulsive behavior, mild to moderate developmental delay, and hypogonadism.

The study of the differences between these two disorders has unraveled a fascinating story of imprinting in this region of chromosome 15. Imprinting refers to the phenomenon of differential epigenetic modification of gene(s), usually methylation, depending on the parent of origin, which subsequently affects gene expression and thereby the phenotype of the patient. The phenotype in AS is caused by the absence of maternal gene(s) in this region either secondary to a maternally derived large deletion of 3 to 4Mb (65–75% of patients), paternal uniparental disomy (UPD; in which the child has two copies of the father's chromosome 15 but is missing the mother's chromosome 15), which is seen in only 2% of patients, or an imprinting mutation so that the patient shows an exclusively paternal methylation pattern on the maternally derived alleles in the 15q11–q13 region (6% of patients; Burger et al., 1997; Saitoh et al., 1994, 1997). The imprinting mutation prevents resetting of imprinting during gametogenesis in the parent. The imprinting mutation is thought to occur upstream of the SNRPN (small nuclear ribonucleoprotein polypeptide N) gene, where a microdeletion has been identified in a few patients with AS or PWS (Burger et al., 1997;

Neurodevelopmental Disorders: Diagnosis and Treatment, by Randi Jenssen Hagerman. New York: Oxford University Press, 1999. © Oxford University Press, Inc.

Saitoh et al., 1997). This region has been named the imprinting center (IC). Recently a candidate gene, E6-AP ubiquitin-protein ligase gene (*UBE3A*), was identified in patients with AS who did not demonstrate the typical deletion nor UPD nor the paternal methylation pattern in peripheral blood studies (Kishino et al., 1997; Matsuura et al., 1997).

The phenotype in PWS is caused by the lack of paternally derived genetic information in the 15q11–13 region. The majority of patients have a large paternally derived deletion of this region (70–75% of patients) or maternal UPD, where two chromosome 15s's come from the mother and the genetic information is missing from the father (20 to 25%). Only a few cases of an imprinting mutation have been reported for PWS (Dittrich et al., 1996; Saitoh et al., 1997). These patients have an exclusively maternal methylation pattern on the paternally derived chromosome. The fathers in these cases were unable to shift the imprint on the chromosome 15 that they had received from their mothers to the male imprint pattern in gametogenesis, so they passed on a chromosome 15 that had a female instead of a male imprint pattern. The IC is thought to encode alternative transcripts of the SNRPN gene; and in three families with PWS and an IC mutation, the *SNRPN* exon 1 is deleted (Dittrich et al., 1996).

Individuals who carry an imprinting mutation (mothers of patients with AS and fathers of patients with PWS) are important to identify because they have a 50% risk of having subsequent children affected by this condition, whereas the recurrence risk is only 1% or less for large deletions or UPD cases. There is also a risk for an imprinting mutation in the same-sex siblings of the carrier parent. If they carry a silent imprint mutation they are also at a 50% risk to have affected offspring (Saitoh et al., 1997; Stalker and Williams, 1998).

A detailed clinical and treatment discussion follows for each disorder, beginning with Angelman syndrome.

ANGELMAN SYNDROME

Angelman syndrome (AS) is a relatively rare disorder with prevalence of approximately 1 in 15,000. It was first described by an English physician, Harry Angelman, in 1965 when he reported three cases with severe mental retardation, ataxia, seizures, and distinctive facial features. The movement problems reminded him of a puppet with the arms on a string. A subsequent paper by Bower and Jeavons (1967) described two additional cases and emphasized the happy temperament with frequent and prolonged bouts of laughter exhibited by these patients, so they suggested the term "happy puppet syndrome."

Most infants with AS look normal at the time of birth, but feeding problems develop soon after birth, including a poor suck, reflux, and regurgitation of feedings or colic in 72% (Clayton-Smith, 1993). Truncal hypotonia is present from birth, although hypertonic extremities are often seen and developmental milestones are delayed. Sitting usually develops by an average age of 20 months, crawling at an average age of 27 months, and walking at an average age of 3.7 years, although the range is 18 months to 12 years (Buntinx et al., 1995; Clayton-Smith, 1993). Because of the spasticity in the lower limbs and ataxia, the gait is usually broad-based and stiff. As the patient grows, features which are typical for the syndrome develop. Williams et al. (1995a) have published the consensus for clinical diagnostic criteria that is outlined in Table 6.1. Problems that are seen in 100% of individuals with AS include severe developmental delay, severe speech impairment, a movement or balance disorder, and a typical behavioral profile that is described herein and in Table 6.1.

TABLE 6.1.   Angelman Syndrome: Clinical Characteristics

Consistent (100%)
  Developmental delay, functionally severe
  Speech impairment, none or minimal use of words; receptive and nonverbal communication
    skills higher than verbal ones
  Movement or balance disorder, usually ataxia of gait and/or tremulous movement of limbs
  Behavioral uniqueness: any combination of frequent laughter/smiling; apparent happy de-
    meanor; easily excitable personality, often with hand-flapping movements; hypermotoric behav-
    ior; short attention span

Frequent (more than 80%)
  Delayed, disproportionate growth in head circumference, usually resulting in microcephaly (ab-
    solute or relative) by age 2
  Seizures, onset usually <3 years of age
  Abnormal EEG, characteristic pattern with large amplitude slow-spike waves (usually 2–3/s), fa-
    cilitated by eye closure

Associated (20–80%)
  Flat occiput
  Occipital groove
  Protruding tongue
  Tongue thrusting; suck/swallowing disorders
  Feeding problems during infancy
  Prognathia
  Wide mouth, wide-spaced teeth
  Frequent drooling
  Excessive chewing/mouthing behaviors
  Strabismus
  Hypopigmented skin, light hair and eye color (compared with family), seen only in deletion
    cases
  Hyperactive lower limb deep tendon reflexes
  Uplifted, flexed arm position especially during ambulation
  Increased sensitivity to heat
  Sleep disturbance
  Attraction to/fascination with water

From C. A. Williams, H. Angelman, J. Clayton-Smith, D. J. Driscoll, J. E. Hendrickson, J. H. M. Knoll, R. E. Magenis, A. Schinzel, J. Wagstaff, E. M. Whidden, and R. Zori (1995), Angelman syndrome: Consensus for diagnostic criteria, American Journal of Medical Genetics 56: 237–8. Reprinted by permission of Wiley-Liss, Inc., a subsidiary of John Wiley & Sons.

Craniofacial and Language Features

The classical features include midface hypoplasia, deep-set eyes, a large mouth, and a prominent chin (Figure 6.1). The tongue is large (macrostomia) in childhood, and tongue protrusion and drooling are common throughout childhood (Buntinx et al., 1995). The prominent chin, or mandibular prognathism, becomes more remarkable as the patient ages; 100% of adults have this finding (Buntinx et al., 1995). The teeth are often widely spaced, and the patients smile frequently.

Many patients have a depression in the occipital bone near the posterior fontanelle which is palpated as a horizontal groove with prominent occipital condyles bilaterally. This finding was originally reported by Angelman, and it influenced his thinking in considering this disorder a syndrome (Williams et al., 1995b).

Otitis media is a frequent problem in early childhood perhaps related to the mid-face hypoplasia and poor drainage of the eustachian tubes (Clayton-Smith, 1993). Language is severely delayed, and there is decreased cooing and babbling

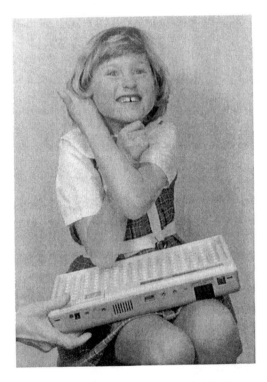

FIGURE 6.1: Seven-year-old girl with AS. Note midface hypoplasia, large mouth, and prominent chin. The Delta Talker is attached by a harness for easy access.

in infants (Williams et al., 1995b). Constant smiling and the initiation of frequent bursts of laughter are usually seen in the first year. A single word such as *mama* may be said at approximately 18 months, but it is usually used without meaning. By 3 years of age, nonverbal communication may be initiated in higher functioning individuals with simple gestures to express their wants and needs (Williams et al., 1995b). In a study of 82 patients with AS in England, 30% were completely nonverbal, and none spoke more than six words (Clayton-Smith, 1993). Children with UPD have higher verbal abilities, with 10 to 20 words used regularly, but conversational speech is usually not achieved (Williams et al., 1995b). Some individuals are able to utilize sign language or picture communication boards, as described in the section on treatment.

Neurological, Cognitive, and Behavioral Features

Seizures usually develop between 18 and 24 months, and they are seen in approximately 86% of individuals with AS. They often begin after a febrile illness, with worsening in the first few years of life and subsequent disappearance during or after adolescence (Clayton-Smith, 1993). Recurrence of seizures after a prolonged silent period can sometimes occur in adulthood (Buntinx et al., 1995). All types of seizures occur in AS, and a characteristic EEG pattern is seen with high-voltage spike-wave discharges ranging from two to six per second. The spikes are more likely to be seen with eye closure. An EEG is often helpful in making the diagnosis because of this characteristic pattern (Boyd et al., 1988).

A recent study by Guerrini et al. (1996) documented a rhythmic myoclonus on EMG involving the hands and face and associated EEG activity of spike-wave discharges over the fronto-rolandic regions, which subsequently generalized. Seven of 11 patients with AS demonstrated myoclonic seizures or myoclonic absences. However, all patients demonstrated multifocal fast jerking and twitching, which was associated with dystonic limb posturing. The EMG pattern showed that the jerks were bursts of activity occurring synchronously in agonist and antagonist muscles at a frequency of 11 Hz. The EEG pattern showed a fast bursting cortical myoclonus, which the authors feel is unique to patients with AS. The authors hypothesize that the cortical myoclonus is reflective of cortical hyperexcitability secondary to loss of GABAergic inhibition (Guerrini et al., 1996). Within the deleted region in AS there is a cluster of gamma-aminobutyric acid (GABA) receptor genes, specifically beta 3, alpha 5, and gamma 3. Furthermore, an autopsy study in a patient with AS has shown marked cerebellar atrophy with loss of Purkinje and granule cells and markedly reduced GABA content (Jay et al., 1991). The loss of inhibitory GABAergic interneurons and Purkinje cells could lead to cortical hyperexcitability and myoclonus (Guerrini et al., 1996).

Further evidence for alterations in GABAergic function comes from studies of plasma GABA levels, which were higher in 9 patients with AS and in 14 patients with PWS than in matched controls (Ebert et al., 1997). These authors postulate that the elevated plasma GABA levels represent a compensatory increase in presynaptic GABA release because of hyposensitivity of a subset of GABA receptors

(Ebert et al., 1997). The *GABRB3* gene, which is located in the deleted segment, may play a role in the AS phenotype, at least in the deletion patients, because it is not imprinted (Kubota et al., 1994).

Patients are usually happy, with frequent smiling, and bouts of laughter begin between 16 months and 3 years of age (Van Lierde et al., 1990). Usually such episodes are precipitated by minimal stimuli, and sometimes they occur with painful experiences, such as venipuncture. These episodes may also be a form of cortical hyperexcitability. Hand-flapping is common, but these patients are particularly well known for the unusual posturing of the hands and arms, with flexion at the wrists and elbows when the arms are raised, such that they resemble a puppet on a string. This posturing in addition to the jerky movements and ataxia in the gait is seen in virtually 100% of patients.

Although hypotonia is usually present in infancy, slightly increased tone in the limbs is usually seen in patients older than 3 years of age. Deep tendon reflexes are usually brisk, but plantar responses are flexor (Robb et al., 1989). Most patients are walking by 3 to 5 years of age, but approximately 10% are non-ambulatory because of more severe spasticity, severe ataxia/hypotonia, or scoliosis complications (Clayton-Smith, 1993). Urinary and fecal continence develops in approximately 60% in childhood and at a mean age of 6½ years (Buntinx et al., 1995).

In a study of 57 patients with AS who underwent CT scanning, 37% were abnormal, and they usually showed mild cerebral atrophy (Clayton-Smith, 1993). Two patients have been reported with cerebellar atrophy, including the autopsy patient described previously (Jay et al., 1991; Williams and Frias, 1982). One patient was reported with partial agenesis of the temporal lobe (Van Lierde et al., 1990) and another with anomalous gyral convolutions on CT studies (Williams et al., 1995b). An autopsy on an infant with AS showed minor perisylvian cerebral gyral abnormalities, partial agenesis of the corpus callosum, and minor foci of neuronal dysplasia and heterotopia in the temporal cortex and hypothalmus (Williams et al., 1995b). Visual problems include strabismus in 42%, nystagmus in an occasional patient, and refraction errors in approximately 10% (Clayton-Smith, 1993).

The behavior problems include severe hyperactivity in childhood, which usually resolves by adulthood. Young children are motorically very hyperactive, with ceaseless activity that includes continually putting things in their mouths and constantly moving from one object to another (Williams et al., 1995b). The attention span is extremely short, and this may interfere with social development because the patient has difficulty in attending to the facial cues of others (Williams et al., 1995b). They also demonstrate impulsive behavior, which sometimes can include pinching, biting, and grabbing (Williams et al., 1995b). Their impulsive behavior and their love of water often leads to jumping into the bathtub or other body of water with their clothes on (Clayton-Smith, 1993). They also demonstrate a fascination for things, such as mirrors or shiny objects. One hyperactive patient had the habit of licking everything that came within his reach, particularly cold smooth metallic objects (Van Lierde et al., 1990). Some of these behaviors and intense interests can be considered obsessive compulsive behavior, which can be treated pharmacologically, as described later in this chapter.

Sleep problems occur in 85 to 90% of patients with AS (Smith et al., 1996). Patients usually are at their worst between 2 and 6 years of age (Clayton-Smith, 1993). They seem to have a reduced need for sleep, with frequent awakenings, and sometimes they are destructive to their rooms at night. Usually the sleep problems have resolved by adolescence (Clayton-Smith, 1993).

Growth and Skeletal Features

The growth parameters at birth, including the head circumference, are normal. However, with age, height growth drops to the third percentile or less in 58% (Smith et al., 1996). In addition, microcephaly develops in just over 50% by 2 years of age (Smith et al., 1996). There is a tendency for obesity in older patients, but this may be related to compulsive eating.

Scoliosis developed in 11% of the 82 patients studied in England (Clayton-Smith, 1993). This was a greater problem in nonambulatory patients, and most required bracing, although one patient underwent spinal fusion. In a study of AS across the life span, 8% of children had scoliosis, but 38% of adults had this problem (Buntinx et al., 1995). Mild cutaneous syndactyly was also found in this study in approximately 60% of patients (Buntinx et al., 1995).

Molecular-Clinical Correlations

Most of the clinical findings in AS, including the facial features, ataxia, severe mental retardation, and seizures, occur in patients with deletions, UPD, and those with an imprinting mutation. An exception to this is hypopigmentation, which is seen in approximately 40% of patients and may occur mainly in those patients with a deletion (Burger et al., 1996; Williams et al., 1995b). Usually the hypopigmentation is mild, creating blue eyes and blonde hair, and it is noticeable when comparing patients to other family members. A rare patient has been reported with oculocutaneous albinism (Smith et al., 1996). The hypopigmentation in AS and in PWS, as discussed later in this section, is related to the deletion of the *P* gene, which codes for a tyrosine transporter protein that is important for making melanin (Lee et al., 1994). The haploinsufficiency in a deletion patient leads to the hypopigmentation, and the presence of an additional mutation on the other allele in 1% of individuals leads to oculocutaneous albinism (Lee et al., 1994). The *P* gene is not deleted in patients with UPD or an imprinting mutation, so they do not have an increased incidence of hypopigmentation (Williams et al., 1995b).

There have been some recent reports of patients with UPD or an imprinting mutation and a mild version of AS with later onset of seizures, more verbalizations, no microcephaly, and/or less ataxia than what is typically seen (Bottani et al., 1994; Burger et al., 1996; Gillessen-Kaesbach et al., 1995a; Saitoh et al., 1997). Smith et al. (1997) have summarized these findings by comparing their 4 patients with 10 previously reported cases of AS resulting from UPD. The head circumference was normal in 72%, the height was normal in 77%, and epilepsy was present in only 42% (Smith et al., 1997). More detailed studies are needed to clarify the full spectrum of involvement in patients with UPD, patients with an imprinting mutation, and patients with a mutation in the candidate gene.

Two laboratories have demonstrated different point mutations in the gene UBE3A which lead to an abnormal or truncated protein from this gene (Kishino et al., 1997; Matsuura et al., 1997). Subsequent studies on the normal expression of UBE3A show that it demonstrates maternal allele-specific expression in the brain but not in lymphocytes or fibroblasts (Rougeulle et al., 1997; Vu and Hoffman, 1997). This means that the maternal imprint occurs in one tissue, brain, which causes the phenotype of AS, but not in other tissues. The UBE3A protein forms a thioester with ubiquitin and transfers ubiquitin to substrate targets. The ubiquitin-mediated proteolytic pathway plays a major role in the regulation of protein turnover. This is important in CNS development, and a related protein in *Drosophila* is needed in the alteration of synaptic connectivity among a subset of neurons (Kishino et al., 1997).

Further studies include the development of a mouse model for AS that has partial paternal disomy that includes the mouse equivalent of the UBE3A gene, *Ube3a*. This mouse model demonstrates mild gait ataxia, EEG, and behavioral abnormalities, a reduction in brain size (especially the cerebellum) and skeletal size, and late-onset obesity (Albrecht et al., 1997). Studies of *Ube3a* expression in the mouse UPD brain have shown absent expression in the hippocampus and in the Purkinje neurons of the cerebellum compared with normal expression in controls (Albrecht et al., 1997). Reduced expression was seen in other areas of the brain, including the cerebral cortex and the olfactory bulb, but the most dramatic differences were seen in the hippocampus and in the Purkinje cells, demonstrating regional differences of the imprint effect within the brain (Albrecht et al., 1997).

Molecular Diagnosis

High-resolution cytogenetic studies will not identify all of the deletion patients with AS or PWS, but they are still recommended because they will also identify rare instances of translocations or other chromosomal problems (ASHG/ACMG, 1996; Butler, 1990). In addition, molecular techniques, including fluorescent in situ hybridization (FISH) studies and methylation analysis, are also recommended. For FISH studies, commercially available probes from the common deletion region, such as the SNRPN probe, are used with a control probe from outside of the deletion region but still on chromosome 15 (ASHG/ACMG, 1996). If a deletion is not found, then molecular methods are used to detect possible UPD. Polymerase chain reaction (PCR) techniques are used to identify short tandem repeats from DNA samples of both parents to detect UPD in the patient (ASHG/ACMG, 1996). In this region of chromosome 15 there is a differential methylation pattern, with most sites methylated on the maternal chromosome and unmethylated on the paternal chromosome. Two such sites are typically utilized for methylation studies; specifically, the *SNRPN* and the *PW71B* probes are used to detect maternal and paternal methylation patterns. If only the maternal pattern is seen, then PWS is confirmed, and if only the paternal pattern is seen, then AS is confirmed (ASHG/ACMG, 1996). A recent report of a PCR-based technique to evaluate the methylation status of the *SNRPN* gene allows rapid diagnosis of PWS and AS (Kosaki et al., 1997). Detection of mutations in the imprinting center or point mutations in *UBE3A* are not carried out in a clinical diagnostic lab, so they can be referred to a research center which specializes in this.

Prenatal diagnosis can detect the deletion, and recently studies by Kubota et al. (1996) suggest that the methylation analysis utilizing the *SNRPN* probe in amniotic cells and CVS tissue may be a safe test for prenatal diagnosis of imprinting defects.

Treatment

Infancy and Early Childhood

Problems with feeding are usually the first difficulties experienced by children with AS. Difficulties in coordinating suck may interfere with breast feeding more than with bottle feeding. Work with an occupational therapist (OT) even in infancy can improve oral motor coordination, sucking, and feeding. Frequent regurgitation of feedings is also common, and gastroesophageal reflux (GER) is seen in 40% (Clayton-Smith, 1993). Sometimes GER will improve or resolve with positioning upright after meals and thickening the feedings with rice cereal. If these interventions do not improve the situation, then medication can be considered to decrease reflux and improve gastric emptying time. Metoclopromide (Reglan), which enhances lower esophageal pressure and improves gastric empty-ing time, and bethanacol, a cholinergic agent which enhances smooth muscle contraction in the intestine, are commonly used to treat GER. Both have side effects, including irritability, and metoclopromide can cause dystonic reactions. Perhaps patients with AS are at greater risk for these problems because of the severity of their CNS dysfunction, which includes motor tone problems. Cisapride (Propulsid) improves gastric emptying time without CNS effects, and therefore may be more helpful in this patient group. However, because cisapride is metabo-lized by the P_{450} cytochrome system, other medications, such as erythromycin, which interfere with this system should be avoided or else cardiac arrhythmias may result (Ward et al., 1999). Recurrent GER can cause a significant esophagitis associated with pain which can be treated with an H2 blocker (i.e., ranitidine or Zantac) or a proton pump inhibitor (omeprazole or Prilosec). If medical treatment fails for GER and problems related to failure to thrive, aspiration, or chronic pain persist, then surgery should be considered to tighten the lower esophageal sphincter area with a Nissen or Thal fundoplication. This surgery was only necessary in 2 of 82 patients with AS studied in England (Clayton-Smith, 1993).

Recurrent otitis media often begins in infancy and persists in early childhood. Aggressive treatment with polyethylene (PE) tubes is recommended because of the frequency of recurrence and the interference with development. Sometimes the adenoids can cause eustachian tube drainage problems and exacerbate mouth breathing, particularly when midface hypoplasia is present. Referral to an ENT physician to evaluate the need for adenoidectomy is occasionally necessary.

Seizures usually develop in the first 2 to 3 years of life and require anticonvulsant therapy. The most commonly used medication is valproic acid (Depakote or Depakene) because it is helpful for partial seizures and generalized seizures, including absence seizures and myoclonic seizures (Brodie and Dichter, 1996). Its mechanism of action is through stimulation of GABA neurotransmission, which is problematic in patients with AS. It is also a mood stabilizer, which may help with the inappropriate bouts of laughter and mood swings. The side effects of valproic acid include appetite changes, especially weight gain; decrease in white blood cell count and platelet number; hair thinning; hepatic toxicity; pancreatitis; and menstrual irregularities, including amenorrhea; and the possible development of polycystic ovarian disease (Brodie and Dichter, 1996). Blood levels, electrolytes, and hepatic function must be followed carefully, especially in young children. Carbamazepine is less helpful in AS because it is usually not effective in patients with absence or myoclonic seizures (Brodie and Dichter, 1996). Benzodiazepines are found to be particularly helpful in AS because of their antimyoclonic and antiabsence properties related to their GABAergic properties (Guerrini et al., 1996). Hutchinson (1997) has recommended the use of lorazepam (Ativan) nasal drops if a prolonged seizure occurs at home. Newer anticonvulsants that also work by enhancing GABAergic inhibition, such as vigabatrin and tiagabine (which blocks GABA uptake), should be helpful in patients with AS, but clinical trials have not yet shown these effects (Guerrini et al., 1996).

Once the diagnosis is made, early intervention in the form of infant stimulation with motor therapy and later speech and language therapy is indicated. Augmentative and alternative communication (AAC) can be helpful, as described later.

Guerrini and colleagues have recommended treatment of the myoclonus with piracetam beginning at a dose of 2.4 g/day and increasing as tolerated until an effect is seen in a range of 114 to 160 mg/kg/day (Guerrini et al., 1996). They saw improvements in the myoclonus, which was stable after 4 to 12 months of treatment in five patients with AS. Piracetam is available in Canada, but in the United States it is only an investigational drug, so it is difficult to give it on a trial basis to patients with AS unless an investigational protocol is in place. Further research regarding the efficacy of piracetam is needed before it can be routinely recommended for AS.

Sleep problems are almost universal in patients with AS, particularly in early childhood. Children usually disrupt their parents' sleep when they get up in the middle of the night, and they may often fall asleep periodically during the day because of sleep deprivation during the night. Summers and colleagues outlined a behavioral program that was coupled with pharmacotherapy, specifically diphenhydramine (Benadryl) at a dose of 25 mg or 0.5 mg/kg 1 hour before bed to treat a 9-year-old boy with AS and sleep disturbance (Summers et al., 1992). The behavioral regimen included (1) not allowing him to fall asleep during the day;

(2) restricting his access to fluids after 7:30 p.m. to reduce night wakenings due to being wet; (3) placing him in bed at a consistent hour every night; (4) not permitting him to get out of bed at night by using gestural or physical prompts; and (5) allowing him to get out of bed in the morning only after a music alarm has sounded, thus establishing the alarm as the discriminative stimulus for rising from bed (Summers et al., 1992). This patient's sleeping time at night improved from 1.9 hours to 8.3 hours on the combined medication and behavior program. After 1 month the medication was discontinued, and his improvements persisted with behavior intervention alone.

A more commonly used medication to induce sleep is melatonin. Studies on over 100 patients with a variety of developmental disabilities have shown improvement of sleep disturbances in over 80% (Jan and O'Donnell, 1996). Melatonin has been given in doses of 1 to 6 mg without significant side effects for over 4 years to individuals with developmental delays, and it can be tried with patients who have AS and sleep problems. A small study found improvement in sleep in 12 of 13 patients with AS who were treated with a low dose of melatonin, 0.3 mg, at bedtime (Zhdanova et al., 1997). Melatonin can be obtained over the counter in 3-mg tablets, but the potency and quality of these products are not monitored as well as is prescription medication.

It is helpful to construct confining bedrooms which are also safe for the child when nighttime wakefulness occurs. For instance, a locking mechanism on the door that prevents wandering throughout the house when children awaken might be helpful.

Patients who have hypopigmentation are also sensitive to the sun and will burn easily because of a lack of melanin. It is therefore essential to use sunscreen for protection from burning (Williams et al., 1995b).

School-Aged Children

By the time children with AS begin school, significant problems with hyperactivity, impulsivity, and a short attention span exist and often lead to a diagnosis of attention deficit hyperactivity disorder (ADHD). Controlled trials of stimulant medication have not been carried out in patients with AS, perhaps because stimulants are not considered to be helpful for individuals with severe mental retardation and ADHD (Aman, 1982). Anecdotal experience, however, has shown that some individuals with AS show improvement in their ADHD symptoms with methylphenidate or pemoline (Williams et al., 1995b). Therefore, stimulant medication is usually worth trying in an effort to improve the severe hyperactivity and impulsivity. Methylphenidate (Ritalin) or Adderall (a mixture of dextro- and levoamphetamine salts) can be tried first to improve ADHD symptoms. Pemoline (Cylert) should be avoided if possible as a first-line treatment for ADHD because of recent reports of rare hepatic failure associated with pemoline's use (Adcock et al., 1998; Berkovitch et al., 1995).

Behavior modification techniques should also be utilized to improve impulsive behavior, which may include pinching or biting. Consultation with a behavioral psychologist is usually helpful to structure a consistent behavior modification program that targets one symptom at a time. This intervention can be initiated in the preschool period or earlier but may also be needed intermittently during the school-age years.

Some children may experience mood fluctuations, irritability, and/or obsessive thinking, which may respond to environmental changes or a behavior modification program. However, if these interventions are not successful, trial of a selective serotonin reuptake inhibitor (SSRI), such as fluoxetine or sertraline, may be considered. SSRIs can improve moodiness, anxiety, irritability, and obsessive-compulsive behavior in individuals with developmental disabilities (Hagerman, 1996; Steingard et al., 1997). SSRIs have few side effects, and they do not require monitoring of blood levels or liver and cardiac function. However, SSRIs inhibit the cytochrome P_{450} enzymes that carry out oxidative metabolism of commonly used medications. Anticonvulsants, particularly phenytoin and carbamazepine, in addition to diazepam, aprazolam, tricyclic antidepressants, and thioridazine, are among the medications that can have significant increases in levels when their metabolic enzymes are inhibited by SSRIs (Preskorn, 1996). There is significant variation among SSRIs regarding the degree to which different P_{450} enzymes are inhibited. Sertraline (Zoloft) has the least inhibition of P_{450} enzymes (Preskorn, 1996; von Moltke et al., 1994), so it should be used first in patients who are taking anticonvulsants, which is the majority of patients with AS. Other side effects of SSRI agents include changes in appetite, nausea, agitation, mania, and the rare occurrence of dystonia, akathisia, and tardive dyskinesia (Leo, 1996; Preskorn, 1996). The movement problems may occur at a higher rate in patients with AS because of their underlying movement abnormalities and CNS pathology.

Augmentative and Alternative Communication (AAC)

The consistent severity of the communication problems in AS (Jolleff and Ryan, 1993) has stimulated the use of both low tech (nonelectrical) and high tech (electrical) assistive technology from preschool through adulthood in individuals with AS. Table 6.2 (Blackstone, 1995) reviews the use of AAC throughout the life span in AS. In the preschool years, communication boards such as the Picture Exchange Communication System (see Appendix 3), which match a picture to objects that the child shows an interest in, can be used for many functions, including making choices, refusing things, requesting things, and expressing emotions (Weitz et al., 1997). Simple systems include the use of cue boards, which are step-by-step sets of pictures, to assist a child in accomplishing a task. A picture schedule can lay out the activities of the day or week or month on a calendar. A symbol or photo or object can represent an activity. If objects or symbols are used, the child can touch or hold it until the end of the activity and then pick up the next one representing the next activity. Pictures or symbols can be put on a key chain or in a wallet for fast and portable communication (Blackstone, 1990). The utilization of body language and signing can also begin with toddlers and advance throughout the school-aged years.

TABLE 6.2. Helping People with AS Communicate Using Assistive Technology

Age and Stage	Description of communication	Desired outcomes	Low-tech strategies (nonelectronic)	High-tech strategies (electronic)
Infancy 0–12 months	Cooing, babbling delayed. Social smiling/laughing atypical. Cognitive delays	Interact with caregivers using recognizable signals. Respond and initiate.	Stable positioning is important for face-to-face communication. Commercially available products applicable.	Shine flashlight on caregiver's face to encourage facial contact and visual attention
Toddler 1–3 years	Lack of speech, oral/speech motor problems. Limited attention span. Cognitive/receptive language delays less severe than expressive delay.	Use simple switches to activate toys, turn on/off appliances, and express simple messages. Begin to attach meaning to objects. Enjoy interaction.	Use objects as symbols to make requests, choices. Present objects on choice boards and encourage child to make choices.	Use simple switches to activate toys, turn on/off appliances, and express simple messages (e.g., coo, babble, or "do it again" using loop tapes, Big Red switch, Voice Pal).
Preschool/Early childhood 3–8 years	Dysarthria precludes functional speech. Difficult to interpret signs, gestures, and facial expressions. Cognitive delays.	Use objects, pictures, communication books, VOCAs, calendar boxes, remnant books to interact with adults and same-age peers.	Begin to pair two-dimensional symbols (photographs, simple pictures) with preferred objects when child shows interest. Use calendar box throughout day.	Caregivers become familiar with simple VOCAs and use with child on a daily basis. Also appropriate computer software can be introduced.
Childhood 8–21 years	Idiosyncratic gestures. Bursts of laughter, drooling, chewing, licking. Behaviors can interfere with using AAC devices.	Use AAC aids and devices (see text) in everyday interaction with adults and peers. Use other tools (e.g., computer) to participate in activities with same-age peers.	Continue to expand functional communication by using objects and context-specific mini-boards and communication books, calendar boxes, remnant books, conversation books. Use them to teach, as well as help child/youth express language.	If the need for messages increases, consider using Macaw, Parrot, AlphaTalker, Walker-Talker, Message Mate, Digivox. These VOCAs offer from nine to hundreds of messages and digitized speech.
Adulthood 22+ years	Little information about communication available.	Have necessary communication skills to reside and work in communities when supported. Have friends.	Depending on representational level, use a combination of communication boards/books, schedule boards/books.	The above devices can be considered. In addition, the phone and computer may be useful.

From Blackstone (1995). Reprinted with permission.

Speech and language therapy can facilitate the use of signing and can gradually introduce the use of AAC devices to facilitate functional communication. Miller surveyed 176 families who are raising children with AS and reported that most children use signs and gestures, 40% use picture boards, and only 20% use electronic communication devices (Miller, 1995). Some of the drawbacks of electronic communication devices include the cost and the fact that children with AS can be hard on these devices, which are damaged frequently. However, they can dramatically enhance the communication abilities of children and adults with AS, particularly voice output communication aids (VOCAs). Some examples are the Alpha Talker, Macaw, and Walker Talker (see Table 6.2 and the Resources at the end of this chapter (Blackstone, 1990; Blackstone, 1995; Weitz et al., 1997).

CASE HISTORY: SARAH

Sarah is a 7-year-11-month-old girl with Angelman syndrome who was diagnosed at 4 years of age when cytogenetic testing demonstrated the classical deletion at 15q11.

Her birth history was normal. Her biological mother was just 17 when she became pregnant. She delivered vaginally; birth weight was 6½ pounds. Sarah received oxygen in the newborn period but subsequently did fine and went home the next day. Her young mother, however, was abusive and neglectful, and at 5 months of age Sarah had a dislocated shoulder and a fracture of her collarbone. Sarah was a very difficult baby to feed, she had a poor suck, and she was also tactilely defensive when held, so she would frequently arch and pull away from holding. At 5 months of age, Sarah's grandmother took over her care and now has legal custody of her. Her grandmother was able to spend the time with her to stimulate sucking, and her weight gain improved. She did not cry excessively, and in fact she was a happy baby who was not particularly fussy. She was, however, very stiff in all of her extremities, and she was diagnosed with cerebral palsy at 10 months of age. Her grandmother felt that her left side was somewhat stiffer than her right, and she was never hypotonic.

Her developmental milestones included sitting at 8 months, crawling at 8 months, but not walking until 2½ years. She has never developed speech, although some of her verbalizations represent words, and those who know her can understand some of her verbalizations. She has also developed her own sign language and signs approximately 15 words.

When she was an infant and up until approximately age 6½, Sarah slept very little and would frequently wake up in the middle of the night and stay awake until morning. This occurred approximately 4 times per week. At the present time she has great difficulty sleeping because it is hard for her to settle down to go to sleep. She was prescribed chloral hydrate within the last 2 years to help with sleep, and she takes 1½ teaspoons approximately once per week for this problem.

She was hyperactive from the time that she could walk, and she has a very short attention span. Her attention will jump from one activity to another in seconds or minutes. She is also quite impulsive and will grab different objects at a fairly fast rate. She was prescribed methylphenidate (Ritalin) at 4 years of age for her hyperactivity, and she responded well to this medication beginning at a dose of 5 mg twice a day. She is presently at a dose of 15 mg in the morning, 15 mg midday, and 5 or 10 mg in the late afternoon. The methylphenidate has decreased her appetite somewhat, but she has not lost weight.

Sarah's past medical history includes recurrent ear infections, with five infections in early childhood. She has also had significant reflux into her ureters bilaterally, and this has caused scarring and loss of volume of her right kidney, secondary to recurrent urinary tract infections. Her ureters were reimplanted at 5 years of age, and she has not had subsequent infections. She had strabismus with a right exotropia, and her treatment included patching of the left eye and surgery at age 2 years. She has done well in follow-up with glasses. She has not had clinical seizures, except between ages 1 and 2 she had an episode of arching of her back, and stiffening which lasted minutes.

Her therapy included physical therapy from 1 year to 3 years of age, and this has helped her increased motor tone remarkably. She became more flexible in her extremities after this intensive therapy. She has also had occupational therapy since she was 4 years old, and they have worked with sensory integration therapy and utilized calming techniques, including swinging, joint compression, and brushing to help her calm her excessive hyperactivity and impulsivity. They have also worked on daily living skills, and she is presently working on putting on her shoes and dressing herself.

She has received intensive speech and language therapy, both at school and through a private therapist. Last year the DeltaTalker, which is a VOCA, was initiated, and she utilizes approximately 15 phrases on a regular basis both at home and at school. A harness was developed to hold the DeltaTalker just below the waist (Figure 6.1). This allows for easy access to use the DeltaTalker both at home and at school. Since she has initiated the DeltaTalker, her frustration level regarding communication has decreased remarkably. Over the last year, her speech and language pathologist has also developed a book that has different sections with approximately 50 pictures in each section. The different categories include breakfast, lunch, and dinner, with pictures representing different foods, and school activities with pictures representing school utensils, such as a backpack, ruler, and painting activities. Also included are pictures of friends and family members and holiday activities. She carries this book with her both at home and at school, and she uses it many times during the day as she makes her wants and needs known.

In general, Sarah has been a very happy child; she has a wonderful sense of humor and she laughs frequently. Her episodes of hyperactivity and out-of-control behavior, which are often stimulated by excessive sensory stimulation, have decreased remarkably with the combination of her methylphenidate and OT sensory-integration therapy.

On examination her weight is at the 40th percentile for age, as is her height, but her head circumference is only 48 cms, which is less than the second percentile for age. She was quite hyperactive, with poor eye contact, intermittent hand flapping, and excessive motor activity throughout the examination. Her head was microcephalic, her ear pinnae were not prominent, and her eyes were normal, although she has blue eyes and light blond hair, demonstrating a mild degree of hypopigmentation. Her teeth were widely spaced, and her mouth was wide. A nose and throat exam was normal. She had increased tone in the upper and the lower extremities, but she did not have contractures. She frequently walked on her toes, but when requested to do so she would walk normally, although her gait was mildly ataxic and wide-based. A heart exam was normal, there was no evidence of scoliosis, and her genitalia demonstrated normal prepubertal development. Deep tendon reflexes were 2+ in all four extremities; she did not have clonus in the lower extremities. She was able to touch my fingers on cerebellar testing without significant ataxia, although her gait demonstrated ataxia. She was unable to hold a pencil well and to draw circles or crosses.

Her treatment program includes continuation of her speech and language therapy and occupational therapy, both through school and at home. It was recommended that she try a 3-mg dose of melatonin at bedtime instead of chloral hydrate, to see if this improves her ability to fall asleep at a reasonable time. Her grandmother states that she does not have problems with mood lability or tantrum behavior, and generally at home she is quite appropriate in her behavior. Her hyperactivity is severe, and she continues to use methylphenidate with a beneficial effect.

Adolescence and Adulthood

Sexual maturation is often delayed in adolescence, but seizures have usually stopped and behavior problems tend to settle down in late adolescence and adulthood. Some patients suffer from severe scoliosis, which can lead to respiratory problems in late adulthood. Although most patients are ambulatory, some find the wheelchair more comfortable in adulthood (Blackstone, 1995). The nonambulatory patients, particularly females, are at highest risk for progressive scoliosis and require careful orthopedic monitoring (Williams et al., 1995b).

AAC technology can continue to be helpful in adolescence and adulthood to enhance peer interactions, facilitate daily living activities, and enhance vocational options by improving and facilitating communication. For many individuals, improvement in communication can decrease frustration and improve behavioral problems (Blackstone, 1995).

PRADER-WILLI SYNDROME

Prader-Willi syndrome (PWS) first came to medical attention in 1956 when Prader, Labhart, and Willi reported a few patients with mental retardation and similar dysmorphic features, including short stature, cryptorchidism, obesity, and poor muscle tone. This disorder has been around for centuries; Cassidy pointed out that the painting titled "La Monstrua," painted in 1680 by Juan Carreno de Miranda, which now hangs in the Prado, is of a 6-year-old girl who certainly had PWS because of her dysmorphic facial features, obesity, and small hands and feet (Cassidy, 1984). Although PWS was initially considered to be very rare, it now is identified far more easily with new molecular techniques as described earlier in this chapter. The prevalence of PWS is approximately 1 per 15,000 (Burd et al., 1990).

Most of the clinical features of PWS are thought to be secondary to hypothalamic insufficiency (Dykens and Cassidy, 1996). In infancy, severe central hypotonia leads to a poor suck, failure to thrive because of feeding difficulties, a weak or unusual cry described as kitten-like or squeaky, absent or weak deep tendon reflexes, frequent breech delivery, and delayed milestones, including sitting independently at 13 months and walking at 28 months on average (Aughton and Cassidy, 1990; Holm et al., 1993). A medical work-up for hypotonia, including nerve conduction studies, electromyography, and muscle enzymes, is normal, and a diagnosis of benign hypotonia is often given (Cassidy, 1984). Hypothalamic insufficiency also leads to genital hypoplasia, which is visible in the majority of males in the newborn period because of cryptorchidism, scrotal hypoplasia, or micropenis, but it is less obvious in the female infants who have labial hypoplasia and/or a small clitoris (Aughton and Cassidy, 1990).

The failure to thrive in infancy may often lead to a prolonged hospitalization and gavage feedings, with a drop in weight and height to less than the third percentile. Between 6 months and approximately 2 years of age the appetite improves, but hyperphagia develops between 2 and 6 years with a lack of normal satiation, leading eventually to severe obesity. Obesity is exacerbated by an inability to vomit and decreased caloric requirements, in addition to an obsession on food (Cassidy, 1984). There is a more global problem with obsessive-compulsive behavior that encompasses other areas besides food and is described later in this section.

Consensus diagnostic criteria were developed for PWS in 1993 to aid in early recognition and research and because at that time not all of the children could be identified by molecular and cytogenetic techniques (Holm et al., 1993). It was anticipated that PWS could be diagnosed by molecular techniques in some individuals who would be excluded by the consensus criteria as more mildly affected cases were identified (Holm et al., 1993).

The consensus criteria include the following major criteria, which are worth 1 point each:

1. Neonatal and infantile central hypotonia with poor suck, gradually improving with age.
2. Feeding problems in infancy with need for special feeding techniques and poor weight gain/failure to thrive.

3. Excessive or rapid weight gain on weight-for-length chart (excessive is defined as crossing two centile channels) after 12 months but before 6 years of age; central obesity in the absence of intervention.
4. Characteristic facial features with dolichocephaly in infancy, narrow face or bifrontal diameter, almond-shaped eyes, small-appearing mouth with thin upper lip, down-turned corners of the mouth (three or more required).
5. Hypogonadism with any of the following, depending on age:
    a Genital hypoplasia (male: scrotal hypoplasia, cryptorchidism, small penis and/or testes for age [<5th percentile]; females: absence or severe hypoplasia of labia minora and/or clitoris).
    b. Delayed or incomplete gonadal maturation with delayed pubertal signs in the absence of intervention after 16 years of age (male: small gonads, decreased facial and body hair, lack of voice change; female: amenorrhea/oligomenorrhea after age 16).
6. Global developmental delay in child younger than 6 years of age; mild to moderate mental retardation or learning problems in older children.
7. Hyperphagia / food foraging / obsession with food.
8. Deletion 15q11–13 on high resolution (>650 bands) or other cytogenetic/molecular abnormality of the Prader-Willi chromosome region, including maternal disomy.

Minor criteria, which are worth 1/2 point each, are as follows:

1. Decreased fetal movement or infantile lethargy or weak cry in infancy, improving with age.
2. Characteristic behavior problems—temper tantrums, violent outbursts, and obsessive compulsive behavior; tendency to be argumentative, oppositional, rigid, manipulative, possessive, and stubborn, perseverating, stealing, and lying (five or more of these symptoms required).
3. Sleep disturbance or sleep apnea.
4. Short stature for genetic background by age 15 (in the absence of growth hormone intervention).
5. Hypopigmentation—fair skin and hair compared to family.
6. Small hands (<25th percentile) and/or feet (<10th percentile) for height and age.
7. Narrow hands with straight ulnar border.
8. Eye abnormalities (estropia, myopia).
9. Thick viscous saliva with crusting at corners of mouth.
10. Speech articulation defects.
11. Skin picking.

Supportive findings that increase the certainty of the diagnosis but are not scored for points include the following:

1. High pain threshold.
2. Decreased vomiting.

3. Temperature instability in infancy or altered temperature sensitivity in older children and adults.
4. Scoliosis and/or kyphosis.
5. Early adrenarche.
6. Osteoporosis.
7. Unusual skill with jigsaw puzzles.
8. Normal neuromuscular studies.

Five points (4 in the major criteria) are required for a clinical diagnosis in children who are 3 years of age or younger, and 8 points (5 in the major criteria) are required for children older than 3 through adulthood (Holm et al., 1993). As more patients are now identified with the biological markers of a deletion, uniparental disomy, or imprint mutation, there is less need for strict consensus criteria, although this information is important for clinicians to consider the diagnosis and order the molecular studies.

Craniofacial and Ophthalmological Features

The typical features of PWS include a small mouth with a thin and downturned upper lip that gives the mouth a triangular shape (Figure 6.2). These features are thought to be related to the severe hypotonia and poor prenatal neuromuscular functioning. The eyes or palpebral fissures are almond-shaped with a mild upslanting laterally. There is a narrow bifrontal diameter that often contrasts with fullness in the cheeks related to the obesity. The skull shape is usually dolicocephalic, and an occasional patient has macrocephaly. Oral pathology includes delayed eruption of teeth, frequent caries, malocclusion in 39%, and enamel hypoplasia in 12% (Cassidy, 1984). The saliva has a sticky viscous quality and often dries on the lips of the patients. Oral motor coordination problems are common and may be related to the hypotonia, in addition to the general CNS impairment (Table 6.3).

Ophthalmologic findings include strabismus in 40 to 75% of patients and myopia in 24% (Butler, 1989; Cassidy, 1984). Hypopigmentation occurs in approximately 50% of patients with PWS and is more common in patients with a deletion than in other molecular subtypes (Butler, 1989; Dykens and Cassidy, 1996). Hypopigmentation includes a lighter hair color and skin pigment than other family members who do not have PWS. The stroma of the iris may also be depigmented, reflecting a scarcity of stromal melanocytes with a radial pattern of translucency of the iris which allows visualization of the lens through an undilated pupil (Cassidy, 1984). The hypopigmentation in the eye and elsewhere in PWS is thought to be related to hemizygosity of the *P* gene, which is located within the 15q11–q13 region and produces a protein that transports tyrosine, a precursor to melanin, across the membrane, as described previously (Lee et al., 1994; Spritz et al., 1997). Approximately 1% of patients with PWS or AS have type-II oculocutaneous albinism, which is secondary to an inherited pathological mutation in the *P* gene on the normal chromosome 15 in addition to the deletion (Lee et al., 1994).

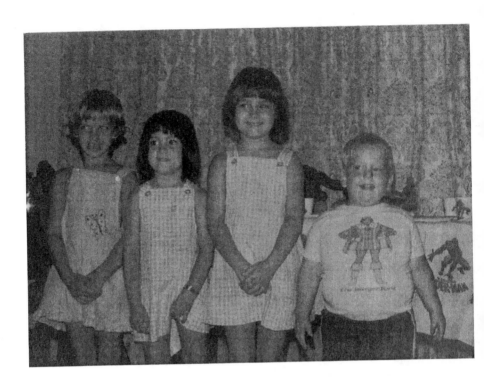

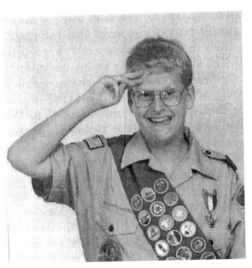

FIGURE 6.2: (a) Young boy with PWS and obesity on the right. (b) Same patient with PWS in young adulthood.

TABLE 6.3. Features of Individuals with Prader-Willi Syndrome (PWS)

Clinical features	Overall %
Gestation	
Reduced fetal activity	76
Nonterm delivery	41
Breech presentation	26
Early infancy	
Developmental delay	98
Hypotonia (weak muscle tone)	94
Feeding problems	93
Low birthweight	30
Face	
Narrow forehead	75
Almond-shaped eyes	75
Strabismus	52
Early dental cavities/enamel hypoplasia	40
Brain function and behavior	
Mental deficiency	97
Obsessive-compulsive disorder	50
Temper outbursts	49
Repetitive actions	88
Compulsions causing adaptive impairment	80
Seizures	20
Skin picking	79
Growth	
Obesity	94
Short stature	76
Delayed bone age	50
Sexual development	
Hypogenitalism/hypogonadism (underdeveloped sex organs)	95
Cryptorchidism (undescended testicles)	88
Menstruation	39
Skeletal	
Small hands and feet	83
Scoliosis	44

Adapted from Thompson et al. (1996), Stein et al. (1994), Dykens et al. (1996), and Dykens and Cassidy (1996).

Individuals with hypopigmentation and PWS have been shown to have misrouting of the optic fibers in central pathways detected by using pattern-onset visual-evoked potentials (Creel et al., 1986). It is thought that the presence of melanin pigment in the retina is important for normal development of optic projections during embryogenesis. Misrouting usually involves excess optic fibers from the temporal retina crossing at the optic chiasm instead of projecting to the ipsilateral hemisphere. This abnormality is common in albinism, and misrouting has catastrophic effects on the organization of the geniculate nucleus of the thalamus and the subsequent organization of the visual cortex (Creel et al., 1986). Misrouting can also predispose to strabismus and nystagmus (Creel et al., 1986).

Growth and Orthopedic Features

Although growth measures are essentially normal at the time of birth, within the first year growth parameters fall off until obesity picks up. Then weight increases dramatically, but height growth only parallels the normal curve during childhood. The prepubertal growth spurt is absent related to hypothalamic insufficiency, and height below the fifth percentile is usually seen in adolescent and adult individuals with PWS (Butler et al., 1991; Cassidy, 1984). Standard growth curves for height, weight and head circumference have been developed for children and young adults with PWS and are useful in following patients long term (Butler and Meaney, 1991). Deficiency of growth hormone (GH) and its mediator insulin-like growth factor (IGF-I), also called somatomedin-C, can usually be demonstrated, and the average untreated adult height is 155 cm for males and 148 cm for females (Dykens and Cassidy, 1996; Lee, 1995). Normally IGF-I and its binding protein IGFBP-3 increase during childhood and puberty, and these levels are also high in non-PWS patients with exogenous obesity; however, in patients with PWS, these levels are invariably below the normal range after 5 years of age (Lee, 1995). Growth of the hands and feet are also slow, and the average adult shoe size in males is 5 (22.3 cm) and in females it is 3 (20.3 cm) (Butler and Meaney, 1991; S. Cassidy, personal communication 1998). The small extremities are even more remarkable because of the contrast with the obesity, which seems to stop at the ankles and wrists (Dykens and Cassidy, 1996). The hands are narrow, with a decrease of the hypothenar bulge so that a straight edge is seen on the ulnar aspect of the hand.

Scoliosis is seen in 25 to 86% of patients, but active orthopedic treatment is needed in only 15 to 20% of those with curves. Osteoporosis is also a frequent problem and may occur throughout life. Both hypogonadism and GH/IGF deficiency contribute to the pathophysiology of osteoporosis in PWS. The obesity, in addition to the osteoporosis and hypotonia, also contributes to the high frequency of scoliosis (Lee, 1995).

Obesity

Obesity is the most severe problem in PWS from both the patient's and the clinician's perspectives because it causes the morbidity and mortality in this disorder and it is the most difficult problem to control. The insatiable desire for food is thought to be secondary to hypothalamic insufficiency in PWS. The parvocellular oxytocin neurons of the paraventricular nucleus of the hypothalamus are thought to be crucial for the regulation of food intake, and both the oxytocin neuron number and the size of the paraventricular nucleus were found on autopsy study to be lower in five patients with PWS than in controls (Swaab et al., 1995). Oxytocin is also important in sexual arousal and orgasm and in inducing the release of insulin and glucagon, so it may be important in the additional problems in PWS that are subsequently described. Swaab et al. (1995) have suggested using nasal oxytocin as a treatment for PWS.

Food hoarding, food stealing, uncontrollable eating without normal satiation, and general obsessions regarding food have led to intensive treatment efforts to control this behavior. The complications of the severe obesity include somnolence and hypoventilation, sometimes leading to a Pickwickian syndrome, which is apnea with sleep. Additional complications include hypertension, type-II diabetes mellitus which is noninsulin dependent and improves with weight loss, and cor-pulmonale or right-heart failure. Diabetes mellitus occurs in approximately 7% of children (Cassidy, 1984; Lofterod and Heiberg, 1992) and in 19% of adults with PWS (Greenswag, 1987). The severe obesity also leads to a poor self-image and to patients' feeling out of control because of their eating behavior. Treatment of obesity is essential to decrease the mortality in PWS. Approaches to treatment are described later in this chapter.

Endocrine Features

Hypothalamic insufficiency leads to underdevelopment of the gonads and delayed or abnormal sexual maturation. Unilateral or bilateral cryptorchidism is seen in over 80% of males, the scrotum is small and poorly rugated, pubic hair is sparse, shaving of the face is rarely needed, the penis is usually small, sexual activity is rare, and infertility is the rule in both sexes (Cassidy, 1984). Basal testosterone and estradiol levels are usually low or borderline, and LH and FSH levels are low (Cassidy, 1984). In females, menarche is usually delayed or may not occur at all, although oligomenorrhea is usually seen. Breast size is commonly small, and the clitoris and labia are hypoplastic (Cassidy, 1984). Precocious adrenarche is not uncommon, and precocious pubarche has rarely been reported (Pardo, 1993). Regardless of the timing of puberty, the subsequent progression will be delayed or arrested, so that treatment of precocious adrenarche or pubarche in PWS is not recommended (Pardo, 1993).

Neurological and Cognitive Features

The most significant neurological problem in PWS is the severe hypotonia and hypothalamic dysfunction. The MRI, however, is usually normal, and autopsy studies have revealed only the abnormalities of the parvoventricular nucleus described previously. Seizures occur in fewer than 20% of patients, are usually precipitated by a fever, and cease by midchildhood (Cassidy, 1984).

There is some evidence for dysfunction of the autonomic nervous system manifested in diminished salivation, an increased tolerance to pain, a diminished metabolic rate, altered sleep control with excessive daytime sleepiness, and abnormal temperature regulation with a reduction in body temperature and an absence of discomfort and shivering in response to cold stress (DiMario et al., 1994). These autonomic problems could also be related to hypothalamic dysfunction. Recent studies have demonstrated diminished parasympathetic activity in individuals with PWS compared with controls, as documented by enhanced pupillary constriction after pilocarpine administration to the eye, higher resting pulse rates, and lower incremental pulse rises after standing (DiMario et al., 1994). These authors speculate that enhancing parasympathetic tone, for instance with pilocarpine treatment, may improve salivary function, gastric motility, and perhaps fat homeostasis in patients with PWS (DiMario et al., 1994).

Intellectual abilities range from an average IQ to profound mental retardation (MR). In a review of intellectual abilities in 575 individuals with PWS, 5% had average IQ, 27% demonstrated borderline IQ, 34% had mild MR, 27% had moderate MR, and 6% had severe to profound MR (Curfs, 1992). The average IQ is 70, but behavioral problems usually interfere with adaptive abilities, although achievement scores are usually higher than overall cognitive abilities (Dykens and Cassidy, 1996; Dykens et al., 1992b). Cognitive strengths include long-term memory, particularly for incidental information, such as what a person wore at a party years ago or what streets to take to the doctor's office. These strengths are similar to what is reported in children with fetal alcohol syndrome and fragile X syndrome. Visual-spatial perceptual abilities and visual memory are also strengths, and some individuals show a great ability with jigsaw puzzles, which is included in the supportive findings for the diagnostic criteria. Academic strengths include reading decoding, acquired information, and vocabulary, whereas math is often an academic weakness (Dykens and Cassidy, 1996; Dykens et al., 1992b; Holm, 1981). Cognitive weaknesses are seen in sequential processing of information, particularly auditory information. Although deficits occur in auditory attention, a diagnosis of attention deficit hyperactivity disorder (ADHD) is rarely made (Gabel et al., 1986). On testing with the Kaufman Assessment Battery for Children, individuals with PWS demonstrated higher Simultaneous than Sequential IQ scores because of sequential processing deficits, and their Achievement scores were higher than their overall Mental Processing Composite scores, a pattern similar to that seen in fragile X syndrome (Bennetto and Pennington, 1996; Dykens et al., 1992b; Kemper et al., 1988). Unlike patients with fragile X syndrome, in patients with PWS IQ scores remain stable over time in longitudinal follow-up studies, and there is no significant association between weight and IQ (Bennetto and Pennington, 1996; Dykens et al., 1992b).

Adaptive functioning as measured by the Vineland Adaptive Behavior Scales was commensurate with cognitive abilities but showed strengths in daily living skills, particularly domestic skills, and weaknesses in socialization and coping skills from adolescence to midadulthood (Dykens et al., 1992a).

Behavioral Problems

Although infants and toddlers with PWS are described as placid and friendly, there is a change in behavior that occurs around 3 to 6 years of age as the insatiable appetite and cravings for food increase (Cassidy, 1984). Stubborn and irritable behavior begins, which is associated with temper tantrums or short-lived episodes of rage. Many of the behavior problems are associated with food restrictions, but they also occur with other issues, and skin picking is usually a constant problem (Cassidy, 1984). Inflexibility in thinking is associated with obsessive and compulsive behavior that does not tolerate change well. Argumentative behavior associated with mood lability and aggression or even violence can sometimes occur (Dykens and Cassidy, 1995). As the child ages, problems develop with peer interactions because of impulsive, immature behavior, inability to read social cues, inflexibility, and the need to be always in control (Cassidy, 1984). Food-related negative behaviors, such as stealing food, hoarding food, and running away to obtain food, and manipulative behaviors are common in childhood and adolescence. In adolescence and adulthood, individuals with PWS feel isolated and are often depressed. Their problems with overeating and obesity lead to a poor self-image and feeling out of control (Cassidy, 1984). In a study of maladaptive behavior in 86 children and adults with PWS, rates of tantrums were equal in children and adolescents, but increasing age was associated with depression and withdrawal, specifically with isolation, negative self-image, and pessimism (Dykens et al., 1995). In a survey of 369 individuals with PWS, 49% had temper outbursts that were rated as moderate or severe and included yelling, angry gestures, breaking objects, and even assault (Stein et al., 1994). In addition, 88% displayed repetitive actions, 67% were perseverative in speech, 75% evidenced skin picking, 12% engaged in hair pulling, 31% had counting compulsions, 34% had arranging or symmetry compulsions, and 22% had hand-washing or cleaning compulsions (Stein et al., 1994).

In a study of non-food-related obsessive-compulsive symptoms in 91 children and adults with PWS, 64% showed a moderate to severe level of distress associated with compulsions and 80% showed adaptive impairment related to compulsions (Dykens et al., 1996). Obsessions are intrusive, recurrent thoughts or images that exceed real-life worries, and compulsions are repetitive behaviors that a person is driven to perform in response to an obsessional thought or set of rigid rules. Symptoms seen in over half of the sample included hoarding a variety of objects such as trash, paper, pens, batteries, and toiletries and the need to know, tell, or ask, leading to persistent telling or questioning (Dykens et al., 1996). One-third of patients had obsessions with ideas of symmetry and exactness, which led to the compulsion to even things out or to order, rewrite, and arrange things. Only 25% showed excessive showering, toileting, and grooming, but 39% showed marked concerns with the care and grooming of their pets (Dykens et al., 1996). Compulsive behavior often led to tantrums, argumentativeness, or anxiety. Approximately half of the subjects had moderate to severe obsessions, and 45% of the subjects had compulsions that took one hour or more each day to carry out (Dykens et al., 1996).

The diagnosis of obsessive-compulsive disorder (OCD) occurs in approximately 50% of patients with PWS, which is higher than in other mental retardation syndromes that have been studied (Dykens and Cassidy, 1996). PWS may also predispose individuals to depression and anxiety, which occur in approximately 25% and 20%, respectively (Dykens and Cassidy, 1996). Although impulsive behavior is common, ADHD is present in only 5 to 7%. Autism or pervasive developmental disorder not otherwise specified is present in 5%, but it has only been reported in individuals who have maternal disomy of chromosome 15 (Dykens and Cassidy, 1996).

Recent reports have suggested an increased incidence of psychosis in individuals with PWS, including those with a deletion or UPD (Clarke et al., 1998). In surveys of patients with PWS, psychotic symptoms were seen in 6.3% of 95 individuals (Clarke, 1998) and in 21.7% of 23 individuals (Beardsmore et al., 1998). There is often an affective and cyclic component to the psychotic symptoms, and treatment with a mood stabilizer such as lithium or valproic acid in addition to an antipsychotic is usually necessary (Verhoeven et al., 1998; Beardsmore et al., 1998).

Molecular-Clinical Correlations

The deletions typically seen in PWS are 4 to 5 megabases (Mb) in size and include more genes than what are imprinted in this region and would be dysfunctional with UPD or an imprinting mutation. Therefore, one would expect that individuals who have deletions would be more severely affected clinically than patients who have UPD or an imprinting mutation. However, UPD most likely arises from an initial trisomy of chromosome 15 with subsequent loss of the only paternal 15. Two cases have been reported with trisomy for 15 on CVS, but a subsequent amniocentesis demonstrated a "normal" karotype with a later diagnosis of PWS and UPD (Cassidy et al., 1992; Purvis-Smith et al., 1992). The early influence of trisomy or perhaps tissue mosaicism for trisomy may have a significant deleterious effect on the fetus above and beyond the effects of UPD, so a subgroup of patients with UPD may have more severe involvement than patients with a deletion (Mitchell et al., 1996). Several studies have been carried out to detect phenotypic differences between the molecular subgroups. Early studies by Butler and colleagues found that hypopigmentation was more common in deletion patients, which is consistent with the *P* gene deletion effects, and that deletion patients had a higher IQ than non-deletion patients (Butler, 1989; Butler et al., 1986). Subsequent studies have better delineated the molecular subgroups because of improvements in molecular technology and have found some differences between the molecular subgroups, including a higher maternal age in mothers of patients with UPD, which is consistent with a possible initial trisomy, and a greater incidence of hypopigmentation in deletion patients, as previously reported (Gillessen-Kaesback et al., 1995b; Mitchell et al., 1996; Spritz et al., 1997). When the molecular subgroups were subdivided by the sex of the patient, females with UPD were found to have a slightly milder phenotype, evidenced by a shorter time spent gavage feeding at birth, and a later onset of hyperphagia than female deletion patients (Mitchell et al., 1996). Recent studies have found further significant differences in the cognitive and behavioral areas. Cassidy et al. (1997) reported that patients with UPD were less likely to show skin picking, skill with jigsaw puzzles, and a high pain threshold than were deletion patients. In addition, patients with UPD were less likely to have "typical" facial features of PWS than were deletion patients. Roof et al. (1998) recently reported more impairment in IQ, social behavior, and independence in patients with a deletion than in those with UPD. The milder phenotype in patients with UPD leads to a later diagnosis (mean age 9.29 years) than in patients with a deletion (mean age 3.76 years) (Gunay-Aygun et al., 1997).

A milder phenotype has also been reported in a 6-year-old girl with PWS and a very small microdeletion of 100 to 200 Kilobases (Kb), which removes the SNRPN gene and two others (Butler et al., 1996). She does not have hyperphagia or behavior problems, although hypotonia in early childhood and typical physical features are present. An additional case of PWS involves a balanced translocation between chromosomes 15 and 19, with the translocation break point at exon 1 of the SNRPN gene (Sun et al., 1996). This patient had a typical PWS phenotype, including hyperphagia and obesity, although cognitive abilities were at the 12th percentile on the Stanford-Binet, and he was tall with normal-sized hands. Surrounding genes to SNRPN showed normal expression. A second case of PWS with a balanced translocation between chromosomes 4 and 15 with break points between SNRPN exons 2 and 3, has a lack of expression of exons 3 and 4 (Kuslich et al., 1999). These cases lend further support to the possibility that the SNRPN gene is responsible for at least part of the phenotype in PWS. SNRPN encodes a protein that plays a role in the splicing of pre-mRNA, and it is expressed at highest levels in brain and heart, but detectable levels are present in most tissues (Glenn et al., 1996). SNRPN is an imprinted gene that is methylated in the maternal allele and unmethylated, and therefore expressed, in the paternal allele (Glenn et al., 1996). SNRPN is expressed equally in all areas of the human brain, including the hypothalamus in normal patients (Glenn et al., 1996). A report of a patient with PWS and a translocation with a breakpoint just below SNRPN and with normal expression of the paternally derived SNRPN gene suggests that another gene is additionally responsible for the PWS phenotype (Schulze et al., 1996).

A recent report has found that the human necdin gene (NDN) is maternally imprinted and is located in the PWS deletion region (Jay et al., 1997). There is a complete absence of this protein in the brain and in fibroblasts of patients with PWS in contrast to normal expression in patients with AS and in normals. The human NDN gene is homologous to the mouse Ndn gene, which is thought to play a role in the establishment or maintenance of growth quiescence in neurons. In addition, the Ndn gene mRNA expression is highest in the hypothalamus of the mouse, which is where the main pathology in PWS is thought to occur (Jay et al., 1997). Further studies of mice deficient in the Ndn gene are needed, in addition to studies of the NDN gene in the rare patient with a PWS phenotype who does not have a deletion, UPD, or an IC mutation to sort out whether deficiency of this gene alone can cause the PWS phenotype.

Treatment

The treatment of PWS requires a team approach because of the combination of medical, nutritional, behavioral, and educational difficulties. Holm has outlined the interaction of such a team both in case management and in coordinating and carrying out treatment programs (Holm, 1995). The following section outlines the treatment issues and approaches at each age of the child with PWS.

After the diagnosis is made, it is also essential for the family to receive genetic counseling to understand the genetic etiology of this disorder and to understand possible recurrence risks. If the molecular studies have demonstrated a typical deletion or UPD, the recurrence risk is less than 1%, because there have been no reports of recurrence in siblings with these molecular findings (Cassidy, 1995). If a chromosomal translocation is present, then the risk is slightly higher than 1% if the translocation is present in one of the parents. The real concern regarding reoccurrence is when an imprinting mutation is present. This is a small deletion or point mutation in the IC which involves a 50% risk for PWS in a subsequent sibling when it is passed on by a father with an IC mutation (Saitoh et al., 1997). There is also the possibility that the brother of the father who carries an IC mutation may also be a carrier (Saitoh et al., 1997). It is important for families to know that prenatal diagnosis for PWS is possible.

Infancy

The most severe problems in infancy are hypotonia and feeding difficulties. Infants have a weak suck and are often listless during the first year. Breast feeding is usually unsuccessful, and bottle feeding requires large holes in a latex nipple and high caloric formulas (Stadler, 1995). Because of the poor suck, feeding takes a prolonged period of time, and parents need lots of encouragement (Cassidy, 1988). An occupational therapist (OT) can help with stimulating an appropriate suck and with finding a nipple that will be helpful in feeding. Frequent feedings are necessary, but if the child is not growing, then a dropper or gavage feedings are needed. Most infants require gavage feedings for several weeks. Consultation with a nutritionist is helpful to avoid failure to thrive (Stadler, 1995). Early transition to cup feedings can also be helpful (Cassidy, 1988).

Thermoregulation is often problematic in infancy, and an isolette to avoid hypothermia may be needed. Thermoregulation problems may also lead to high fevers periodically in childhood which require prompt use of acetaminophen to reduce fever.

The OT or physical therapist (PT) can provide motor therapy, which is important in the newborn period to prevent disuse atrophy and contractures that can occur with severe hypotonia and inactivity. In addition, the OT or PT can facilitate the development of motor milestones that are usually delayed. Initiation of an infant stimulation program that includes both motor and language therapy is helpful. The hypotonia gradually improves, and between the first and second year the child has appropriate musculature and tone to feed well and thrive (Stadler, 1995). Although the parents now breathe a sigh of relief, they must be prepared for the second phase of behavior, which includes an insatiable appetite and obesity begining between 2 and 4 years of age.

Toddlers and Preschoolers

Controlling obesity and behavioral management dominate the treatment needs at this time. It is important to start strict behavioral management of food intake at 2 years of age before the problems intensify. Eating should only occur at mealtimes, and access to food at other times must be prevented. To restrict food accessibility refrigerators, freezers, cabinets, pantries, and even kitchens should be locked. Leftover food should be disposed of immediately, and pet food and garbage cans should be inaccessible (Stadler, 1995). It is important to educate everyone in the family and school personnel about the importance of restricting food intake or the child will obtain food from others. Food restriction and dieting must be coupled with positive reinforcement strategies so that the child gains a positive self-image and feels in control of his intake.

The caloric needs of children with PWS are lower than those of the normal population. Weight maintenance occurs with a diet that provides 8 to 11 kcal/cm of height/day (20 to 28 kcal/inch), and weight loss occurs with an energy-restricted diet of 7 kcal/cm/day (18 kcal/inch) in children with PWS (Stadler, 1995). Normal children achieve weight maintenance with an intake of 12 to 22 kcal/cm/day (Cassidy, 1984). These dieting parameters usually mean an intake of 600 to 800 kcal/day among young children and 1000 to 1300 kcal/day among older children and adults with PWS (Stadler, 1995). Because weight management is difficult and requires constant supervision, the family should meet on a regular basis with a nutritionist (Stadler, 1995).

A weight management program must also include a daily exercise component. Children with PWS have decreased physical activity, so starting daily exercise and sports in the preschool period will counteract this tendency and improve the self-image when coupled with positive behavioral reinforcers. A practical goal for daily exercise in patients with PWS is 30 minutes per day (Cassidy, 1997).

In general, a behavior management program must be utilized in all aspects of the child's life because mood lability, tantrums, and obstinate behavior do not occur only with food issues. The basic principles of a behavior program include a focus on the positive, with a concrete reward that is given many times in a day. Examples of rewards include stars, stickers, cards, pictures, movies or videos, and games, but food should be avoided as a reward except in special circumstances for patients with PWS. A negative behavior is either ignored or followed by a negative consequence, such as time-out. If behavior problems are severe in the preschool period, then the family should work with a behavioral psychologist who can give ongoing guidance on a weekly basis and organize an overall behavioral program. Behavioral management for patients with PWS is reviewed by Whitman and Greenswag (1995) and Luiselli (1988).

After 2 years of age, a developmental preschool program should be utilized; it should include both motor and language therapy, most preferably in an integrated setting that includes normally developing children.

A micropenis or small penis with a stretched penile length of <1.5 to 2.0 cm is likely to cause problems with upright urination and difficulties with peer relationships. Therefore, treatment with a short course of low-dose testosterone such as depot testosterone (cypionate or enanthate) 25 mg IM every 3 to 4 weeks for 3 to 6 months will improve the appearance and function of the penis (Lee, 1995).

The evaluation of cryptorchidism, which is common in PWS, includes the use of chorionic gonadotropin, which can often stimulate descent of the testes. Gonadotropin can be given IM, subcutanously, or intranasally. Spontaneous descent of the testes can occur prepubertally or during puberty, perhaps related to an increase in adrenal androgens (Lee, 1995). The need for an orchiopexy (surgical relocation of the testes to the scrotum) to avoid a tumor is controversial in PWS because only one case of a testicular tumor has been reported and because infertility is the rule (Lee, 1995). However, it may be psychologically beneficial for a high-functioning patient to have testicles in the scrotum. If surgery reveals very small testicles, a prosthesis may be placed in the scrotum (Lee, 1995).

School-Aged Children

Obesity control measures and behavior management must continue throughout childhood and adolescence and even into adulthood. Sometimes the behavior problems may intensify during this period, particularly if early intervention was not carried out because of a late diagnosis. Food stealing is a common problem and can be a focus in behavioral management. For instance, by giving positive reinforcers for not stealing at each mealtime, such as poker chip tokens that can later be exchanged for prizes or even low-calorie food items, the frequency of food stealing can dramatically decrease (Luiselli, 1988). An overall weight reduction program for older children and adults can also include cognitive control strategies such as (1) *self-monitoring*, having the individual write down the types of food and the time and place of eating; (2) *stimulus control*, having the individual eat in one location only and stocking the house with only low calorie foods; (3) *controlling consummatory responses*, having the individual put the utensil down between bites and counting every bite; (4) *reinforcement* for adherence to the program with tokens or prizes; and (5) *cognitive restructuring* techniques to change negative self-statements such as "I'm fat and I'll never lose weight" to "losing weight is difficult but I can do it if I try hard" (Luiselli, 1988).

Medical follow-up includes vitamin supplementation, including vitamin D and calcium to help avoid osteoporosis. Patients need to be periodically monitored for anemia because significant food restrictions may lead to iron deficiency. Obese adolescents and adults need to have periodic urinalyses to check for proteinuria or glucosuria, and blood pressure should be monitored along with weight checks (Alexander and Greenswag, 1995). To screen for diabetes mellitus, the level of glycohemoglobin in the blood can be periodically checked (S. Cassidy, personal communication 1998).

Type II diabetes mellitus occurs in approximately 7% of children and 19% of adults with PWS. It is caused by obesity. The treatment for this problem is weight reduction through calorie restriction and exercise. Oral hypoglycemic agents have only limited efficacy unless they are used with a weight control regimen (Lee, 1995). Insulin treatment can compound the tendency for weight gain, but in limited cases it may be useful (Lee, 1995).

Endocrine follow-up for children includes treatment for short stature that is secondary to GH and IGF-I (somatomedin-C) deficiency (Lee, 1995). This deficiency can be documented by measuring levels of IGF-I and IGFBP-3 and by studying GH secretion through standard stimulation procedures, such as using clonidine or glucagon or insulin (Lee, 1995). If deficiency of GH/IGF is documented, treatment with GH is indicated in children with open epiphyses. Several studies have shown that children with PWS have a good response to standard GH doses, 0.3 mg/kg/wk or 0.05 mg/kg/day (Angulo et al., 1996; Lee, 1995; Lindgren et al., 1997, 1998). The side effects of GH therapy include an insulin counter regulatory effect, which can theoretically worsen insulin resistance, so monitoring patients for fasting hyperglycemia and glucosuria is important during GH therapy (Lee, 1995). The benefits of GH therapy include enhanced growth, improvement in osteoporosis, and improvement in the ratio of nonbone lean mass to adipose tissue. In addition, parents report improved energy level, appetite control, mental concentration, and overall behavior in their children with PWS during treatment with GH (Lee, 1995; Lindgren et al., 1997). A recent report of 17 children with PWS treated for 2 to 5 years with GH therapy demonstrated improvement in penile length in all children, the onset of puberty in six of seven children after 12 years of age, and premature adrenarche in three subjects (Angulo et al., 1997). The authors conclude that GH therapy facilitates maturation of both adrenal and testicular tissue, even in cases of hypothalamic hypogonadism.

To help increase saliva flow, sugarless gum and an over-the-counter toothpaste and mouthwash called Biotene has been beneficial (S. Cassidy, personal communication 1998).

MEDICATIONS   Psychopharmacological intervention can be a helpful adjunct in treatment of obsessive-compulsive behavior, depression, outburst behavior, aggression, and overeating in patients with PWS. In a survey of 347 families with a member who had PWS, Stein and colleagues found that 19% of the patients were on psychotropic medication (Stein et al., 1994). Most of the patients (40%) were taking fluoxetine (Prozac), and the remaining were on antipsychotics (23%), stimulants (21%), or anticonvulsants (15%). Fluoxetine has been used to treat compulsive eating disorders, and, when used in combination with behavior therapy, patients lost significantly more weight than controls (Marcus et al., 1990). Dech and Budow (1991) were among the first to report the anecdotal use of fluoxetine in a case of PWS to control behavior problems, appetite, and trichotillomania. Fluoxetine has also been found to be useful for severe skin picking, which is on the spectrum of obsessive compulsive behavior (Warnock and Kestenbaum, 1992). In one case report, a 35-year-old woman did not respond to 20 mg/day but responded well to 60 mg/day of fluoxetine (Warnock and Kestenbaum, 1992). In a similar case, a 36-year-old man demonstrated improvement in hoarding and explosive outbursts with 60 mg of fluoxetine (Hellings and Warnock, 1994). In another case, a 9-year-old boy was treated with fluoxetine at a dose of 60 mg/day and a strict behavioral program, which included a 900 kcal diet, and he lost considerable weight (Benjamin and Buot-Smith, 1993). However, improvement in skin picking and foraging for food did not occur until naltrexone was added and gradually increased to a dose of 50 mg/day. Naltrexone is an opoid antagonist, and there is some evidence that obesity may be related to excessive beta endorphins (Benjamin and Buot-Smith, 1993).

It is not unexpected that selective serotonin reuptake inhibitors (SSRIs) would be the most widely used medications in PWS, because they are effective in treatment of obsessive-compulsive behavior and depression, which are common problems in PWS, as already described. Some individuals experience a decrease in appetite with fluoxetine, which was the first SSRI to be introduced. Fluvoxamine (Luvox) is a more recently introduced SSRI that is targeted specifically for obsessive-compulsive symptoms; it has demonstrated efficacy for these problems in childhood and adolescence (Apter et al., 1994; Goodman et al., 1997; Riddle et al., 1996). Controlled studies are needed to evaluate the efficacy of fluvoxamine and fluoxetine for the eating and behavior problems in PWS.

Other psychotropic medications may also be helpful in PWS. Mood stabilizers have been used for outburst behavior. A 15-year-old boy with PWS and Klinefelter's syndrome made significant improvements in hyperphagia, outburst behavior, and weight loss on carbamazepine and a behavior program (Tu et al., 1992). Individuals with severe mood instability may require lithium, valproic acid, or carbamazepine, which are described in more detail in chapters 2 and 3. If psychotic features are present, then antipsychotics, such as risperidone and olanzepine (also described in chapter 2) may be utilized, although weight gain is a significant side effect. Verhoeven et al. (1998) and Beardsmore et al. (1998) describe the treatment of patients with PWS with both antipsychotics and mood stabilizers. Stimulant medication may be helpful in improving a short attention span or decreasing impulsive behavior, but hyperactivity and ADHD are not typically seen in patients with PWS. Stimulants may decrease appetite, but they should always be combined with a behavior program and dieting to induce weight loss. A stimulant medication, mazindol, which is not used in ADHD but which causes anorexia, has recently been shown to be helpful in promoting weight loss in three patients with PWS. Mazindol is an imidazoline derivative; it was given in a dose of 1 to 2 mg/day in one or two doses to 11-year-old and 15-year-old girls and to a 23-year-old man with insulin dependent diabetes mellitus and PWS (Inui et al., 1997; Itoh et al., 1995). The mazindol was also helpful in controlling blood glucose levels in the last patient (Inui et al., 1997). Mazindol deserves further study in the treatment of obesity in PWS.

Fenfluramine (Pondimin), a serotonin-reducing agent, has been marketed as an appetite suppressant, but it was removed from the market along with dexfenfluramine (Redux) in September 1997. Many cases of people developing valvular heart disease or pulmonary hypertension while taking these medications have been reported (Connolly et al., 1997; Mark et al., 1997). This complication, combined with the potential for neurotoxicity in humans because of long-term serotonin depletion, as has been noted in animals treated with fenfluramine (reviewed by Aman et al., 1997; Gillberg et al., 1998), leads to the recommendation to avoid these medications with patients who have PWS.

The recent discovery of the *ob* gene and its protein product leptin, which is produced in the adipose tissue and gives feedback inhibition to the appetite and satiety centers in the hypothalamus, and the identification of appetite stimulants such as neuropeptide Y, may lead to new treatments for obesity that could stimulate satiety factors and decrease expression of appetite stimulants in the future (Rosenbaum et al., 1997). Butler et al. (1998) studied leptin levels in 19 obese and 14 nonobese patients with PWS and found that leptin levels were generally high but comparable to obese controls. They speculated that a defect in transporting leptin into the hypothalamus in PWS could lead to overproduction of neuropeptide Y with subsequent hyperphagia and hypogonadism.

EDUCATIONAL INTERVENTION   The educational issues in the school-age period include the need for special education support. Most children with PWS can be mainstreamed in the regular classroom, but they require support for language and motor deficits, in addition to educational supports. The cognitive deficits may be mild to severe, but the behavior problems, including perseveration, mood lability, and tantrums, may interfere most with the educational process. A behavior modification program can be organized by the school psychologist and followed by the teacher and therapists. Control of food acquisition must occur in all environments in the school, particularly the cafeteria. Peers must also be educated not to share food with the patient.

The learning strengths for children with PWS include long-term memory; receptive language; the ability to learn visually through the use of pictures, illustrations, videos, and computer technology; the ability to learn through hands-on experiences; and reading abilities (Levine and Wharton, 1995). Learning weaknesses include short-term auditory memory problems, which make it difficult to learn from verbal instructions or explanations. Repeating information, writing it down, or using visual information to supplement instruction or explanations is usually helpful. Fine motor deficits and motor planning problems interfere with drawing and writing. In addition, motor underactivity and arousal problems causing sleepiness in sedentary or boring situations can also be a problem. Children with PWS can get stuck on certain issues because of their obsessive-compulsive behavior, and they frequently perseverate and ask the same question over and over again, as is seen in fragile X syndrome. Teachers can direct the child to write the answers to a perseverative question on a card to which they can refer to when they ask again (Levine and Wharton, 1995). The OT can provide therapy in an individual or group setting to address the motor deficits. Regular exercise with a positive behavior reinforcement program can improve self-image and help with weight reduction. School personnel should be given information regarding the educational needs of children with PWS; Levine and Wharton's (1993) handbook is particularly valuable.

Use of a computer to enhance written language and to improve language and learning skills should begin in kindergarten. Computers combine visual input with auditory feedback in learning programs that can enhance math, along with other academic areas. Math problems can begin with preschool concepts such as size, shape, and amount and advance through addition, subtraction, division, word problems, geometry, and algebra. Favorite math software programs include Millie's Math House and Math Blaster (see Appendix 2 for further information on software). A talking word processor, such as Write: Outloud, can provide auditory feedback, and Co:Writer, a word prediction program, can guess what word the child is trying to type from the first few letters. These programs can be helpful for the young child with early writing skills but significant visual motor coordination problems. An evaluation by a computer specialist can test out a variety of software to see what computer program will fit the child's abilities and needs. More information regarding software suggestions can be found in Appendix 2.

Children with PWS usually have more significant expressive language deficits than receptive deficits because of hypotonia, hypernasality of speech, oral motor coordination problems, vocabulary deficits, word retrieval problems, grammatical errors, use of incomplete sentence structure, and pragmatic deficits (Downey and Knutson, 1995). They benefit from both individual and group language therapy throughout their schooling. A great area of need is social communication, which includes pragmatics, or the ability to use acquired language in a socially acceptable way. Group therapy focused on pragmatic and social skills can address how to initiate peer communication, how to take turns in communication, and how to read verbal and nonverbal cues appropriately (Downey and Knutson, 1995). Materials that can be used in pragmatic language training can be found in Appendix 3 of this book.

Adolescence and Adulthood

Some patients with PWS have severe problems that are difficult to manage at home when the parents become exhausted and eating is out of control. For these patients, an out-of-home placement may be the best option for improved control of the behavior and weight problems. The most optimal residential setting is a small-group home situation that is specifically designed for patients with PWS. Approximately 50 such programs have been developed in the last decade throughout the United States and in some international locations. They have demonstrated efficacy in improving weight control (Greenswag et al., 1995). They have multidisciplinary staff who usually cover nutrition, nursing, psychology, and education with consulting physicians. An intense behavioral program is typical, and control of food access and nutritional programming is continuous. Programming may also focus on daily living skills and vocational skills. One of the great difficulties is the weight gain that often occurs once an individual leaves such a program. However, it is possible to maintain a behavior and dietary program with appropriate education and case management even outside such a residential setting, although many patients remain in such a program long term (Greenswag et al., 1995).

Endocrine follow-up in adolescence includes the use of hormonal replacement to stimulate pubertal changes, since patients with PWS rarely progress beyond Tanner stage 2 or 3. Although such a decision is based on each patient's individual needs, individuals with mild to moderate mental retardation or higher functioning abilities may benefit socially and perhaps cognitively from such intervention. For males who are 14 or 15 years old, a low-dose IM testosterone injection of 100 mg can be initiated every 2 to 4 weeks and gradually increased to a dose of 200 mg and coupled with psychological counseling and behavioral monitoring (Lee, 1995). For females, estrogen replacement can be helpful for improving osteoporosis, in addition to having psychological and cognitive benefits (Lee, 1995; McEwen et al., 1997). Low-dose estrogen contraceptives are perhaps most convenient because they usually include a progestin to minimize cancer risks (Lee, 1995).

Adolescent patients with PWS can benefit from counseling that addresses several psychosexual issues (Greenswag, 1995). They need to understand that PWS is associated with a lack of normal sexual development and that hormonal replacement can treat many of these problems. Prior to hormonal replacement, they need to be aware of both the benefits and the side effects of this treatment. Changes which will happen both physically and mentally need to be discussed before they occur. Honest, sensitive, and uncomplicated sex education is also important for the adolescent and can be addressed in counseling. A discussion of sexually transmitted diseases and sex abuse also needs to be included in counseling (Greenswag, 1995).

Vocational training is essential in the educational setting of the adolescent with PWS. Typical vocational programs have an opportunity for on-the-job training before graduation so that the individual is ready to make the transition to the working world by the time of graduation. Prior to graduation from high school, the state vocational rehabilitation professionals should be contacted so that vocational services are not delayed after graduation. Vocational opportunities relate to cognitive abilities, which have a broad spectrum in PWS. Individuals with PWS usually do well in an office setting with clerical work, in a library with cataloging or computer work, in a laboratory (because they are usually precise and persistent), or carrying out horticulture work, which requires the nurturing of plants that helps to build their self-esteem (Saporito, 1995). Work in the food industry may not be successful because weight control is difficult when tempting food is present throughout the day. Lower-functioning individuals or those with severe behavioral problems may require a sheltered workshop setting where intensive supervision is available throughout the day.

In a recent study of 52 adults with PWS with a mean IQ of 69, 21% lived with their families, 75% lived in group homes, many of which were specifically for PWS, and one person lived in a supervised apartment (Greenswag et al., 1997). Although 82% were reported to be good-natured, skin picking occurred in 65%, sleep disturbances in 42%, stubborn behaviors in 98%, food stealing in 80%, and food belligerence in 76%. Hospitalization for physical problems occurred in the current year for 67%, and 15% required hospitalization for aberrant behaviors (Greenswag et al., 1997). Clearly problems related to obesity and behavior continue throughout the life span in individuals with PWS.

CASE HISTORY: AARON

Aaron is now a 23-year-old man with Prader-Willi syndrome who was diagnosed at 4 years of age when cytogenetic testing demonstrated the classical deletion at 15q associated with Prader-Willi syndrome.

His mother did not notice any significant movement in utero throughout her pregnancy. She delivered 3½ weeks early; it was a breech presentation, and the birth weight was 6 pounds, 8 ounces. Aaron had significant respiratory problems immediately after delivery, which precipitated a transport to the university's intensive care unit. He had full life support for the first 3 days of life, including a respirator, then he was in intermediate care until he was sent home at 16 days of age. He had severe hypotonia, he was gavage fed, and a muscle biopsy was done in the newborn period, which was abnormal. When home, his mother gavage-fed him every 4 hours until he was 8 months old, and then he was spoon-fed. He did not suck well on a nipple (soft nipple with large holes) until 18 months of age.

He was extremely weak, with poor stamina, and his developmental milestones were severely delayed. He sat at 11 months, but did not crawl until he was 2 years old, when he was motivated to crawl to catch a new kitten that the family obtained. He had physical therapy beginning at 2 years of age, and by 2 years 4 months he was able to walk independently and the physical therapy was discontinued. He did not speak in words until 5 years of age, but it was not until age 12 that he spoke five words, and it was not until he was 15 years old that he put together sentences. Bed-wetting was also a continuing problem for him until age 16; he would wet at least seven to eight times during the night, and he would also wet during naps.

At 1 year old, he weighed 13 pounds; by 2 years, he weighed 18 pounds; and between 2 and 3 years, hyperphagia developed. By 3 years of age he had gained 45 pounds, and he weighed 75 pounds when he was 4 years old. He was clearly obese until age 6, when he weighed 86 pounds. He was foraging in the garbage at 3 years, and the family needed to institute very tight structure for weight management 24 hours a day. After his diagnosis was made at 4 years of age, the family knew what they had to do, and both school and extended family members helped in maintaining his behavior program for eating. The family had to lock cupboards and even lock the whole kitchen to avoid food stealing or overeating. At times the refrigerator also was padlocked. He would roam around at least three to four times each evening searching for food. When he was obese, he fell asleep easily during the day and would usually go to sleep for the night at 3:30 p.m. He would always sleep when riding in cars, but he was able to wake up with the smell or sounds of food, and he was even able to eat with his eyes closed or partially sleeping. His structured weight program made a difference in his weight after age 7, and he maintained a reasonable weight until age 21, when he finished with his school program.

Aaron's behavior problems also included severe skin picking, and one mosquito bite was an open lesion for 8 years. The family uses whirlpool therapy with

Betadine on a daily basis and Silvadine cream on the lesions at bedtime with bandages. Also, Neosporin is put on the lesions during the day. Weekly massage therapy, which began at 23 years, has dramatically improved his skin picking and healing of lesions. He does not feel pain, heat, or even cold very well, and so he did not experience appropriate pain associated with picking the lesions. Although he had some temper tantrums in early childhood, they were not allowed at home, so he never really got started into a tantrum behavior routine. On the occasion when he would have an aggressive or violent outburst, a family member simply sat on him. Some of his tantrums were more problematic at school, where they were handled poorly at times because of staff and teacher changes.

Aaron was in a private school for exceptional children from age 6 to age 21. He received speech and language therapy two to three times per week, and he also received motor therapy there, although he has never received sensory integration occupational therapy.

Cognitive testing at approximately 18 years of age showed an IQ of 75 on the WAIS-R. In earlier childhood, his IQ scores were lower because of his severe speech delays. Since his speech and language therapy was discontinued after he finished with school, he went downhill in his language abilities. His mother has only been able to obtain 6 weeks of therapy over the last year, and she is fighting to receive more services through adult programming.

His medical problems included undescended testicles, and at 4 years old an orchiopexy with a bilateral hernia repair was carried out. He was also diagnosed with Legg Perthe's disease, which required orthopedic intervention and surgery at 6 years of age. Surgery included an internal support with bracing; this was removed at age 15 years. Osteoporosis was recently diagnosed, and he will be treated with Fosmax. He has never received hormonal replacement, and the family has decided against testosterone treatment at this time because of concern for complications, including acne and perhaps an increase in aggression or behavior problems. He developed pubic hair at 20 years of age, and he also has underarm hair and a mustache at this time. He has severe facial scars from repeated skin picking.

He is very social, he participates in an Eagle Scout program, and he is an usher at the local church. He goes to a social group at least three times a week with his peers. He does not do well independently, and he has never been alone for more than an hour. He basically does not have good control of his eating, and he still will periodically steal food. Other types of impulsive behavior, such as turning on the shower with scalding hot water, can also occur. In social situations he still needs guidance periodically.

He has always demonstrated strengths in working puzzles, and he used to fill out a puzzle book 24 hours a day. Hoarding is not a problem for him at this time, but he enjoys collecting movies. He is now 5' tall and weighs 136 pounds. His shoe size is a boy's size 4, and his foot is quite wide.

He presently works in a veteran's hospital, where he cleans mouse cages for a 4-hour period twice a week. He is also self-employed and has developed a business in which he makes calendars and cards on the computer. He had extensive vocational training in high school, and he also worked in the community in a local plant. His mother does not feel that he will ever be able to live independently.

ACKNOWLEDGMENTS   I thank Suzanne Cassidy, Merlin Butler, and Joseph Wagstaff for their detailed review of chapter 6 and their helpful suggestions. I also thank Mrs. Delmarmol and Jacqueline Johnston for their helpful information. This work was partially supported by MCH grant no. MCJ089413.

REFERENCES

Adcock, K. G., MacElroy, D. E., Wolford, E. T., Farrington, E. A. (1998) Pemoline therapy resulting in liver transplantation. Annals of Pharmacotherapy 32: 422–4.

Albrecht, U., Sutcliffe, J. S., Cattanach, B. M., Beechey, C. V., Armstrong, D., Eichele, G., Beaudet, A. (1997) Imprinted expression of the murine Angelman syndrome gene, Ube3a, in hippocampal and Purkinje neurons. Nature Genetics 17: 75–8.

Alexander, R. C., and Greenswag, L. R. (1995) Medical and nursing interventions. In: Management of Prader-Willi syndrome. Greenswag, L. R., and Alexander, R. C. (eds.). 2nd ed. Springer-Verlag, New York, pp. 66–87.

Aman, M. G. (1982) Stimulant drug effects in developmental disorders and hyperactivity. Journal of Autism and Developmental Disorders 12: 385–98.

Aman, M. G., Kern, R. A., Osborne, P., Tumuluru, R., Rojahn, J., del Medico, V. (1997) Fenfluramine and methylphenidate in children with mental retardation and borderline IQ: Clinical effects. American Journal on Mental Retardation 101 (5): 521–34.

Angelman, H. (1965) "Puppet" children: A report on three cases. Developmental Medicine and Child Neurology 7: 681–8.

Angulo, M., Castro-Magana, M., Mazur, B., Canas, J. A., Vitollo, P. M., Sarrantonio, M. (1996) Growth hormone secretion and effects of growth hormone therapy on growth velocity and weight gain in children with Prader-Willi syndrome. Journal of Pediatric Endocrinology and Metabolism 9 (3): 393–400.

Angulo, M. A., Castro-Magana, M., Canas, J. A., Prakasam, G., Vitollo, P. (1997) Penile length and sexual maturation in Prader-Willi syndrome (PWS) children on growth hormone (GH) therapy [Abstract]. American Journal of Medical Genetics 73: 396.

Apter, A., Ratzoni, G., King, R. A., Weizman, A., Iancu, A., Binder, M., Riddle, M. (1994) Fluvoxamine open-label treatment of adolescent inpatients with obsessive-compulsive disorder or depression. Journal of the American Academy of Child and Adolescent Psychiatry 33 (3): 342–8.

ASHG/ACMG (1996) Diagnostic testing for Prader-Willi and Angelman syndromes: Report of the ASHG/ACMG test and technology transfer committee. American Journal of Human Genetics 58: 1085–8.

Aughton, D. J., and Cassidy, S. B. (1990) Physical features of Prader-Willi syndrome in neonates. American Journal of Diseases of Children 144 (11): 1251–4.

Beardsmore, A., Dorman, T., Cooper, S.-A., Webb, T. (1998) Affective psychosis and Prader-Willi syndrome. Journal of Intellectual Disability Research 42 (6): 463–71.

Benjamin, E., and Buot-Smith, T. (1993) Naltrexone and fluoxetine in Prader-Willi syndrome. Journal of the American Academy of Child and Adolescent Psychiatry 32 (4): 870–3.

Bennetto, L., and Pennington, B. (1996) The neuropsychology of fragile X syndrome. In: Fragile X syndrome: Diagnosis, treatment and research. Hagerman, R. J., and Cronister, A. (eds.). 2nd ed. Johns Hopkins University Press, Baltimore, pp. 210–48.

Berkovitch, M., Pope, E., Phillips, J., Koren, G. (1995) Pemoline-associated fulminant liver failure: Testing the evidence for causation. Clinical Pharmacology and Therapeutics 57 (6): 696–8.

Blackstone, S. W. (1990) Equipment: A full range of options for persons with severe and profound mental challenges. Augmentative Communication News 3 (3): 1–6.

Blackstone, S. W. (1995) Angelman syndrome and AAC. Augmentative Communication News 8 (3): 1–8.

Bottani, A., Robinson, W. P., DeLozier-Blanchet, C. D., Engel, E., Morris, M. A., Schmitt, B., Thun-Hohenstein, L., Schinzel, A. (1994) Angelman syndrome due to paternal uniparental disomy of chromosome 15: A milder phenotype? American Journal of Medical Genetics 51: 35–40.

Bower, B. D., and Jeavons, P. M. (1967) The "happy puppet" syndrome. Archives of Diseases of Childhood 42: 298–302.

Boyd, S. C., Harden, A., Patton, M. A. (1988) The EEG in early diagnosis of Angelman's (happy puppet) syndrome. European Journal of Pediatrics 147: 508–13.

Brodie, M. J., and Dichter, M. A. (1996) Antiepileptic drugs. New England Journal of Medicine 334 (3): 168–75.

Buntinx, I. M., Hennekam, R. C. M., Brouwer, O. F., Stroink, H., Beuten, J., Mangelschots, K., Fryns, J. P. (1995) Clinical profile of Angelman syndrome at different ages. American Journal of Medical Genetics 56: 176–83.

Burd, L., Vesely, B., Martsolf, J., Kerbeshian, J. (1990) Prevalence study of Prader-Willi syndrome in North Dakota. American Journal of Medical Genetics 37 (1): 97–9.

Burger, J., Kunze, J., Sperling, K., Reis, A. (1996) Phenotypic differences in Angelman syndrome patients: Imprinting mutations show less frequent microcephaly and hypopigmentation than deletions. American Journal of Medical Genetics 66: 221–6.

Burger, J., Buiting, K., Dittrich, B., Grob, S., Lich, C., Sperling, K., Horsthemke, B., Reis, A. (1997) Different mechanisms and recurrence risks of imprinting defects in Angelman syndrome. American Journal of Human Genetics 61: 88–93.

Butler, M. G. (1989) Hypopigmentation: A common feature of Prader-Labhart-Willi syndrome. American Journal of Human Genetics 45 (1): 140–6.

Butler, M. G. (1990) Prader-Willi syndrome: Current understanding of cause and diagnosis. American Journal of Medical Genetics 35 (3): 319–32.

Butler, M. G., and Meaney, F. J. (1991) Standards for selected anthropometric measurements in Prader-Willi syndrome. Pediatrics 88 (4): 853–60.

Butler, M. G., Meaney, F. J., Palmer, C. G. (1986) Clinical and cytogenetic survey of 39 individuals with Prader-Labhart-Willi syndrome. American Journal of Medical Genetics 23: 793–809.

Butler, M. G., Christian, S. L., Kubota, T., Ledbetter, D. H. (1996) A five-year-old white girl with Prader-Willi syndrome and a submicroscopic deletion of chromosome 15q11q13. American Journal of Medical Genetics 65: 137–41.

Butler, M. G., Moore, J., Morawiecki, A., Nicolson, M. (1998) Comparison of leptin protein levels in Prader-Willi syndrome and control individuals. American Journal of Medical Genetics 75: 7–12.

Cassidy, S. B. (1984) Prader-Willi syndrome. Current Problems in Pediatrics 14 (1): 1–55.

Cassidy, S. B. (1988) Management of the problems of infancy: Hypotonia, developmental delay, and feeding problems. In: Prader-Willi syndrome: Selected research and management issues. Caldwell, M. L., and Taylor, R. L. (eds.). Springer-Verlag, New York, pp. 43–51.

Cassidy, S. B. (1995) Genetics of Prader-Willi syndrome. In: Management of Prader-Willi syndrome. Greenswag, L. R., and Alexander, R. C. (eds.). 2nd ed. Springer-Verlag, New York, pp. 18–31.

Cassidy, S. B. (1997) Prader-Willi syndrome. Journal of Medical Genetics 34 (11): 917–23.

Cassidy, S. B., Li-Wen, L., Erickson, R. P., Magnuson, L., Thomas, E., Gendron, R., Herrmann, J. (1992) Trisomy 15 with loss of the paternal 15 as a cause of Prader-Willi syndrome due to maternal disomy. American Journal of Human Genetics 51: 701–8.

Cassidy, S. B., Forsythe, M., Heeger, S., Nicholls, R. D., Schork, N., Benn, P., Schwartz, S. (1997) Comparison of phenotype between patients with Prader-Willi syndrome due to deletion 15q and uniparental disomy 15. American Journal of Medical Genetics 68 (4): 433–40.

Clarke, D., Boer, H., Webb, T., Scott, P., Frazier, S., Vogels, A., Borghgraef, M., Curfs, L. M. G. (1998) Prader-Willi syndrome and psychotic symptoms: 1. Case descriptions and genetic studies.

Journal of Intellectual Disability Research 42 (6): 440–50.

Clarke, D. (1998) Prader-Willi syndrome and psychotic symptoms: 2. A preliminary study of prevalence using the psychopathology assessment schedule for adults with developmental disabilities checklist. Journal of Intellectual Disability Research 42 (6): 451–4.

Clayton-Smith, J. (1993) Clinical research on Angelman syndrome in the United Kingdom: Observations on 82 affected individuals. American Journal of Medical Genetics 46: 12–15.

Connolly, H. M., Crary, J. L., McGoon, M. D., Hensrud, D. D., Edwards, B. S., Edwards, W. D., Schaff, H. V. (1997) Valvular heart disease associated with fenfluramine-phentermine. New England Journal of Medicine 337 (9): 581–8.

Creel, D. J., Bendel, C. M., Wiesner, G. L., Wirtschafter, J. D., Arthur, D. C., King, R. A. (1986) Abnormalities of the central visual pathways in Prader-Willi syndrome associated with hypopigmentation. New England Journal of Medicine 314 (25): 1606–9.

Curfs, L. G. (1992) Psychological profile and behavioral characteristics in Prader-Willi syndrome. In: Prader-Willi and other 15q deletion disorders. Cassidy, S. B. (ed.). Springer-Verlag, Berlin, pp. 211–22.

Dech, B., and Budow, L. (1991) The use of fluoxetine in an adolescent with Prader-Willi syndrome. Journal of the American Academy of Child and Adolescent Psychiatry 30: 298–302.

DiMario, J., Francis J., Dunham, B., Burleson, J. A., Moskovitz, J., Cassidy, S. B. (1994) An evaluation of autonomic nervous system function in patients with Prader-Willi syndrome. Pediatrics 93 (1): 76–88.

Dittrich, B., Buiting, K., Korn, B., Rickard, S., Buxton, J., Saitoh, S., Nicholls, R. D., Poustka, A., Winterpacht, A., Zabel, B., Horsthemke, B. (1996) Imprint switching on human chromosome 15 may involve alternative transcripts of the SNRPN gene. Nature Genetics 14: 163–70.

Downey, D. A., and Knutson, C. L. (1995) Speech and language issues. In: Management of Prader-Willi syndrome. Greenswag, L. R., and Alexander, R. C. (eds.). 2nd ed. Springer-Verlag, New York, pp. 142–55.

Dykens, E. M., and Cassidy, S. B. (1995) Correlates of maladaptive behavior in children and adults with Prader-Willi syndrome. American Journal of Medical Genetics (Neuropsychiatric Genetics) 60: 546–9.

Dykens, E. M., and Cassidy, S. B. (1996) Prader-Willi syndrome: Genetic, behavioral, and treatment issues. Mental Retardation 5 (4): 913–27.

Dykens, E. M., Hodapp, R. M., Walsh, K., Nash, L. J. (1992a) Adaptive and maladaptive behavior in Prader-Willi syndrome. Journal of the American Academy of Child and Adolescent Psychiatry 31 (6): 1131–6.

Dykens, E. M., Hodapp, R. M., Walsh, K., Nash, L. J. (1992b) Profiles, correlates, and trajectories of intelligence in Prader-Willi syndrome. Journal of the American Academy of Child and Adolescent Psychiatry 31 (6): 1125–30.

Dykens, E. M., Leckman, J. F., Cassidy, S. B. (1996) Obsessions and compulsions in Prader-Willi syndrome. Journal of Child Psychology and Psychiatry and Allied Disciplines 37 (8): 995–1002.

Ebert, M. H., Schmidt, D. E., Thompson, T., Butler, M. D. (1997) Elevated plasma gamma-aminobutyric acid (GABA) levels in individuals with either Prader-Willi syndrome or Angelman syndrome. Journal of Neuropsychiatry 9: 75–80.

Gabel, S., Tarter, R. E., Gavaler, J.,

Golden, W. L., Hegedus, A. M., Maier, B. (1986) Neuropsychological capacity of Prader-Willi children: General and specific aspects of impairment. Applied Research in Mental Retardation 7: 459–66.

Gillberg, C., Aman, M. G., Reiss, A. (1998) Fenfluramine. In: Psychtropic medications and developmental disabilities: The international consensus handbook. Reiss, S., and Aman, M. G. (eds.). Ohio State University, Nisonger Center, Columbus, Ohio.

Gillessen-Kaesbach, G., Albrecht, B., Passarge, E., Horsthemke, B. (1995a) A further patient with Angelman syndrome due to paternal disomy of chromosome 15 and a milder phenotype. American Journal of Medical Genetics 56: 328–9.

Gillessen-Kaesback, G., Robinson, W., Lohmann, D., Kaya-Westerloh, S., Passarge, E., Horsthemke, B. (1995b) Genotype-phenotype correlations in a series of 167 deletion and non-deletion patients with Prader-Willi syndrome. Human Genetics 96: 638–43.

Glenn, C. C., Saitoh, S., Jong, M. T., Filbrandt, M. M., Surti, U., Driscoll, D. J., Nicholls, R. D. (1996) Gene structure, DNA methylation, and imprinted expression of the human SNRPN gene. American Journal of Human Genetics 58 (2): 335–46.

Goodman, W. K., Ward, H., Kablinger, A., Murphy, T. (1997) Fluvoxamine in the treatment of obsessive-compulsive disorder and related conditions. Journal of Clinical Psychiatry 58(Suppl. 5): 32–49.

Greenswag, L. R. (1987) Adults with Prader-Willi syndrome: A survey of 232 cases. Developmental Medicine and Child Neurology 29: 145–52.

Greenswag, L. R. (1995) Understanding psychosexuality. In: Management of Prader-Willi syndrome. Greenswag, L. R., and Alexander, R. C. (eds.). 2nd ed. Springer-Verlag, New York, pp. 181–94.

Greenswag, L. R., Singer, S. L., Condon, N., Bush, H. H., Omrod, S., Mulligan, M. M., Shaw, P. L. (1995) Residential options for individuals with Prader-Willi syndrome. In: Management of Prader-Willi syndrome. Greenswag, L. R., and Alexander, R. C. (eds.). 2nd ed. Springer-Verlag, New York, pp. 214–47.

Greenswag, L. R., Alexander, R. C., Boyt, M., Whitman, B. Y. (1997) A current physical and mental health profile of persons with Prader-Willi syndrome age 35 and over: Description of preliminary data [Abstract]. American Journal of Medical Genetics 73: 397.

Guerrini, R., De Lorey, T. M., Bonanni, P., Moncla, A., Draver, C., Suisse, G., Livet, M. O., Bureau, M., Malzac, P., Genron, P., Thomas, P., Sartucci, F., Simi, P., Serratosa, F. (1996) Cortical myoclonus in Angelman syndrome. Annals of Neurology 40: 39–48.

Gunay-Aygun, M., Heeger, S., Schwartz, S., Cassidy, S. B. (1997) Delayed diagnosis in patients with Prader-Willi syndrome due to maternal uniparental disomy 15. American Journal of Medical Genetics 71 (1): 106–10.

Hagerman, R. J. (1996) Medical follow-up and pharmacotherapy. In: Fragile X syndrome: Diagnosis, treatment, and research. Hagerman, R. J., and Cronister, A. (eds.). 2nd ed. Johns Hopkins University Press, Baltimore, pp. 283–331.

Hellings, J. A., and Warnock, J. K. (1994) Self-injurious behavior and serotonin in Prader-Willi syndrome. Psychopharmacology Bulletin 30 (2): 245–50.

Holm, V. A. (1981) The diagnosis of Prader-Willi syndrome. In: Prader-Willi syndrome. Holm, V., Sulzbacher, S., Pipes, P. (eds.). University Park Press, Baltimore, pp. 27–40.

Holm, V. A. (1995) A team approach to case management. In: Management of Prader-Willi syndrome. Greenswag, L. R., and Alexander, R. C. (eds.). 2nd ed. Springer-Verlag, New York, pp. 61–5.

Holm, V. A., Cassidy, S. B., Butler, M. G., Hanchett, J. M., Greenswag, L. R., Whitman, B. Y., Greenberg, F. (1993) Prader-Willi syndrome: Consensus diagnostic criteria. Pediatrics 91 (2): 398–402.

Hutchinson, T. (1997) Seizures—Diagnosis and treatment. Angelman Syndrome Foundation International Conference, Seattle, Wash.

Inui, A., Uemoto, M., Takamiya, S., Shibuya, Y., Baba, S., Kasuga, M. (1997) A case of Prader-Willi syndrome with long term mazindol treatment. Archives of Internal Medicine 157: 464.

Itoh, M., Koeda, T., Ohno, K., Takeshita, K. (1995) Effects of mazindol in two patients with Prader-Willi syndrome. Pediatric Neurology 13: 349–51.

Jan, J. E., and O'Donnell, M. E. (1996) Use of melatonin in the treatment of paediatric sleep disorders. Journal of Pineal Research 21: 193–9.

Jay, P., Rougeulle, C., Massacrier, A., Moncla, A., Mattei, M.-G., Malzac, P., Roeckel, N., Taviaux, S., Lefranc, J. L. B., Cau, P., Berta, P., Lalande, M., Muscatelli, F. (1997) The human necdin gene, NDN, is maternally imprinted and located in the Prader-Willi syndrome chromosomal region. Nature Genetics 17: 357–61.

Jay, V., Becker, L. E., Chan, F.-W., Perry, T. L. (1991) Puppet-like syndrome of Angelman: A pathologic and neurochemical study. Neurology 41: 416–22.

Jolleff, N., and Ryan, M. M. (1993) Communication development in Angelman's syndrome. Archives of Disease in Childhood 69 (1): 148–50.

Kemper, M. B., Hagerman, R. J., Altshul-Stark, D. (1988) Cognitive profiles of boys with the fragile X syndrome. American Journal of Medical Genetics 30: 191–200.

Kishino, T., Lalande, M., Wagstaff, J. (1997) UBE3A/E6-AP mutations cause Angelman syndrome. Nature Genetics 15: 70–73.

Kosaki, K., McGinniss, M. J., Veraksa, A. N., McGinnis, W. J., Jones, K. L. (1997) Prader-Willi and Angelman syndromes: Diagnosis with a bisulfite-treated methylation-specific PCR method. American Journal of Medical Genetics 73 (3): 308–13.

Kubota, T., Niikawa, N., Jinno, Y., Ishimaru, T. (1994) GABAA receptor beta 3 subunit gene is possibly paternally imprinted in humans [Letter to the editor]. American Journal of Medical Genetics 49 (4): 452–3.

Kubota, T., Aradhya, S., Macha, M., Smith, A. C., Surh, L. C., Satish, J., Verp, M. S., Nee, H. L., Johnson, A., Christan, S. L., Ledbetter, D. H. (1996) Analysis of parent of origin specific DNA methylation at SNRPN and PW71 in tissues: Implication for prenatal diagnosis. Journal of Medical Genetics 33 (12): 1011–14.

Kuslich, C. D., Kobori, J. A., Mohapatra, G., Gregorio-King, C., Dolon, T. A. (1999) Prader-Willi syndrome is caused by disruption of the SNRPN gene. American Journal of Human Genetics (64): 70–6.

Lee, P. D. K. (1995) Endocrine and metabolic aspects of Prader-Willi syndrome. In: Management of Prader-Willi syndrome. Greenswag, L. R., and Alexander, R. C. (eds.). 2nd ed. Springer-Verlag, New York, pp. 32–65.

Lee, S. T., Nicholls, R. D., Bundey, S., Laxova, R., Musarella, M., Spritz, R. A. (1994) Mutations of the P gene in oculocutaneous albinism, ocular albinism, and Prader-Willi syndrome plus albinism. New England Journal of Medicine 330 (8): 529–34.

Leo, R. J. (1996) Movement disorders associated with serotonin selective reuptake inhibitors. Journal of Clinical Psychiatry 57 (10): 449–54.

Levine, K., and Wharton, R. H. (1993) Children with Prader-Willi syndrome: Information for school staff. Visible Ink, New York.

Levine, K., and Wharton, R. H. (1995) Educational considerations. In: Management of Prader-Willi syndrome. Greenswag, L. R., and Alexander, R. C. (eds.). 2nd ed. Springer-Verlag, New York, pp. 156–69.

Lindgren, A. C., Hagenas, L., Muller, J., Blichfeldt, S., Rosenborg, M., Brismar, T., Ritzen, E. M. (1997) Effects of growth hormone treatment on growth and body composition in Prader-Willi syndrome: A preliminary report. Swedish National Growth Hormone Advisory Group. Acta Paediatrica (Suppl. 423): 60–62.

Lindgren, A. C., Hagenas, L., Muller, J., Blichfeldt, S., Rosenborg, M., Brismar, T., Ritzen, E. M. (1998) Growth hormone treatment of children with Prader-Willi syndrome affects linear growth and body composition favourably. Acta Paediatrica 87: 28–31.

Lofterod, B., and Heiberg, A. (1992) Prader-Willi syndrome in Norway: An epidemiological and sociomedical study. In: Prader-Willi syndrome and other chromosome 15q deletion disorders. Cassidy, S. B. (ed.). Springer-Verlag, Berlin, pp. 131–6.

Luiselli, J. K. (1988) Behavior management and intervention. In: Prader-Willi syndrome: Selected research and management issues. Caldwell, M. L., and Taylor, R. L. (eds.). Springer-Verlag, New York, pp. 52–72.

Marcus, M., Wing, R., Ewing, L., Kern, E., McDermott, M., Gooding, W. (1990) A double-blind, placebo-controlled trial of fluoxetine plus behavior modification in the treatment of obese binge eaters and non-binge eaters. American Journal of Psychiatry 147: 876–81.

Mark, E. J., Patalas, E. D., Chang, H. T., Evans, R. J., Kessler, S. C. (1997) Fatal pulmonary hypertension associated with short-term use of fenfluramine and phentermine. New England Journal of Medicine 337 (9): 602–6.

Matsuura, T., Sutcliffe, J. S., Fang, P., Galjaard, R.-J., Jiang, Y.-H., Benton, C. S., Rommens, J. M., Beaudet, A. L. (1997) De novo truncating mutations in E6-AP ubiquitin-protein ligase gene (UBE3A) in Angelman syndrome. Nature Genetics 15: 74–7.

McEwen, B. S., Alves, S. E., Bulloch, K., Weiland, N. G. (1997) Ovarian steroids and the brain: Implications for cognition and aging. Neurology 48 (suppl. 7): S8–S15.

Miller, L. W. (1995) Angelman syndrome: A parent's guide. Angelman Syndrome Foundation, Gainesville, Fla.

Mitchell, J., Schinzel, A., Langlois, S., Gillessen-Kaesbach, G., Schuffenhauer, S., Michaelis, R., Abeliovich, D., Lerer, I., Christian, S., Guitart, M., McFadden, D. E., Robinson, W. P. (1996) Comparison of phenotype in uniparental disomy and deletion Prader-Willi syndrome: Sex specific differences. American Journal of Medical Genetics 65 (2): 133–6.

Pardo, J. M. (1993) Central precocious puberty in a girl with Prader-Labhart-Willi syndrome. International Pediatrics 8 (4): 443–5.

Prader, A., Labhart, A., Willi, H. (1956) Ein Syndrom von Adipositas, Kleinwuchs, Kryptorchismus, and Oligophrenie nach Myotonicartigem Zustand in Neugeborenalter. Schweizerische Medizinische Wochenschrift 86: 1260–61.

Preskorn, S. H. (1996) Clinical pharmacology of selective serotonin reuptake inhibitors. Professional Communications, Caddo, Okla.

Purvis-Smith, S. G., Saville, T., Manass, S., Yip, M.-Y., Lam-Po-Tang, P. R. L., Duffy, B., Johnston, H., Leigh, D., McDonald, B. (1992) Uniparental disomy 15 resulting from 'correction' of an ini-

tial trisomy 15. American Journal of Human Genetics 50: 1348–50.

Riddle, M. A., Claghorn, J., Gaffney, G. (1996) A controlled trial of fluvoxamine for OCD in children and adolescents. Biological Psychiatry 39 (7): 568.

Robb, S. A., Pohl, K. R., Baraitser, M., Wilson, J., Brett, E. M. (1989) The 'happy puppet' syndrome of Angelman: Review of the clinical features. Archives of Disease in Childhood 64 (1): 83–86.

Roof, E., Feurer, I., Thompson, T., Stone, W., Butler, M. (1998) Psychological and behavioral characteristics of Prader-Willi syndrome. Paper presented at the 31st Annual Gatlinburg Conference on Research and Theory in Mental Retardation and Developmental Disabilities, Charleston, S.C., March 12–14, 1998.

Rosenbaum, M., Leibel, R. L., Hirsch, J. (1997) Obesity. New England Journal of Medicine 337 (6): 396–407.

Rougeulle, C., Glatt, H., Lalande, M. (1997) The Angelman syndrome candidate gene, UBE3A/E6-AP, is imprinted in brain. Nature Genetics 17: 14–15.

Saitoh, S., Harada, N., Jinno, Y., Hashimoto, K., Imaizumi, K., Kuroki, Y., Fukushima, Y., Sugimoto, T., Renedo, M., Wagstaff, J., et al. (1994) Molecular and clinical study of 61 Angelman syndrome patients. American Journal of Medical Genetics 52 (2): 158–63.

Saitoh, S., Buiting, K., Cassidy, S., Conroy, J. M., Driscoll, D. J., Gabriel, J. M., Gellessen-Kaesbach, G., Glenn, C. C., Greenswag, L. R., Horsthemke, B., Kondo, I., Kuwajima, K., Nikkawa, N., Rogan, P. K., Schwartz, S., Seip, J., Williams, C. A., Nicholls, R. D. (1997) Clinical spectrum and molecular diagnosis of Angelman and Prader-Willi syndrome patients with an imprinting mutation. American Journal of Medical Genetics 68: 195–206.

Saporito, A. M. (1995) Vocational concepts in Prader-Willi syndrome. In: Management of Prader-Willi syndrome. Greenswag, L. R., and Alexander, R. C. (eds.). 2nd ed. Springer-Verlag, New York, pp. 248–64.

Schulze, A., Hansen, C., Skakkebaek, N. E., Brondum-Nielsen, K., Ledbeter, D. H., Tommerup, N. (1996) Exclusion of SNRPN as a major determinant of Prader-Willi syndrome by a translocation breakpoint. Nature Genetics 12 (4): 452–4.

Smith, A., Wiles, C., Haan, E., McGill, J., Wallace, G., Dixon, J., Selby, R., Colley, A., Marks, R., Trent, R. J. (1996) Clinical features in 27 patients with Angelman syndrome resulting from DNA deletion. Journal of Medical Genetics 33: 107–12.

Smith, A., Marks, R., Haan, E., Dixon, J., Trent, R. J. (1997) Clinical features in four patients with Angelman syndrome resulting from paternal uniparental disomy. Journal of Medical Genetics 34 (5): 426–9.

Spritz, R. A., Bailin, T., Nicholls, R. D., Lee, S., Park, S., Mascari, M. J., Butler, M. G. (1997) Hypopigmentation in the Prader-Willi syndrome correlates with p gene deletion but not with haplotype of the hemizygous p allele. American Journal of Medical Genetics 71: 57–62.

Stadler, D. D. (1995) Nutritional management. In: Management of Prader-Willi syndrome. Greenswag, L. R., and Alexander, R. C. (eds.). 2nd ed. Springer-Verlag, New York, pp. 88–114.

Stalker, H. J., and Williams, C. A. (1998) Genetic counseling in Angelman syndrome: The challenges of multiple causes. American Journal of Medical Genetics 77: 54–59.

Stein, D. J., Keating, J., Zar, H. J., Hollander, E. (1994) A survey of the phenomenology and pharmacotherapy of compulsive an impulsive-aggressive symptoms in Prader-Willi syndrome.

Journal of Neuropsychiatry and Clinical Neurosciences 6: 23–29.

Steingard, R. J., Zimnitzky, B., DeMaso, D. R., Bauman, M., Bucci, J. P. (1997) Sertraline treatment of transition-associated anxiety and agitation in children with autistic disorder. Journal of Child and Adolescent Psychopharmacology 7 (1): 9–15.

Summers, J. A., Lynch, P. S., Harris, J. C., Burke, J. C., Allison, D. B., Sandler, L. (1992) A combined behavioral/ pharmacological treatment of sleep-wake schedule disorder in Angelman syndrome. Journal of Developmental and Behavioral Pediatrics 13: 284–7.

Sun, Y., Nicholls, R. D., Butler, M. G., Saitoh, S., Hainline, B. E., Palmer, C. G. (1996) Breakage in the SNRPN locus in a balanced 46XY,t(15;19) Prader-Willi syndrome patient. Human Molecular Genetics 5: 517–24.

Swaab, D. F., Purba, J. S., Hofman, M. A. (1995) Alterations in the hypothalamic paraventricular nucleus and its oxytocin neurons (putative satiety cells) in Prader-Willi syndrome: A study of five cases. Journal of Clinical Endocrinology and Metabolism 80 (2): 573–9.

Thompson, T., Butler, M. G., MacLean, W. E., Joseph, B. (1996) Prader-Willi syndrome: Genetics and behavior. Peabody Journal of Education 71 (4): 187–212.

Tu, J.-B., Hartridge, C., Izawa, J. (1992) Pharmacogenetic aspects of Prader-Willi syndrome. Journal of the American Academy of Child and Adolescent Psychiatry 31 (6): 1137–40.

Van Lierde, A., Atza, M. G., Giardino, D., Viani, F. (1990) Angelman syndrome in the first year of life. Developmental Medicine and Child Neurology 32: 1005–21.

Verhoeven, W. M. A., Curfs, L. M. G., Tuinier, S. (1998) Prader-Willi syndrome and cycloid psychoses. Journal of Intellectual Disability Research 42 (6): 455–62.

von Moltke, L. L., Greenblatt, D. J., Harmatz, J. S., Shader, R. I. (1994) Cytochromes in psychopharmacology. Journal of Clinical Psychopharmacology 14 (1): 1–2.

Vu, T. H., and Hoffman, A. R. (1997) Imprinting of the Angelman syndrome gene, UBE3A, is restricted to brain. Nature Genetics 17: 12–13.

Ward, R. M., Lemons, J. A., Molteni, R. A. (1999) Cisapride: A survey of the frequency of use and adverse events in premature newborns. Pediatrics 103 (2): 469–72.

Warnock, J. K., and Kestenbaum, T. (1992) Pharmacologic treatment of severe skin-picking behaviors in Prader-Willi syndrome. Archives of Dermatology 128: 1623–5.

Weitz, C., Dexter, M., Moore, J. (1997) AAC and children with developmental disabilities. In: The handbook of augmentative and alternative communication. Glennen, S. L., and DeCoste, D. C. (eds.). Singular, San Diego, pp. 395–431.

Whitman, B. Y., and Greenswag, L. R. (1995) Psychological and behavioral management. In: Management of Prader-Willi syndrome. Greenswag, L. R., and Alexander, R. C. (eds.). Springer-Verlag, New York, pp. 125–41.

Williams, C. A., and Frias, J. I. (1982) The Angelman (happy puppet) syndrome. American Journal of Medical Genetics 11: 453–60.

Williams, C. A., Angelman, H., Clayton-Smith, J., Driscoll, D. J., Hendrickson, J. E., Knoll, J. H. M., Magenis, R.E ., Schinzel, A., Wagstaff, J., Whidden, E. M., Zori, R. (1995a) Angelman syndrome: Consensus for diagnostic criteria. American Journal of Medical Genetics 56: 237–8.

Williams, C. A., Zori, R. T., Hendrickson, J., Stalker, H., Marum, T., Whidden, E., Driscoll, D. J. (1995b) Angelman syndrome. Current problems in pediatrics 25: 216–31.

Zhdanova, I. V., Lynch, H. J., Wurtman, R. J. (1997) Melatonin: A sleep-promoting hormone. Sleep 20: 899–907.

RESOURCES

Angelman Syndrome Support Groups

Angelman Syndrome Foundation
P.O. Box 12437
Gainesville, FL 32604
telephone: (800) IF-ANGEL
international telephone: (713) 354-7192

Angelman Syndrome Support Group
15 Place Cresent
Waterlooville, Hants, PO75UR
United Kingdom
telephone: 011-70-526-4224; 011-70-538-5566

Canadian Angelman Syndrome Society
P.O. Box 37
Priddis, Alberta, TOL1WO, Canada
telephone: (403) 931-2415

National Angelman Syndrome Association
P.O. Box 554
Sutherland, 2232 New South Wales, Australia
telephone: 02 587 24 44

Word Wide Web Sites for Information on Angelman Syndrome

---

http://shell.idt.net/~julhyman/angel.htm
http://asclepius.com/angel/

http://www.algonet.se/~soomus/angel/

http://home.sol.no/hevo/angel.htm

http://www.concentric.net/~sggirb/index.html

http://members.aol.com/miller566/as_paper.htm

http://people.zeelandnet.nl/fhof/angelman.htm

http://www.interserf.net/fruitcake/AS_home.html

http://usrwww.mpx.com.au/~altona/index.html

http://www.netgroup.it/medico/orsa/

General Reading

Evans, A., and Hyman, J. (1997)
Angelman syndrome from A to
Z—Everything you wanted to know
about Angelman Syndrome and then
some. Gainseville, FL. Angelman
Syndrome Foundation An easy to read
compilation of tips, hints, and ideas of
how to survive and enjoy life with a
child with Angelman syndrome.

Miller, L. W. (1995) Angelman syndrome:
A parent's guide. Gainseville, FL:
Angelman Syndrome Foundation. See
contact numbers above.

Angelman Project Videos

1. Cetarra's First IEP

2. Interview with Child Psychologist,
Timothy Freedman, Ph.D.

3. Three Portraits of Angelman Syndrome

4. Portrait of Joey H. (age 23)

To order any of these four videos, contact
Louise Tiranoff Productions, 488 14th
Street, Brooklyn, NY 11215. Telephone:
(718) 788-6403; fax: (718) 369-2387; e-
mail: Tiranoff@aol.com

Manufacturers of Assistive Technology Devices (Table 6.2): Voice Output Communication Aids (VOCAs)

Speak Easy, Big Red Switch
AbelNet
1081 Tenth Avenue, S.E.
Minneapolis, MN 55414
telephone: (800) 322-0956

Voice Pal with Taction Pads
Adaptech, Inc., ISU Research
2501 N. Loop Dr.
Amens, IA 50010
telephone: (800) 723-2783

WalkerTalker, Alpha Talker
Prentke Romich Co.
1022 Heyl Road
Wooster, OH 44691
telephone: (800) 262-1984

Digivox
Sentient Systems
2100 Wharton Street, Suite 630
Pittsburgh, PA 15203
telephone: (800) 394-1778

SwitchMate 4, Scan Mate
TASH, Inc.
Unit 1, 91 Station Street
Ajax, Ontario, LIS 3H2, Canada
telephone: (905) 686-4129

Cheap Talk 4, Say It Switch Plate
Toys for Special Children
385 Warburton Avenue
Hasting-On-Hudson, NY 01706
telephone: (800) 832-8697

Message Mates
Word +, Inc.
40015 Sierra Highway, B-145
Palmdale, CA 93550
telephone: (800) 869-8521

Macaw
Zygo Industries Inc.

P.O. Box 1008
Portland, OR 97207
telephone: (503) 684-6006; (800) 234-6006
fax: (503) 684-6011

Prader-Willi Syndrome Support Groups

Prader-Willi Syndrome Association (PWSA)
5700 Midnight Pass Road, Suite #6
Sarasota, FL 34242
telephone: (800) 926-4797
fax: (941) 312-0142
http://www.pwsausa.org
e-mail: pwsausa@aol.com

The Prader-Willi Foundation, Inc.
223 Main Street
Port Washington, NY 11050
telephone: (800) 253-7993
fax: (516) 484-7154
http://www.prader-willi.org
e-mail: foundation@prader-willi.org

Prader Willi Perspectives Newsletter
Visible Ink Incorporated
40 Holly Lane

Roslyn Heights, NY 11577
telephone: (800) 358-0682
fax: (516) 484-7154
e-mail: pwsforum@aol.com

World Wide Web Sites for Information on Prader-Willi Syndrome

Prader-Willi Syndrome Association (USA)
http://www.pwsausa.org

Prader-Willi Foundation
http://www.prader-willi.org

The Prader Willi Connection
http://www.pwsyndrome.com

General Reading

Butler, M. G. (1995) Prader-Willi syndrome: A guide for parents and professionals. Prader-Willi Perspectives and Visible Ink. Roslyn Heights, New York.
Greensway, L. R., and Alexander, R. C. (eds.). (1995) Management of Prader-Willi syndrome. New York: Springer-Verlag.

7

22q Deletion Syndromes

The 22q deletion syndromes include DiGeorge syndrome (DGS), which was first reported in 1965 (DiGeorge, 1965) and is associated with thymic aplasia, T-cell mediated immune defects, hypoparathyroidism, cardiac defects, and characteristic facial anomalies; conotruncal anomaly face syndrome (CTAFS), reported in 1976 (Kinouchi et al., 1976), when the characteristic facial features, conotruncal anomalies, and developmental delays were linked; and Shprintzen syndrome, or velocardiofacial syndrome (VCFS), which was reported in 1978 by Shprintzen and colleagues (1978) in a group of patients with characteristic facial features, learning problems, cardiac anomalies, and cleft palate, or velopharyngeal incompetence. Although these three disorders were originally thought to be separate entities, their clinical overlap was noted as patients with DGS survived their immunological problems and grew up to look like patients with Shprintzen syndrome (Thomas and Graham, 1997).

In 1981, the first report of a visible deletion at 22q11 was seen in cytogenetic studies of patients with DGS (de la Chapelle et al., 1981). This was followed by reports of microdeletions at 22q11 in patients with DGS (Scambler et al., 1991), Shprintzen syndrome or VCFS (Scambler et al., 1992), and CTAFS (Burn et al., 1993) seen with molecular probes in individuals who may look normal in cytogenetic studies. Only 20% of patients have a visible deletion on high-resolution cytogenetic studies, so FISH testing, or fluorescent in situ hybridization studies that utilize a molecular probe for this region of deletion, will detect the great majority of patients with VCFS. The overall incidence of the three disorders that make up the 22q deletion syndromes is approximately 1 per 3,000 to 4,000 in the general population (Thomas et al., 1997). It is estimated that 8% of patients

Neurodevelopmental Disorders: Diagnosis and Treatment, by Randi Jenssen Hagerman. New York: Oxford University Press, 1999. © Oxford University Press, Inc.

with cleft palates have VFCS and 5% of newborns with cardiac defects have VCFS, so it is the single most important cause of cardiac problems after Down syndrome (Thomas et al., 1997). In addition, 6 of 16 (38%) patients with velopharyngeal insufficiency alone, without cleft palate, have the 22q11 deletion (Zori et al., 1998).

The acronym CATCH 22 (cardiac abnormalities, abnormal facies, thymic hypoplasia, cleft palate, hypocalcemia, and deletion on chromosome 22) has been proposed as a new name to remember the main clinical and cytogenetic features, but it is not well accepted by family members because of the negative literary connotations: Joseph Heller's book *Catch-22* depicts a no-win situation (Leana-Cox et al., 1996). The term VCFS has been used to encompass the three syndromes, although those with significant immune defects are still labeled DGS.

Approximately 25% of cases have a familial deletion, which is relatively high compared with other deletion syndromes. The rest of the cases represent de novo or new deletions in the patient, but they are subsequently passed on in an autosomal dominant fashion with a 50% risk of transmitting the deletion to offspring. In familial cases, the parent with the deletion is usually less affected than his or her children, probably related to a selection bias for less affected individuals that reproduced (Leana-Cox et al., 1996). There is an equal rate of maternal versus paternal deletions, although in many studies the mother has been more available for FISH studies (Ryan et al., 1997). It is recommended that FISH studies be routinely carried out on both parents when this deletion is detected in the patient.

PHYSICAL FEATURES

Craniofacial Features

The classical facial phenotype of VCFS includes a pear-shaped nose which has a built-up nasal bridge, a bulbous tip, and deficient alae. The eyes are somewhat narrow and sometimes downturned, there is a wide space between the eyes (hypertelorism), the jaw is posteriorly displaced (termed *retrognathia*), the cheeks are flat, and the ears are usually small, with helical thickening, and are sometimes prominent (Figures 7.1 and 7.2). These features are often not noticeable at birth, but they become more noticeable in early childhood. Over 90% of patients with VCFS have some of these typical facial features, even patients identified because of their cardiovascular abnormalities in a cardiology clinic.

Over 90% of patients identified as having Shprintzen syndrome or VCFS through an ENT or craniofacial clinic have cleft palate without cleft lip (Goldberg et al., 1993). This number is significantly reduced in a broad European survey of 558 patients identified with the deletion at 22q11 (Ryan et al., 1997). Ryan and colleagues (1997) found that only 14% had a cleft palate or submucous cleft, although an additional 32% had velopharyngeal insufficiency. Velopharyngeal insufficiency is usually diagnosed when the voice is hypernasal, but it can be documented by video fluoroscopic studies that show poor motion in the lateral pharyngeal walls or in the soft palate and inadequate closure of the posterior

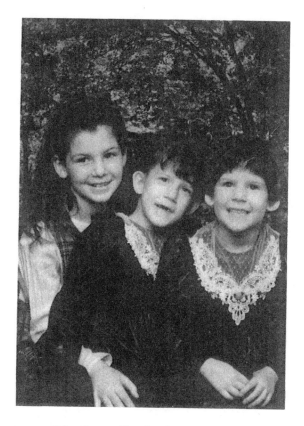

FIGURE 7.1:   7-year-old girl with VCFS flanked by her two normal sisters. Note prominent ears and nasal bridge and narrow eyes.

pharynx. Children with VCFS also have a hypotonic pharynx, a wide pharyngeal width, and adenoidal hypoplasia, which all add to the velopharyngeal insufficiency (Thomas et al., 1997). The presence of a cleft palate or velopharyngeal insufficiency causes a hypernasal voice and the frequent occurrence of ear infections and conductive hearing loss. A bifid uvula may be a marker for an occult or submucous cleft palate. The examination of the palate should be thorough in these patients. A rare patient with VCF has been reported with a subglottic web, which can cause a hoarse voice (Marble et al., 1998).

Less frequent facial features include microcephaly in 40%, ocular coloboma (missing segment usually of the retina) in 3%, and a nasal dimple at the tip of the nose in an occasional patient (Gripp et al., 1997; Thomas et al., 1997). Choanal stenosis or atresia (narrowing or underdevelopment of the nasal passages) is seen in only 1% of patients with VCFS, but both the coloboma and choanal problems relate to the occasional presence of this deletion in patients diagnosed

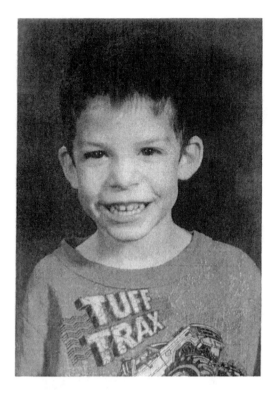

FIGURE 7.2:   Young boy with VCFS. Note
mildly prominent ears and broad nasal bridge.

with the CHARGE association (coloboma, heart anomalies, atresia of the choanae,
retarded growth and development, genital anomalies, and ear anomalies). Other
problems such as laryngeal web (1%) and tracheomalasia (2%) are also seen in
patients with VCFS (Ryan et al., 1997).

The presence of retrognathia is related to a flattening of the cranial base
(platybasia) in VCFS. Retrognathia may subsequently lead to the Pierre Robin
sequence, which includes a large tongue, U-shaped cleft, and feeding problems
in infancy. Goldberg and colleagues (1993) have reported that 17% of individuals
with VCFS have Pierre-Robin sequence and, conversely, that 13% of patients
with Pierre-Robin sequence have VCFS.

Three patients with the autosomal dominant Opitz GBBB syndrome (capital
letters represent the first letter of the last name of the four families originally
reported), which is characterized by hypertelorism, downslanting palpebral fissures, epicanthal folds, hypospadius, and laryngotracheoesophageal defects, have
also been reported with a deletion at 22q11.2 detected by FISH studies (Goldberg
et al., 1993). The laryngeal, tracheal, and esophageal abnormalities all share the

same origin of cephalic neural crest cells which migrate into the brachial arches 3 through 6. Abnormal or absent migration of neural crest cells also tie in the defects of cardiac, thymic, and parathyroid development seen in VCFS.

Immunological and Endocrine Features

Although the immune deficiency was often severe in patients diagnosed with complete DGS who had marked deficiency of T-cell numbers, thymic aplasia, and a severe susceptibility to infections, a partial DGS has low T-cell counts only in infancy and eventually the numbers increase and problems with infections decrease (Thomas et al., 1997). However, hypergammaglobulinemia and problems with autoantibodies relate to the deficits in T-cell development, and an occasional patient may have autoantibody-related disease, such as juvenile rheumatoid arthritis or Raynaud's phenomenon, and B-cell dysfunction with a poor antibody response (Thomas et al., 1997). From the larger perspective of patients with a deletion at 22q11, the immunological problems are relatively uncommon. The European survey had immunological information on 218 patients with a deletion. Only two patients had severe immunodeficiency, both of whom had died; one of these had an absent thymus (Ryan et al., 1997). Only an additional 10 patients had minor problems with infection.

The lack of neural cell migration in pharyngeal pouches 2 and 3 also causes problems with the development of the parathyroid gland or hypoparathyroidism. The survey by Ryan et al. (1997) found that 60% of 340 patients with the deletion had hypocalcemia, which usually presented in the newborn period. Other studies have found a lower incidence of hypocalcemia, and Thomas et al. (1997) report hypocalcemia in 10 to 20% of patients. If it is unrecognized, it may present with seizures; this occurred in 39% (Ryan et al., 1997). Replacement of calcium is necessary, although calcium homeostasis usually normalizes (in 70%) if some parathyroid tissue is present (Ryan et al., 1997; Thomas et al., 1997). Rarely, hypocalcemia may present in adolescence, so surveillance of calcium levels should continue until adulthood, especially during times of stress (Thomas et al., 1997).

The lack of migration of neural crest cells to the pharyngeal pouches may on rare occasion affect the function of the thyroid gland, in addition to the parathyroid gland, leading to hypothyroidism (Wilson et al., 1993).

Cardiovascular Anomalies

After the typical facial features, the cardiovascular anomalies are the most common physical findings in VCFS. The European survey compiled cardiovascular information on 545 patients and found 20% with normal hearts, 5% with insignificant problems including aberrant subclavian arteries and right-sided aortic arches, and 75% with significant cardiac pathology (Ryan et al., 1997) (see Table 7.1). The most common problem is tetrology of Fallot (17%), followed by ventricular septal defect (14%) and interrupted aortic arch (14%). Multiple cardiac anomalies are seen in the majority of patients; for instance, a right-sided aortic arch is seen in

TABLE 7.1. Clinical Features of Velocardiofacial Syndrome

Clinical feature	Percentage with this feature
Craniofacial Abnormalities	
cleft palate/or submucous cleft	14–85
retrognathia	80
prominent nose with squared nasal root	76
minor ear anomalies	60–70
microcephaly	40
velopharyngeal insufficiency	32
tracheomalasia/laryngomalasia	2
choanal stenosis/atresia	1
Cardiovascular	
significant cardiac pathology	75
tetrology of Fallot	17
ventricular septal defects	14
interrupted aortic arch	14
pulmonary atresia/ventricular septal defect	10
truncus arteriosis	9
pulmonary valve stenosis	2
other significant abnormalities	9
Genital/Urinary Abnormalities	
genital/urinary abnormalities overall	36
abnormal kidneys	17
obstructive abnormalities	10
Musculoskeletal Abnormalities	
slender tapered digits	60
umbilical hernia	5
talipes equinovarus	4
scoliosis	3
Ocular Abnormalities	7
Central Nervous System	
learning problems	100
hypotonia	70–80
ADHD in children	60–80
mild to moderate mental retardation	40–50
psychosis	10–20
Endocrine/Immunological	
hypocalcemia	10–60
seizures	21
absent or small thymus	10
growth hormone deficiency	4

Data derived from Thomas and Graham (1997), Ryan et al. (1997), and Wein-zimer et al. (1998).

80% of patients with tetrology and 30% of patients with a VSD (Thomas et al., 1997). In the European survey, 8% of patients had died, all except one from cardiovascular causes. Eighty-six percent of the deaths occurred in the first 6 months of life (Ryan et al., 1997).

Many patients with VCFS present initially to the cardiologist because of the life-threatening aspects of the cardiac problems. The additional dysmorphic features may not be recognized at the time of presentation. Mehraein et al. (1997) found that 22.5% of children with complex cardiovascular disease demonstrated the 22q11 deletion by FISH studies. After the deletion was identified, the typical facial dysmorphology was identified in 92%, hypocalcemia was found in 62%, and borderline low T-lymphocyte numbers were found in 41%.It is therefore recommended that all cardiac patients, especially those with conotruncal defects, should be studied by FISH analysis for the 22q11 deletion (Goldmuntz et al., 1993; Mehraein et al., 1997).

Growth and Skeletal Features

Growth retardation is a common finding in patients with VCFS. Ryan and colleagues (1997) found heights and/or weights below the third percentile in 36% and below the 50th percentile in 83% of 158 patients studied. Although severe cardiovascular disease can lead to poor growth, 29% of patients without cardiovascular disease had growth parameters below the third percentile. Growth hormone (GH) deficiency has been found in 4% of patients with the 22q11 deletion, and in 10% of deletion patients who also have short stature (Weinzimer et al., 1998). The GH deficiency may be related to a migration problem of oral ectoderm into the anterior pituitary and into the palate, since individuals with cleft palate have a higher incidence of GH deficiency than the general population (Weinzimer et al., 1998). Two of three patients with GH deficiency and the 22q11 deletion who underwent an MRI demonstrated anatomical abnormalities, including anterior pituitary hypoplasia and abnormal insertion of the infundibular stalk (Weinzimer et al., 1998). The third patient had evidence of hypogonadotropic hypogonadism.

The majority of patients with VCFS have long, slender, tapered, and hyperextensible fingers (Thomas et al., 1997). Additional minor skeletal abnormalities were seen in 17% of 548 patients with VCFS surveyed in the European study (Ryan et al., 1997). These problems included talipes equinovarus (clubfoot) in 4% and scoliosis in 3%. Only 1% or fewer had abnormal vertebrae, or polydactyly, syndactyly, or craniosynostosis.

Genitourinary Features

Although previous studies report genitourinary findings only occasionally, the European survey received information on 136 patients; 36% reported abnormalities, including absent, dysplastic, or multicystic kidneys in 17% and obstructive abnormalities of the urinary tract in 10%. Undescended testes were present in

8% of males (Ryan et al., 1997). Umbilical hernias occur in 5% of patients, and inguinal hernias are reported in 20 to 30% of patients (Thomas et al., 1997).

NEUROLOGICAL, COGNITIVE, AND BEHAVIORAL FEATURES

Most patients with VCFS are hypotonic in childhood. The face may be so hypotonic that it is reminiscent of myotonic dystrophy. Lipson and colleagues (1991) have hypothesized that the typical facial features in this syndrome are secondary to the weak facial muscles in utero. For instance, the narrow palpebral fissures and retrognathia are similar to patients with Prader-Willi syndrome who have severe hypotonia, and the Pierre-Robin sequence may be secondary to the hypotonia of the mandible and tongue. When the tongue falls back it obstructs the closure of the hard and soft palate. The occurrence of the Pierre-Robin sequence and cleft palate is also occasionally seen in fragile X syndrome, which presents with hypotonia in early childhood (Hagerman, 1996; Lachiewicz et al., 1991).

Seizures occur in approximately 21% of patients with VCFS (Ryan et al., 1997). Most seizures are secondary to hypocalcemia. Structural brain abnormalities are far less common and occur in only 3% of patients (Ryan et al., 1997). They include cerebellar vermal hypoplasia, cerebral atrophy, cerebral vascular abnormalities, hydrocephalus, hypoplastic corpus callosum, enlarged ventricles, and a rare neural tube defect (Nickel and Magenis, 1996). However, an MRI study of 11 patients with VCF who were scheduled for pharyngeal flap surgery demonstrated abnormalities in 9 (Mitnick et al., 1994). Five of the patients had small cerebellar vermis, four had small posterior fossa, and three had small cysts adjacent to the anterior horns. No abnormalities were found in the cerebral cortex. A subsequent study of 17 subjects with deletion of 22q11 discovered enlargement of the Sylvian fissures in 10 patients, which was more prominent at a younger age and more prominent on the left than the right (Bingham et al., 1997). The age effect suggests delayed growth of the opercular cortex, and preliminary evidence suggests that the abnormal prenatal growth in this region is associated with bulbar incoordination, causing feeding problems and oral motor coordination problems in infancy and childhood (Bingham et al., 1997). A rare patient may present with a seventh-nerve palsy and asymmetric facies with crying (Ryan et al., 1997).

Mild to moderate mental retardation is present in approximately 40 to 50% of patients with VCFS; however, all patients have some degree of learning difficulties, even when their IQs are in the normal range (Swillen et al., 1997; Thomas et al., 1997). When mental retardation occurs, it is usually mild. Most patients with mental retardation have familial deletion (70.5%), whereas the majority of nonretarded patients have de novo deletion (90%) (Swillen et al., 1997). This is probably related to background gene effects and environmental influences, because parents with the deletion are affected cognitively, and through assortative mating the other parent usually has a lower IQ. Socioeconomic status is lower in families with familial deletion than in those with de novo deletion (Swillen et al., 1997). The presence of cardiac defects has no significant effect on IQ (Swillen et al., 1997). Occasional patients may have more severe cognitive deficits, and VCFS has been reported in a severely autistic patient (Kozma, 1998).

Patients usually present in early childhood with mild language and motor delays, hypotonia, and sometimes feeding problems or constipation (Swillen et al., 1997; Thomas et al., 1997; Wang et al., 1998). On the WISC-III, the Verbal IQ is usually higher than the Performance IQ, although exceptions exist when severe language problems exist (see the second case history, in this chapter). Language deficits are common in both receptive and expressive areas, and overall language skills averaged more than 2 SD below the mean (Moss et al., 1999). Language scores are usually lower than the Verbal IQ. Almost half of the patients show a Verbal IQ–Performance IQ split of over 10 points (Moss et al., 1995; Wang et al., 1998). There is also limited evidence of an IQ decline over time in some patients with VCFS, especially those with significant language deficits (Golding-Kushner et al., 1985; McCandless et al., 1998). Reading and spelling achievement is significantly better than math achievement, and they are usually commensurate with the Verbal IQ (Moss et al., 1999). However, phonemic awareness problems, difficulties with problem solving, difficulties with inferential comprehension, and problems in drawing conclusions are seen in most children with VCFS (Kok et al., 1995). Typically these children are two or more years behind academically compared with their peers even when their IQ is in the normal range (Kok and Solman, 1995).

Language development is usually delayed in early childhood, and velopharyngeal insufficiency with recurrent ear infections further complicates the picture. In addition, a clinical picture of attention deficit hyperactivity disorder (ADHD) is combined with auditory processing and attentional problems, which further exacerbate language development. Attentional problems and ADHD behaviors were first noted by Golding-Kushner et al. (1985) in patients with VCFS, and further studies by Carlson and colleagues (1997) show that the majority of children with VCFS have ADHD. Swillen et al. (1997) found on a behavioral checklist that social problems, particularly withdrawn behavior combined with attentional problems, were common in childhood. This clinical picture appears to be part of a broader psychological phenotype of bipolar spectrum disorders. Up to 70% of cases of VCFS are on this spectrum (Carlson et al., 1997). This fits with the frequent clinical reports of mood lability or moodiness in these patients. Sometimes ADHD symptoms co-occur with bipolar disorder in childhood, and sometimes the symptoms of ADHD evolve into bipolar disorder in adolescence or adulthood. Shprintzen et al. (1992) have reported that 30% of patients with VCFS demonstrated psychotic symptoms in adolescence. However, these symptoms may also be part of the bipolar spectrum. Some schizophrenic patients with VCFS reported by Pulver and colleagues (1994) have been rediagnosed with bipolar disorder (Lachman et al., 1996). The screening of 100 patients with schizophrenia yielded two patients with the 22q11 deletion consistent with VCFS (Lindsay et al., 1995). A separate study of 53 children with childhood-onset schizophrenia or variants revealed one patient with 22q11 deletion (Yan et al., 1998).

Within the deleted segment in patients with VCFS is the gene for catechol-O-methyltransferase (COMT), which inactivates dopamine at the synapse. Approximately 20 to 25% of Caucasians have a low-activity form of this enzyme, whereas the majority of people have a high-activity form of this enzyme (Lachman et al., 1996). A significant association was found in patients with VCFS between the presence of bipolar disorder, particularly the rapid cycling form (BPII), and the presence of the low-activity form of COMT (Lachman et al., 1996). Because these patients have only one allele for COMT, the low-activity form may lead to high levels of dopamine, which in turn may be related to the clinical picture of bipolar disorder. These patients are said to respond to mood stabilizers, discussed later in this chapter (see also Lachman et al., 1996). In addition, two patients treated with methylphenidate for their ADHD developed rapid cycling bipolar disorder within days of treatment (Lachman et al., 1996). Perhaps excessive dopamine levels from hemizygosity of the low-activity form of COMT were exacerbated by methylphenidate, which inhibits the dopamine transporter at the synapse and enhances the dopamine levels even further.

MOLECULAR STUDIES

High-resolution cytogenetic studies are able to identify only 25 to 30% of the deletion at 22q11.2. The use of FISH probes or other molecular techniques, however, can identify a deletion in 83% of patients with the clinical phenotype of VCFS (Carlson et al., 1997). Over 90% of the patients with a deletion have a large 3-Mb deletion, and most of the remaining cases have a 1.5-Mb deletion. There is no correlation between the deletion size and the degree of clinical involvement. There is an occasional patient who has a unique smaller deletion, and Carlson et al. (1997) have identified a 480-Kb critical region for this syndrome, which contains five genes identified so far, including the goosecoid-like GSCL gene. The GSCL gene is a homeobox gene that is expressed in early fetal development, and it functions as a transcription factor. When the mouse goosecoid homologue to this gene is knocked out, craniofacial defects occur because of disruption in cephalic neural crest cells (Gottlieb et al., 1997). This gene is a likely candidate for causing many of the clinical features of VCFS that involve disruption of neural crest cell migration. However, some of the other genes in this region may also be involved in the phenotype when there is only one copy or haploinsufficiency. These genes include the clathrin D gene, which is important for muscle function and a deficiency of which may be related to muscle weakness or hypotonia; a catenin gene (ARVCF), which is important for cell-to-cell interactions and communication; a citrate transport protein (CTP), which moves citrate across the mitochondrial inner membrane; and the COMT gene, which is important for dopamine function related to the problems of ADHD and bipolar disorder

(Carlson et al., 1997). The overall phenotype in VCFS is likely related to dysfunction in more than one gene, and it is therefore a contiguous gene syndrome (Schmickel, 1986).

FISH studies typically use two probes for chromosome 22, one located within the deletion region at 22q11.2 and one a control probe more distal to the deleted region. The normal FISH signal pattern is two fluorescent signals for each chromosome 22. A patient with a deletion at 22q11 will show two signals on the normal chromosome and only one signal on the deleted chromosome. The hybridization efficiency for these probes is more than 99%, so the test is accurate for detecting a deletion covered by the probe (Crifasi et al., 1995). Approximately 17% of patients with the phenotype of VCFS do not have a detectable deletion at 22q11. It is possible that they may have a point mutation, which is as yet unidentified, or a different mutation. Deletions at 10p13, 18p, and several other locations can cause a similar phenotype to VCFS (Greenberg, 1993). In addition, teratogenic exposures, such as retinoic acid or alcohol, and exposure to maternal diabetes can lead to a similar phenotype to VCFS (Driscoll and Emanuel, 1996).

CASE HISTORY: SUSIE

Susie is a 7-year-old girl who was diagnosed at age 4 with VCFS when high-resolution cytogenetic studies, along with FISH probing, demonstrated the deletion at 22q11. Her mother's pregnancy was associated with high blood pressure, and Susie was delivered by repeat C-section, although she had some significant fetal distress. She was given oxygen for a few days because of rapid breathing, and her birth weight was 6 lbs., 10 oz. Her Apgar scores were 6 and 8. She had hypocalcemia in the newborn period, which was treated in the nursery. At home, she vomited frequently, but this improved when her formula was changed. Eventually she was fed by cup at 1 year of age, and the vomiting no longer persisted.

Her developmental milestones were essentially normal, with sitting at 7 to 8 months, walking at 13 months, riding a tricycle at 3½ years, and riding a bicycle at 5 years. She also said words in the first year and sentences by age 2, but significant hypernasality in her speech, combined with severe articulation problems, made most of what she said incomprehensible. Speech and language therapy was initiated at 2½ years of age on a twice weekly basis and continues to the present time in school. Occupational therapy was started at 3½ years of age because of mild motor delays and was discontinued after 1 year. She now is described as well coordinated and very active. She plays soccer and t-ball on a regular basis. She has never been hyperactive at school, but her teacher states that attention can be a problem for her in the classroom. This has been treated with significant structure in the school, and she has not required medication. She is very social and well liked by most of her peers.

Susie's medical history has included recurrent upper respiratory tract infections associated with sinus infections. These have occurred throughout most of her life on a once-monthly basis. She has never had ear infections. A CT scan was carried out early on in her development, and it was read as normal. She was evaluated by cardiology after her diagnosis of VCFS, and she had a normal examination. She has had problems with enamel dysplasia, which was a severe problem for her baby teeth, although her permanent teeth are better.

At age 4 years, she had pharyngeal flap surgery because of the severity of her velopharyngeal incompetence and hypernasal speech. This surgery improved her hypernasality, and her speech has continued to improve in therapy.

Susie has just finished the first grade, where she received special education 1 hour per day to help with written language problems. She uses computers to help with academic progress and also to help with word processing and written language. She has kept up with her class, and her reading level is in the top part of her class. Her main difficulties academically are in the written language area, particularly with formulating sentences. She will continue to receive special education support for this in the second grade.

Her parents were studied with FISH testing, and they do not carry the deletion.

TREATMENT

Infancy

Infants with VCFS may not show obvious dysmorphic facial features initially. However, the diagnosis should be considered in any child with congenital cardiac disease and/or cleft palate. These children often present with feeding problems, particularly regurgitation through the nose. Calcium levels, parathyroid hormone levels, and immunological function studies should be done as soon as the diagnosis is made, because seizures and infections are common. Mortality is secondary to severe heart disease or severe infections. For the rare patient with thymic aplasia or complete DGS, bone marrow transplantation or thymic transplantation have been shown to be effective (Goldsobel et al., 1987). For the patients with partial DGS, T-cell numbers, including CD3 (pan T), CD4 (T helper), and CD8 (T supressor) marker cells are below the normal range in infancy, although lymphocyte proliferation responses and immunoglobulin levels are usually normal (Junker and Driscoll, 1995). Responses to immunizations are usually normal, although the killed polio vaccine should be substituted for the live polio vaccine. Before the measles/mumps/rubella vaccine in the second year, immunological studies should be repeated to make sure the immunological status has not deteriorated (Junker and Driscoll, 1995). Most patients with partial DGS have frequent infections in the first 1 to 3 years, and then they usually do fine from an immunological perspective (Thomas et al., 1997).

Calcium supplementation is usually only needed transiently during the first year; only a rare patient requires long-term supplementation over years. Vitamin D supplementation can also be given to enhance calcium levels. Thyroid function studies should also be carried out in patients diagnosed with VCFS; hypothyroidism occurs rarely, but if it is present, early supplementation prevents additional cognitive deficits. An endocrine consultation is helpful for both hypoparathy-roidism and hypothyroidism to guide treatment.

All patients with this diagnosis require a cardiology consult in the newborn period because of the high rate of complex cardiovascular disease. An EKG and cardiac X-rays should be done prior to the consultation. Many of these children require shunting and subsequent surgical repair.

The cleft palate and velopharyngeal insufficiency require surgical intervention usually toward the end of the first year. Recurrent otitis media (ear infections) is common, and hearing should be tested at diagnosis and regularly in follow-up. Lipson et al. (1991) make the point that those patients without cleft palate often have a delayed diagnosis of VCFS and velopharyngeal incompetence or submucus cleft. The expressive language deficits, combined with hypernasal speech and poor intelligibility, lead to social withdrawal over time. There is a poor response to speech and language therapy until repair of the velopharyngeal insufficiency is carried out. The earlier this surgery is done, the better the response in terms of subsequent speech development and the quality of the speech sounds (Lipson et al., 1991).

These patients should be followed by a craniofacial team who will also avoid unnecessary surgery. An example of inappropriate surgery is the removal of the adenoids, which usually makes velopharyngeal insufficiency and hypernasal speech worse. This mistake occurs when hypernasal speech is confused with hyponasal speech. The initial evaluation includes cinefluoroscopy to study palatal movement and palate length to assess the need for surgery. For those patients who require surgery, magnetic resonance angiography is recommended to identify ectopic internal carotid arteries that may be cut during surgery (Mitnick et al., 1994). Obstructive apnea occasionally occurs after surgery, particularly in infancy, so patients should be monitored for this postoperatively (Shprintzen et al., 1981).

If significant short stature is present, referral to an endocrinologist is indicated for evaluation of GH deficiency. This problem occurs in approximately 10% of individuals with a 22q11 deletion and short stature (Weinzimer et al., 1998). For information regarding GH replacement, the reader is referred to chapter 5, which discusses GH replacement in Turner syndrome in detail.

Approximately 7% of patients with VCFS have ocular abnormalities, which may include colobomas, cataracts, microophthalmia, strabismus, and small optic discs (Ryan et al., 1997). Therefore, an ophthalmological evaluation is recommended at the time of diagnosis, with at least yearly follow-up if problems exist (Thomas et al., 1997).

Beginning in the first year, these children can benefit from infant stimulation programs that include early language and motor therapy. This therapy can intensify after 2 years of age as children move into the preschool environment. If failure to thrive or feeding problems occur, an evaluation should include a barium swallow to rule out gastroesophageal reflux or a vascular ring which may require surgery. An occupational therapist can help with oral motor coordination problems that may interfere with feeding. More complex problems can be evaluated by a craniofacial or feeding team.

Childhood and Adolescence

In the preschool and school-aged period, children with VCFS continue to benefit from speech and language therapy and motor therapy typically provided by an occupational therapist. Most children with VCFS who have been studied in detail require some form of additional special education support in school. Often this can be given in an inclusion setting in the regular classroom, but sometimes pull out remediation or a self-contained setting is necessary. Kok and Solman (1995) have written about the remarkable gains that occur when microcomputers are used to enhance the learning environment in school. They studied six children with VCFS who all demonstrated poor learning strategies and had difficulty in learning independently through reading or other modalities. They also had difficulty in focusing their attention and were described as generally unmotivated to learn. The computer system they used was the World Institute of Computer Assisted Teaching (WICAT) instructional system, which provided an individualized program with auditory feedback so that students could immediately correct their responses. Significant gains were seen in phonemic awareness, sight word recognition, reading decoding, fluency, and mathematics. Most important, gains were seen in self-esteem, and the students developed learning strategies and applied them to the learning of spelling, reading comprehension, and math (Kok and Solman, 1995). For more information regarding computer software, see Appendix 2 of this book.

Medication may be helpful in improving the attention and concentration problems of children with VCFS, but adverse effects have been reported, and controlled studies have not been carried out. The preliminary report of Lachman et al. (1997) documented two children who had an adverse response to methylphenidate, specifically the development of rapid cycling bipolar disease. However, McCandless et al. (1998) described a 12-year-old boy with VCFS and ADHD who demonstrated improvement when treated with methylphenidate, and several other patients have done well on stimulants (P. Wang, personal communication 1998). If stimulants are used, they should be tried cautiously and at low dose. Perhaps they may be better utilized after a mood stabilizer such as valproate, carbamazepine, gabapentin, or lithium. The mood stabilizers are indicated when significant mood lability occurs, leading to aggression, manic symptoms, depression, or fluctuations in mood (McElroy and Weller, 1997). (For more information on mood stabilizers, see Chapters 1, 2, and 3.) The bipolar symptoms may not develop until adolescence or adulthood. These patients are at greater risk for developing bipolar symptoms not only with stimulants but also with tricyclics and selective serotonin reuptake inhibitors (SSRIs) such as fluoxetine (Prozac), which more commonly precipitate mania compared to methylphenidate.

Because stimulants may be problematic for treating ADHD behavior, non-medical interventions should be undertaken first, including structure in the environment, positive behavioral reinforcement techniques, and therapy that emphasizes cognitive techniques for improving impulsivity and inattention, such as self-talk or the Think Aloud program (Bloomquist, 1996; Howard, 1996). An interesting tool that can be used in therapy is the Stop, Relax & Think game, which is designed to teach children self-control, particularly when ADHD or impulsivity is a problem (see the Resources in this chapter and Appendixes 2 and 3 at the end of the book).

The late-onset psychosis requires the use of antipsychotic medication if patients do not respond to mood stabilizers. Chow et al. (1998) recently reported a 32-year-old man with schizophrenia and 22q11 deletion who did well on haloperidal 10 mg per day. In addition, some antipsychotics may further help to stabilize mood when used in addition to a mood stabilizer. Risperidone is a new-generation antipsychotic that blocks both dopamine and serotonin pathways and has a lower incidence of extrapyramidal symptoms (EPS) compared to other antipsychotics (Kapur and Remington, 1996). For more information regarding risperidone, see chapter 3. Controlled trials comparing antipsychotics have not been carried out in patients with VCFS.

CASE HISTORY: DAN

Dan is a 9½-year-old boy who was diagnosed with VCFS at age 8 when FISH testing demonstrated the deletion on chromosome 22 at q11.2, consistent with VCFS (figure 7.2).

His mother's pregnancy was normal, and she delivered by a planned, repeat C-section at 38 weeks. Dan's birth weight was 8 pounds 1¾ ounces, and his Apgar scores were 8 and 8. He was treated with oxygen for the first 4 days of life because of mild breathing problems, but he subsequently went home with his mother when she was discharged from the hospital. As a newborn, he had significant feeding problems, which involved vomiting after most of his meals. Gastroesophageal reflux was diagnosed in the first month, and after many formula switches he finally did well on a soy formula. He had mild problems with colic, and he appeared to be very sensitive to stimuli. He hated baths and was somewhat tactilely defensive.

His early developmental milestones included walking at 18 months, saying words in the first year, and putting two words together just after the first year. His recurrent ear infections caused significant language delays and articulation problems, and polyethylene tubes were placed when he was 18 months old, with a second set at 3 years of age and a third set at 8 years of age. Over the last year he has had fewer problems with infections, but velopharyngeal incompetence continues, and his voice has significant nasality.

Other surgeries included a bilateral hernia operation at 8 weeks and a tonsillectomy and adenoidectomy at 4 years. This improved his ear infections, and the quality of his voice did not worsen after this surgery. After his diagnosis of VCFS, a thorough cardiology evaluation did not demonstrate cardiac pathology.

At 2 years of age, he was described as hyperactive, because he climbed all over and seemed to be always on the go. His hyperactivity was a mild problem in preschool, but his teacher was quite structured and gave significant positive reinforcement, and he did well.

Dan was held back 1 year in preschool before entering kindergarten, but he subsequently did well in kindergarten with the addition of speech and language therapy and occupational therapy and the support of an aide. When the family moved, the new public school system refused to give him special education support or the help of an aide. He had limited speech and language therapy each week, but the parents opted to place him in a private school with a smaller number of children so he could receive more individualized attention. His teacher in his private school program accommodates his attentional and auditory processing problems and gives him additional educational support. He loves playing on the computer, and he utilizes software programs to enhance his academics and also to do word processing. He continues to receive speech and language therapy twice a week through the public school program.

Intellectual testing carried out through his public school demonstrated a Verbal IQ of 58 and a Performance IQ of 79 on the WISC-III. He has severe language delays, verbal planning problems, and difficulties with penmanship and reading.

Dan's family has noted moodiness in him since he was approximately 6 years of age; this has been associated with frequent frustration, which can make him angry, sometimes leading to a tantrum. He most commonly has tantrums after school, and such an episode may involve yelling, stomping of his feet, slamming doors, and pouting. This most frequently happens toward the end of the school year and before holidays. He is generally happy and well adjusted, he has not had problems with aggression, and his ADHD symptoms are improving with age.

On examination at 9 years of age, his height was at the 40th percentile, weight at the 25th percentile, and head circumference at the 50th percentile for age. His facial features are slightly coarse, with mildly low-set ears which are cupped, a high arched palate, and crowding of his lower teeth. His speech demonstrates a mild degree of oral motor incoordination with hypernasality. Heart exam demonstrates a regular rhythm without murmur, he has mild pectus excavatum, genitalia is normal, and extremities show long and tapering fingers. His gait is normal and his reflexes are symmetrical.

The family history is significant in that the mother's first pregnancy resulted in a boy who was diagnosed with tetrology of Fallot at birth. He subsequently died at 8½ months after undergoing surgical repair of his tetrology, which led to complications, including hypotension, brain damage, and coma. A subsequent pregnancy after Dan resulted in a molar pregnancy. FISH testing was also carried out on the mother, who has a history of learning difficulties, including attentional problems, auditory processing difficulties, and reading problems. She also had a history of sinus and ear infections throughout childhood. Emotionally she has had problems with intermittent depression. The mother's FISH testing was also positive for the deletion at 22q11.

The family found that knowing about the diagnosis of VCFS and reading the newsletter of the VCFS Foundation was remarkably helpful in better understanding their problems.

FUTURE DIRECTIONS

VCFS is a broad-spectrum disorder with multiple manifestations that have only recently been found to be caused by the same deletion. The genes responsible for this multifaceted disorder are now being identified so that the molecular mechanisms that cause the psychological and physical problems can be delineated. VCFS is an interesting medical/molecular model for ADHD and bipolar disorder. Further psychopharmacological studies are necessary to clarify the response rates to stimulants or alternative medications for ADHD and to determine when to initiate mood stabilizers.

ACKNOWLEDGMENTS   I want to thank Janet Thomas, Paul Wang, and David Manchester for reviewing this manuscript and providing helpful suggestions on chapter 7. This work was partially supported by the MCH training grant no. MCJ-089413. I am indebted to the Developmental Psychobiology Research Group (DPRG) from the University of Colorado Health Sciences Center for helpful discussions.

REFERENCES

Bingham, P. M., Zimmerman, R. A., Mc-Donald-McGinn, D., Driscoll, D., Emanuel, B. S., Zackai, E. (1997) Enlarged Sylvian fissures in infants with interstitial deletion of chromosome 22q11. American Journal of Medical Genetics (Neuropsychiatric Genetics) 74 : 538–43.

Bloomquist, M. L. (1996) Skills training for children with behavior disorders: A parent and therapist guidebook. Guilford, New York.

Burn, J., Takao, A., Wilson, D., Cross, I., Momma, K., Wadey, R., Scambler, P., Goodship, J. (1993) Conotruncal anomaly face syndrome is associated with a deletion within chromosome 22q11. Journal of Medical Genetics 30 (10): 822–4.

Carlson, C., Papolos, D., Pandita, R. K., Faedda, G. L., Veit, S., Goldberg, R., Shprintzen, R., Kucherlapati, R., Morrow, B. (1997) Molecular analysis of velo-cardio-facial syndrome patients with psychiatric disorders. American Journal of Human Genetics 60 (4): 851–9.

Chow, L. Y., Waye, M. M. Y., Garcia-Barcelo, M., Chiu, H. F. K., Fung, K. P., Lee, C. Y. (1998) Velo-cardio-facial syndrome, schizophrenia, and deletion at chromosome 22q11. Journal of Intellectual Disability Research 42 (2): 184–8.

Crifasi, P., Michaels, V. V., Driscoll, D. J., Jalal, S. M., Dewald, G. W. (1995) DMA fluorescent probes for diagnosis of velocardiofacial and related syndromes. Mayo Clinical Proceedings 70: 1148–52.

de la Chapelle, A., Herva, R., Koivisto, M., Aula, P. (1981) A deletion in chromosome 22 can cause DiGeorge syndrome. Human Genetics 57 (3): 253–6.

DiGeorge, A. M. (1965) Discussions on a new concept of the cellular basis of immunology. Journal of Pediatrics 67: 907.

Driscoll, D. A., and Emanuel, B. S. (1996) DiGeorge and velocardiofacial syndromes: The 22q11 deletion syndrome. Mental Retardation and Developmental Disabilities Research Reviews 2 (3): 130–8.

Goldberg, R., Motzkin, B., Marion, R., Scambler, P. J., Shprintzen, R. J. (1993) Velo-cardio-facial syndrome: A review of 120 patients. American Journal of Medical Genetics 45 (3): 313–9.

Golding-Kushner, K. J., Weller, G., Shprintzen, R. J. (1985) Velo-cardio-facial syndrome: Language and psychological profiles. Journal of Craniofacial Genetics and Developmental Biology 5 (3): 259–66.

Goldmuntz, E., Driscoll, D., Budarf, M. L., Zackai, E. H., McDonald-McGinn, D. M., Biegel, J. A., Emanuel, B. S. (1993) Microdeletions of chromosomal region 22q11 in patients with congenital conotruncal cardiac defects. Journal of Medical Genetics 30: 807–12.

Goldsobel, A. B., Haas, A., Stiehm, E. R. (1987) Bone marrow transplantation in DiGeorge syndrome. Journal of Pediatrics 111 (1): 40–44.

Gottlieb, S., Emanuel, B. S., Driscoll, D.A., Sellinger, B., Wang, Z., Roe, B., Budarf, M. L. (1997) The DiGeorge syndrome minimal critical region contains a goosecoid-like (GSCL) homeobox gene that is expressed early in human development. American Journal of Human Genetics 60 (5): 1194–1201.

Greenberg, F. (1993) DiGeorge syndrome: An historical review of clinical and cytogenetic features. Journal of Medical Genetics 30 (10): 803–6.

Gripp, K. W., McDonald-McGinn, D. M., Driscoll, D. A., Reed, L. A., Emanuel, B. S., Zackai, E. H. (1997) Nasal dimple as part of the 22q11.2 deletion syndrome. American Journal of Medical Genetics 69 (3): 290–2.

Hagerman, R. J. (1996) Physical and behavioral phenotype. In: Fragile X syndrome: Diagnosis, treatment and research. Hagerman, R. J., and Cronister, A. (eds.). 2nd ed. Johns Hopkins University Press, Baltimore, pp. 3–87.

Howard, B. J. (1996) Advising parents on discipline: What works. Pediatrics 98 (4): 809–17.

Junker, A. K., and Driscoll, D. A. (1995) Humoral immunity in DiGeorge syndrome. Journal of Pediatrics 127 (2): 231–7.

Kapur, S., and Remington, G. (1996) Serotonin-dopamine interaction and its relevance to schizophrenia. American Journal of Psychiatry 153 (4): 466–76.

Kinouchi, A., Mori, K., Ando, M., Takao, A. (1976) Facial appearance of patients with conotruncal anomalies. Pediatrics Japan 17: 84.

Kok, L. L., and Solman, R. T. (1995) Velocardiofacial syndrome: Learning difficulties and intervention. Journal of Medical Genetics 32: 612–18.

Kozma, C. (1998) On cognitive variability in velocardiofacial syndrome: Profound mental retardation and autism. American Journal of Medical Genetics (Neuropsychiatric Genetics) 81: 269–70.

Lachiewicz, A. M., Hoegerman, S. F., Holmgren, G., Holmberg, E., Arinbjarnarson, K. (1991) Association of the Robin sequence with the fragile X syndrome. American Journal of Medical Genetics 41 (3): 275–8.

Lachman, H. M., Morrow, B., Shprintzen, R., Veit, S., Parsia, S. S., Faedda, G., Goldberg, R., Kucherlapati, R., Papolos, D. F. (1996) Association of codon 108/158 catechol-O-methyltransferase gene polymorphism with the psychiatric manifestations of velocardio-facial syndrome. American Journal of Medical Genetics 67 (5): 468–72.

Lachman, H. M., Kelsoe, J. R., Remick, R. A., Sadovnick, A. D., Rapaport, M. H., Lin, M., Pazur, B. A., Roe, A. M., Saito, T., Papolos, D. F. (1997) Linkage studies suggest a possible locus for bipolar disorder near the velo-cardio-facial syndrome region on chromosome

22. American Journal of Medical Genetics 74 (2): 121–8.

Leana-Cox, J., Pangkanon, S., Eanet, K. R., Curtin, M. S., Wulfsburg, E. A. (1996) Familial DiGeorge/velocardiofacial syndrome with deletions of chromosome area 22q11.2: Report of five families with a review of the literature. American Journal of Medical Genetics 65: 309–16.

Lindsay, E. A., Morris, M. A., Gos, A., Nestadt, G., Wolyniec, P. S., Lasseter, V. K., Shprintzen, R. (1995) Schizophrenia and chromosomal deletions within 22q11.2. American Journal of Human Genetics 56: 1502–3.

Lipson, A. H., Yuille, D., Angel, M., Thompson, P. G., Vandervoord, J. G., Beckenham, E. J. (1991) Velocardiofacial (Shprintzen) syndrome: An important syndrome for the dysmorphologist to recognise. Journal of Medical Genetics 28 (9): 596–604.

Marble, M., Morava, E., Tsien, F., Amedee, R., Pierce, M. (1998) Subglottic web in a mother and son with 22q11.2 deletion. American Journal of Medical Genetics 75: 537.

McCandless, S. E., Scott, J. A., Robin, N. A. (1998) Deletion 22q11: A newly recognized cause of behavioral and psychiatric disorders. Archives of Pediatric and Adolescent Medicine 152: 481–4.

McElroy, S. L., and Weller, E. (1997) Psychopharmacological treatment of bipolar disorder across the life span. In: Psychopharmacology across the life span. McElroy, S. L. (ed.). American Psychiatric Press, Washington, D.C., pp. 31–85.

Mehraein, Y., Wippermann, C. F., Michel-Behnke, I., Nhan Ngo, T. K., Hillig, U., Giersberg, M., Aulepp, U., Barth, H., Fritz, B., Rehder, H. (1997) Microdeletion 22q11 in complex cardiovascular malformations. Human Genetics 99 (4): 433–42.

Mitnick, R. J., Bello, J. A., Shprintzen, R. J. (1994) Brain anomalies in velocardio-facial syndrome. American Journal of Medical Genetics 54 (2): 100–106.

Moss, E. M., Wang, P. P., McDonald-McGinn, D. M., Gerdes, M., DaCosta, A. M., Christensen, K. M., Driscoll, D. A., Emanuel, B. S., Batshaw, M. L., Zackai, E. H. (1995) Characteristic cognitive profile in patients with a 22q11.2 deletion: Verbal IQ exceeds nonverbal IQ. American Journal of Human Genetics 57 (suppl.): A20.

Moss, E. M., Wang, P. P., Solot, C. B., Gerdes, M., McDonald-McGinn, D. M., Driscoll, D. A., Emanuel, B. S., Zackai, E. H., Batshaw, M. L. (1998) Psychoeducational profile of the 22q11.2 microdeletion: A complex pattern. Journal of Pediatrics.

Nickel, R. E., and Magenis, R. E. (1996) Neural tube defects and deletions of 22q11. American Journal of Medical Genetics 66: 25–27.

Pulver, A. E., Nestadt, G., Goldberg, R., Shprintzen, R. J., Lamacz, M., Wolyniec, P. S., Morrow, B., Karayiorgou, M., Antonarakis, S. E., Housman, D., et al. (1994) Psychotic illness in patients diagnosed with velo-cardio-facial syndrome and their relatives. Journal of Nervous and Mental Disease 182 (8): 476–8.

Ryan, A. K., Goodship, J. A., Wilson, D. I., Philip, N., Levy, A., Seidel, H., Schuffenhauer, S. (1997) Spectrum of clinical features associated with interstitial chromosome 22q11 deletions: A European collaborative study. Journal of Medical Genetics 34: 798–804.

Scambler, P. J., Carey, A. H., Wyse, R. K., Roach, S., Dumanski, J. P., Nordenskjold, M., Williamson, R. (1991) Microdeletions within 22q11 associated with sporadic and familial DiGeorge syndrome. Genomics 10 (1): 201–6.

Scambler, P. J., Kelly, D., Lindsay, E., Williamson, R., Goldberg, R., Shprintzen, R., Wilson, D. I., Goodship, J. A.,

Cross, I. E., Burn, J. (1992) Velo-cardio-facial syndrome associated with chromosome 22 deletions encompassing the DiGeorge locus. Lancet 339 (8802): 1138–9.

Schmickel, R. D. (1986) Contiguous gene syndromes: A component of recognizable syndromes. Journal of Pediatrics 109 (2): 231–41.

Shprintzen, R. J., Goldberg, R. B., Lewin, M. L., Sidoti, E. J., Berkman, M. D., Argamaso, R. V., Young, D. (1978) A new syndrome involving cleft palate, cardiac anomalies, typical facies, and learning disabilities: Velo-cardio-facial syndrome. Cleft Palate Journal 15 (1): 56–62.

Shprintzen, R. J., Goldberg, R. B., Young, D., Wolford, L. (1981) The velo-cardio-facial syndrome: A clinical and genetic analysis. Pediatrics 67 (2): 167–72.

Shprintzen, R. J., Goldberg, R., Golding-Kushner, K. J., Marion, R. W. (1992) Late-onset psychosis in the velo-cardio-facial syndrome [Letter to the editor]. American Journal of Medical Genetics 42 (1): 141–2.

Swillen, A., Devriendt, K., Legins, E., Eyskens, B., Dumoulin, M., Gewillig, M., Fryns, J. P. (1997) Intelligence and psychosocial adjustment in velocardiofacial syndrome: A study of 37 children and adolescents with VCFS. Journal of Medical Genetics 34: 453–8.

Thomas, J. A., and Graham, J. M., Jr. (1997) Chromosomes 22q11 deletion syndrome: An update and review for the primary pediatrician. Clinical Pediatrics 36 (5): 253–66.

Wang, P. P., Solot, C., Moss, E. M., Gerdes, M., McDonald-McGinn, D. M., Driscoll, D. A., Emanuel, B. S. (1998) Developmental presentation of 22q11.2 deletion (DiGeorge/Velo-cardio-facial syndrome). Journal of Developmental and Behavioral Pediatrics 19 (5): 342–5.

Weinzimer, S. A., McDonald-McGinn, D. M., Driscoll, D. A., Emanuel, B. S., Zackai, E. H., Moshang, T. (1998) Growth hormone deficiency in patients with a 22q11.2 deletion: Expanding the phenotype. Pediatrics 101: 929–32.

Wilson, T. A., Blethen, S. L., Vallone, A., Alenick, D. S., Nolan, P., Katz, A., Amorillo, T. P., Goldmuntz, E., Emanuel, B. S., Driscoll, D. A. (1993) DiGeorge anomaly with renal agenesis in infants of mothers with diabetes. American Journal of Medical Genetics 47 (7): 1078–82.

Yan, W., Jacobsen, L. K., Krasnewich, D. M., Guan, X., Lenane, M. C., Paul, S. P., Dalwadi, H. N., Zhang, H., Long, R. T., Kumra, S., Martin, B. M., Scambler, P. J., Trent, J. M., Sidransky, E., Ginns, E. I., Rapoport, J. L. (1998) Chromosome 22q11.2 interstitial deletions among childhood-onset schizophrenics and "multidimensionally impaired". American Journal of Medical Genetics (Neuropsychiatric Genetics) 81: 41–43.

Zori, R. T., Boyar, F. Z., Williams, W. N., Gray, B. A., Bent-Williams, A., Stalker, H. J., Rimer, L. A., Nackashi, J. A., Driscoll, D. J., Rasmussen, S. A., Dixon-Wood, V., Williams, C. A. (1998) Prevalence of 22q11 region deletions in patients with velopharyngeal insufficiency. American Journal of Medical Genetics 77: 8–11.

RESOURCES

Velo-Cardio-Facial Syndrome Educational Foundation
SUNY Health Science Center at Syracuse
750 East Adams Street
Jacobsen Hall, Room 707
Syracuse, NY 13210
telephone: (315) 464-6590
fax: (315) 464-5321
e-mail: vcfsef@hscsyr.edu
http://www.hscsyr.edu/~vcfsef

Velo-Cardio-Facial Syndrome Research Institute
Albert Einstein College of Medicine
1300 Morris Park Avenue
Bronx, NY 10461
telephone: (718) 430-2568
fax: (718) 430-8778
e-mail: rgoldberg@aecom.yu.edu

22q and You
Department of Clinical Genetics
Children's Hospital of Philadelphia
One Children's Center
34th Street and Civic Center Boulevard
Philadelphia, PA 19104
telephone: (215) 590-2920
e-mail: lunny@email.chop.edu
http://cbil.humgen.upenn.edu/VCFS/index.html

American Academy of Otolaryngology-Head and Neck Surgery
One Prince Street
Alexandria, VA 22314
telephone: (703) 836-4444

American Cleft Palate Cranial Facial Association
1218 Grandview Avenue
Pittsburgh, PA 15211
telephone: (412) 481-1376;
    (800) 242-5338

American Heart Association
7272 Greenville Avenue
Dallas, TX 75231-4596

telephone: (214) 373-6300;
    (800) 242-8271
e-mail: inquire@amhrt.org
http://www.amhrt.org

American Speech-Language-Hearing Association
10801 Rockville Pike
Rockville, MD 20852
telephone: (301) 987-5700 (voice, TTY/TDD/TT); toll free: (800) 638-8255
fax: (301) 571-0457

The ARC of the United States
500 East Border Street, S-300
Arlington, TX 76010
telephone: (817) 261-6003

Children's Craniofacial Association (CCA)
9441 LBJ FRWY, Suite #115
Dallas, TX 75243
telephone: (214) 994-9902;
    (800) 535-3643
fax: (214) 994-9831

FACES: The National Craniofacial Association
P.O. Box 11082
Chattanooga, TN 37401
telephone: (423) 266-1632;
    (800) 332-2373
fax: (423) 267-3124
e-mail: faces@mindspring.com

March of Dimes Birth Defects Foundation
National Headquarters
1275 Mamaroneck Avenue
White Plains, NY 10605
telephone: (888) MO-DIMES;
    (206) 624-1373

NIH/National Oral Health Information Clearinghouse
1 NOHIC Way
Bethesda, MD 20892-3500

telephone: (301) 402-7364
e-mail: nidr@aerie.com
http://www.aerie.com/nohicweb/

National Organization for Rare Disorders, Inc. (NORD)
P.O. Box 8923
New Fairfield, CT 06812-8923
telephone: (203) 746-6518;
(800) 999-6673; TDD: (203) 746-6927
fax: (203) 746-6481

e-mail: orphan@nord-rdb.com
http://www.nord-rdb.com/~orphan

Tools

Stop, Relax and Think
Child's Work, Child's Play
The Fourth St. Company
Center for Applied Psychology
telephone: (800) 962-1141

8

Williams Syndrome

Williams, Barratt-Boyes, and Lowe (1961) first described a syndrome of infantile hypercalcemia, supravalvular aortic stenosis, mental retardation, and distinctive facies in four children in 1961. Beuren and colleagues (1964) expanded the syndrome to include peripheral pulmonary artery stenosis and dental anomalies. Black and Bonham Carter (1963) recognized the similarity of the dysmorphic features in the patients reported by Williams to those in patients with Fanconi-type idiopathic infantile hypercalcemia. The coexistence of hypercalcemia and supravalvular aortic stenosis was established by Garcia and colleagues (1964). The syndrome subsequently became known as Williams-Beuren syndrome, or simply Williams syndrome (WS). It is relatively rare, with an estimated incidence of 1 per 20,000 live births, but it is an interesting disorder with a well-delineated behavioral phenotype and molecular-cognitive brain associations that are worth describing here. WS is associated with many cognitive strengths, including a good vocabulary, enhanced expressive language skills, and emotionally enriched narratives that are far better than those of cognitively matched controls (Bellugi et al., 1996, 1999; Reilly et al., 1990). They represent a significant contrast to individuals with autism because of their strengths in social interaction, including their abilities to use affective information to enrich their expressive vocabulary (Courchesne et al., 1995). These language abilities are described as chatty, with stereotypic phrases, but they are able to carry on conversations that are not reflective of their intellectual deficits, and they are usually charming and engaging.

Detailed studies have been carried out to better understand gene, brain, and behavior relationships, and the advances in molecular biology have revealed a submicroscopic deletion of the elastin gene (*ELN*) at 7q11.23 which can be

Neurodevelopmental Disorders: Diagnosis and Treatment, by Randi Jenssen Hagerman. New York: Oxford University Press, 1999. © Oxford University Press, Inc.

detected by fluorescent in situ hybridization (FISH) studies in greater than 96% of patients with the classical Williams syndrome phenotype (Lowery et al., 1995; Osborne et al., 1996).

PHYSICAL FEATURES

The typical facial features in Williams syndrome include a short upturned nose, puffy eyes or periorbital fullness, bitemporal narrowness, wide mouth, long filtrum, prominent ears, full cheeks, prominent lips, and small widely spaced teeth with frequent malocclusion and small jaw (micrognathia). The overall gestalt of these features has been termed "elfin facies" (Figure 8.1). Hovis and Butler (1997) have carried out detailed photoanthropometric studies of craniofacial traits in 29 individuals with WS and found prominent ears, posteriorally rotated ears, broad palpebral fissure (opening of the eye) width, broad nasal bridge, small chin, broad interalar distance (breadth of nose at the nostrils), and a long philtrum compared with controls, which supports the clinical impressions. The eyes have a lacy, stellate iris pattern in over 50% of WS patients. This is easy to distinguish in blue-eyed patients, but it is harder to see in dark-eyed patients (Holmstrom et al., 1990). Strabismus is seen in 54%, and almost all of these patients had esotropia (eye turned in; Winter et al., 1996). In 152 patients assessed with a detailed ophthalmological exam, 22% demonstrated retinal vascular tortuosity, three had cataracts, and two had ptosis, but no patient had ocular manifestations of hypercalcemia (Winter et al., 1996).

Supravalvular aortic stenosis, peripheral pulmonic stenosis, or other arterial stenoses (such as renal, mesenteric, or coronary arteries) and hypertension are common (Table 8.1). The supravalvular aortic stenosis (SVAS) is a congenital narrowing of the aorta above the take-off of the coronary arteries. Most patients with WS do not have a structural defect of the heart but instead have discrete or diffuse arterial stenoses related to the elastin gene (*ELN*) deletion described later in this chapter. Approximately 20% of individuals with the *ELN* deletion do not have arterial stenoses. In those patients with arterial stenoses, there is a progression of the degree of stenosis in one-third which requires surgical intervention (Pober and Dykens, 1996). A rare complication in WS is sudden death. Two anatomical abnormalities predispose individuals to sudden death: coronary artery stenosis and severe biventricular outflow tract obstruction (Bird et al., 1996). These problems can lead to myocardial ischemia, decreased cardiac output, and arrhythmia. A cardiology evaluation at the time of diagnosis can identify the individuals who are at higher risk for sudden death.

Most of the physical findings associated with Williams syndrome are thought to be secondary to the deletion of *ELN* at 7q11.23. Further evidence that the elastin deletion causes the supravalvular aortic stenosis came from a study by Curran et al. (1993) in which a pedigree with familial supravalvular aortic stenosis was found with a mutation, specifically a break in the middle of the elastin gene, leading to premature termination of this gene; all individuals with this defect had

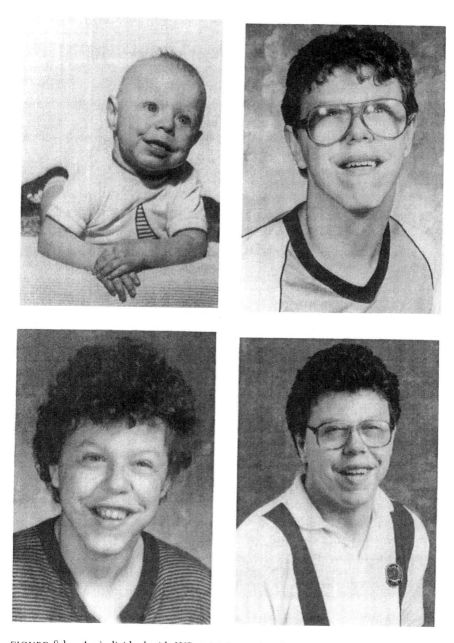

FIGURE 8.1: An individual with WS at (a) 6 months, (b) 12 years, (c) 17 years, and (d) 29 years of age. Note full cheeks, wide mouth, and puffiness around the eyes.

TABLE 8.1. Phenotypic Features in Williams Syndrome

Feature/problem	Present (%)
Physical and Behavioral Features	
Developmental delay	96
Supravalvular aortic stenosis	53
Any congenital or vascular heart disease	74
Hoarse voice	98
Williams syndrome personality	88
Wide mouth	96
Broad forehead	92
Long filtrum	96
Bitemporal narrowness	88
Periorbital fullness	92
Hypercalcemia	15
Medical Problems in Childhood	
Feeding difficulties	71
Failure to thrive	81
Vomiting	40
Constipation	43
Colic	67
Umbilical hernia	14
Inguinal hernia	38
Esotropia	50
Chronic otitis media	43
Enamel hypoplasia	48
Malocclusion	85
Hypertension	17
Enuresis	52
Joint limitation	50
Kyphosis	21
Lordosis	38
Scoliosis	12
Renal anomalies	18
Medical Problems in Adulthood	
Hypertension	47
Urinary tract infections	29
Constipation	41
Peptic ulcer disease	18
Cholelithiasis	12
GI diverticulitis	12
Obesity	29
Prematurely gray hair	60

Adapted from Joyce et al. (1996), Mervis et al. (1999), Morris et al. (1988), and Pankau et al. (1996).

SVAS. Therefore, this cardiac disorder can occur in isolation or in a dominant inheritance pattern in families that is separate from the full Williams syndrome. In a study by Joyce and colleagues (1996) in which seven patients with SVAS or peripheral pulmonic stenosis were referred for DNA analysis, one out of the seven (14%) showed a deletion at *ELN*.

Other manifestations of the elastin defect include umbilical or inguinal hernias, which lead to surgery in 38% of patients (Morris et al., 1988), and bowel or bladder diverticula, which are more common in adulthood (Table 8.1). Recurrent otitis media is a problem for 38% of children, and 19% required polyethylene tube placement (Morris et al., 1988). Patients usually have loose joints in childhood, but progressive joint stiffness or joint limitation is common, and adolescents or adults often have a stiff and awkward walk. Scoliosis, kyphosis, and lordosis are not uncommon and are likely related to the elastin defect and the joint stiffness. The puffy cheeks and eyelids that are part of the "elfin facies" are considered secondary to the elastin defect influencing soft tissue. It is also possible that the hoarse voice is due to the abnormalities in elastin fibers affecting the larynx (Mervis et al., 1999). The hemizygosity of *ELN* may result in abnormal production of elastin protein needed for elastin fibers. These fibers are fragmented and disorganized in SVAS. The stenosis is caused by fibrosis and results from blood pressure impinging on a relatively inelastic arterial wall (Mervis et al., 1999). SVAS often gets worse with age, whereas the peripheral pulmonic stenosis that is not exposed to high arterial pressures usually improves with age. The abnormal elastin fibers also cause premature aging of the skin (Mervis et al., 1999).

The dental problems in WS may also be related to the *ELN* deletion. Patients usually have small teeth with wide spacing, malocclusion, and occasional missing teeth (Pober and Dykens, 1996). Enamel hypoplasia is also common. Most of the dental problems can be corrected by orthodontia (Hertzberg et al., 1994).

Seizures occasionally occur in WS, but consistent EEG abnormalities have not been reported. It is likely that background genes influence the presence of seizures in WS; a family history of epilepsy was seen in two patients with infantile spasms and WS (Tsao and Westman, 1997).

In a study by Chapman and colleagues (1995) of 24 children and adults with Williams syndrome, a detailed neurological examination revealed that 41% of the children had hypotonia, whereas 29% had hypertonia; 85% of the adults had hypertonia. Fine motor coordination problems were seen in over 60% of the overall group. There appears to be a pattern of hypotonia which is remarkable in the younger patients and may exacerbate feeding problems in infancy, but this problem may evolve to hypertonia as the patients age. Joint contractures can develop in the adolescent and adult, and radioulnar synostosis (fusion of the upper end of the radius and ulna arm bones) is occasionally seen (Pober and Dykens, 1996). Gait abnormalities were seen in 70% of the younger children and 85% of the adults (Chapman et al., 1995). Praxis problems were present in 70% of the children and 71% of the adults, but cranial nerve abnormalities or cerebellar findings were not present. Prolonged clonus (more than three beats) and brisk reflexes were seen in 11 of 17 young patients and 6 of 7 older patients (Chapman et al. 1995).

Developmental delays are typical, and walking occurs at an average age of 21 months, talking at 21.6 months, and toilet training at 39 months (Morris et al., 1988). By the first grade children with WS have recognizable academic delays (Morris et al., 1988).

Morris et al. (1988) studied the growth of 80 patients with WS and found that the growth disturbance was greatest in early childhood, perhaps related to the feeding problems, hypotonia, and hypercalcemia, but growth often recovered after 4 years of age. Growth curves are available for WS, and they should be used in following growth for these patients (Morris et al., 1988; Pankau et al., 1992). The mean head circumference is at the fourth percentile in the first 4 years and subsequently increases to the 25th percentile. Only 16% of the 80 patients studied had microcephaly (Morris et al., 1988).

A recent report by Perez Jurado and colleagues (1996) studied 39 families in which the parent of origin of the deletion was known. All of the deletions were de novo; 18 were paternally derived and 21 were maternally derived. There was significantly more severe growth retardation and microcephaly in the maternal deletion group than in the paternal deletion group, suggesting an imprinted locus that is silent on the paternal chromosome and that contributes to statural and head circumference growth (Perez Jurado et al., 1996).

Pankau and colleagues (1996) surveyed the kidneys and urinary tract by ultrasound of 130 patients with WS (mean age 5.5 years for females and 6.4 years for males). The incidence of renal anomalies was 17.7%, and they ranged from mild problems (bladder diverticula) to severe malformations, such as renal hypoplasia (5/130). A duplicated kidney was found in nine patients, but nephrocalcinosis was not seen. Renal ultrasound studies are recommended at the time of diagnosis, because there is a 12- to 36-fold increase in structural abnormalities of the urinary system compared with the normal population (Pankau et al., 1996).

In a study of 41 patients with WS, 32% were noted to have genitourinary symptoms, including urinary frequency and daytime wetting (Schulman et al., 1996). Four of these patients had bladder diverticula and uninhibited detrusor contractions on urodynamic studies. Bladder training and anticholinergic medication can improve the patients' voiding pattern (Schulman et al., 1996).

Precocious puberty has been reported in a girl with WS who developed breasts and pubic hair at 7½ years and subsequently began menstruating at 8½ years (Scothorn and Butler, 1997). These authors report that anecdotal information from discussions with families suggest that precocious puberty is not an unusual finding in children with WS.

BEHAVIORAL FEATURES

Attentional problems associated with impulsivity and sometimes hyperactivity that are consistent with a diagnosis of attention deficit hyperactivity disorder (ADHD) were seen in 70% of the younger children and 40% of the older patients (Chapman et al., 1995). Morris et al. (1988) identified ADHD in 84% of 25 patients between the ages of 4 and 16 years, but only three patients were being medicated with stimulants (all were on methylphenidate). ADHD is a significant component of the WS personality, and it may add to the impulsive verbalizations and impulsive friendliness that characterizes the personality of these patients.

Their language is phonologically and syntactically well developed, and they have an ability to elaborate with unusual descriptive responses in their stories (Bellugi et al., 1999). To enrich their narratives, they may also use fluctuations in the tone and emotions of their speech and mimicry to a greater extent than normal control patients of the same mental age or patients with Down syndrome (Bellugi et al., 1996; Bellugi et al., 1999). Studies of their narratives are reflective of their sociability and emotional sensitivity, which are in stark contrast to individuals with autism (Courchesne et al., 1995).

Despite verbal skills that are better developed than visual perceptual skills, a follow-up study of 119 late adolescent and adult individuals with WS demonstrated significant difficulties with social and adaptive skills (Udwin, 1990). Two-thirds of the patients were described as socially isolated, and they had great difficulty in initiating and maintaining friendships. Only 14% were currently in a steady relationship, and only 1 of the 119 individuals was married (Udwin, 1990). Only 3% could be left alone at home for the weekend, and only 22% could be left alone for an evening. An occasional patient has even been reported with autism (a total of six cases of autism with WS have been reported; Pober and Dykens, 1996; Reiss et al., 1985).

Hyperacusis

An unusual feature of Williams syndrome is patients' sensitivity to sound, which is described as hyperacusis. They have an aversion to loud noises and can experience discomfort with many noises, such as a vacuum cleaner, a hairdryer, or the sound of an elevator, which may not necessarily be loud. They may also experience anxiety in anticipation of such noises. Younger children may cry or become irritable, and older children usually cover their ears and verbalize pain with some noises. As the individual ages, an attraction may develop to the noises that previously caused discomfort (U. Bellugi, personal communication 1998). For instance, the individual may become obsessed with vacuum cleaners or lawn mowers.

There is no evidence of peripheral auditory pathology in individuals with Williams syndrome (Marriage, 1995). However, Bellugi and colleagues (1999) have found evidence for abnormalities in auditory evoked potential studies, including a lack of the attenuation of the N_{100} response to rapidly presented stimuli and an abnormally large P_{200} response. These abnormalities may represent the hyperexcitability in the primary auditory cortex in individuals with Williams syndrome (Neville et al., 1994). The auditory brainstem-evoked responses are normal. Therefore, the hyperexcitability does not appear to be in the brainstem but within the cortical areas that are important for processing auditory information.

Psychiatric Problems

Psychiatric problems beyond ADHD are beginning to be deciphered in both children and adults with WS. Anxiety is a significant problem when compared with controls matched on Verbal IQ (Einfeld et al., 1997; Udwin and Yule, 1991; Udwin et al., 1987). Anxiety is often described as a pervasive problem, with excessive worrying about new situations, preoccupations, fearfulness, and somatic complaints (Pober and Dykens, 1996; Davies et al., 1998). In addition to hyperacusis, other sensory sensitivities have been noted, such as tactile defensiveness (Mervis et al., 1999), but the severity of sensory dysfunction and its association with anxiety have not been studied. Obsessive-compulsive behavior, mood lability, depression, and aggression associated with ADHD may also occur, but these problems have not been adequately studied, and therefore they are often not treated (Davies et al., 1998).

Patients with WS have a significant difficulty in identifying fear, in contrast to their ability to recognize other emotions (Lai, 1998). They can approach strangers indiscriminately, and in the laboratory they have an abnormally high approach rating for unfamiliar faces, just as do patients with bilateral amygdala damage (Cassady et al., 1997).

NEUROCOGNITIVE FEATURES

There is a broad spectrum of involvement in Williams syndrome, ranging from normal intellectual abilities to severe mental retardation, although the mean IQ is in the range of 50 to 60 (Pober and Dykens, 1996; Udwin et al., 1987; Howlin et al., 1998). The study by Joyce et al. (1996) included a patient with a normal IQ and relatively few behavioral and physical features of Williams syndrome, in addition to another patient who had severe mental retardation, no speech, and most of the physical features of Williams syndrome. In studies by Bellugi et al. (1999), the mean IQ was 60, with a characteristic profile of cognitive strengths and weaknesses. The defects include impaired spatial cognition and difficulties with constructive visual-spatial tasks, but strengths are seen in lexical knowledge, in facial processing, and recognizing affective states. Weaknesses are most dramatic in visual-spatial tasks, and there is typically great difficulty in organizing an overall drawing or in processing visual information (Figure 8.2; Bellugi et al., 1996, 1999; Crisco et al., 1988). Often their pictures look fragmented with no overall gestalt compared with individuals with Down syndrome (Bellugi et al., 1994). Children with WS tend to focus on the local details of a picture and miss the overall design. When asked to copy a diamond shape made up of small + signs, they perseverated on the + signs and missed the overall diamond shape, whereas the patients with Down syndrome drew the overall diamond shape but did not notice the local

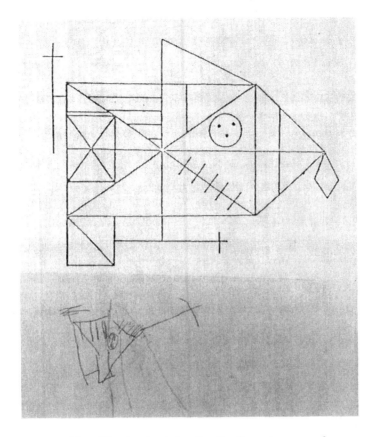

FIGURE 8.2:   The drawing below the Rey figure is a copy of
the Rey drawn by a 29-year-old man with Williams syndrome.
This was copied while looking at the sample Rey figure.

detail of the plus signs (Wang and Bellugi, 1993). When complex visual-spatial
copying tasks are presented with a small amount of spacing between the blocks
or the components, performance was significantly more accurate than it was
without the spacing for 21 adults with WS (Mervis et al., 1999).

Although the verbal strengths usually lead to a significant verbal and performance IQ descrepancy, this difference is less apparent in lower functioning
individuals (Jarrod et al., 1998). In late adolescence and adulthood, IQ does not
decline. A recent study of 62 adults with WS found only 4.8% with an IQ below
50, 87.1% with an IQ between 50 and 69, and 8.1% with an IQ above 70
(Howlin et al. 1998). Although the IQ is maintained, academic performance
was disappointingly low, with age-equivalent scores in reading comprehension,
spelling, and math at the 7- to 8-year age level (Howlin et al. 1998).

Even though most individuals with WS have IQs in the mentally retarded
range, 73% score in the normal range on a test for auditory short-term memory,

and 42% score in the normal range on the Peabody Picture Vocabulary Test (PPVT-R) (Mervis et al., 1999). The excellent auditory memory of individuals with WS contributes to their strength in vocabulary development. In addition, the syntactical complexity of speech improves in WS as the mean length of utterance (MLU) increases with age, unlike in other developmental disorders, such as Down syndrome, autism, or fragile X syndrome (Scarborough et al., 1991). Although patients with WS have significant language and motor delays in early childhood that are comparable to children with Down syndrome, their language development excels in complex grammatical structures, vocabulary development, comprehension, and emotional enrichment as they grow older, in contrast to individuals with Down syndrome (Bellugi et al., 1996; Singer Harris et al., 1997).

Patients with Williams syndrome show strengths in discrimination of unfamiliar faces, immediate recall of unfamiliar faces, and perception of facial contours. Patients with Williams syndrome perform significantly better in these facial processing tasks than age- and IQ-matched patients with Down syndrome or mental-age-matched normal patients (Bellugi et al., 1994).

There are two streams involved in the processing of visual information: the dorsal stream, which goes from the occipital area to the parietal lobe and encodes information regarding location and locomotion, and the ventral stream, which goes from the occipital area to the temporal lobe structures and is involved with the recognition of faces and objects (Atkinson et al., 1997). Patients with WS have significant impairments on tasks that involve the dorsal stream but not the ventral stream because of their strengths in facial recognition (Atkinson et al., 1997; Wang et al., 1995). The unique profile of cognitive strengths and weaknesses in WS can be further understood by studying the neuroimaging and neuroanatomical changes in this disorder.

Neuroimaging and Neuroanatomical Studies

Studies of neuroimaging, particularly volumetric MRI studies, have shown some significant neuroanatomical correlates to the cognitive strengths and weaknesses which have been documented in Williams syndrome. Most patients with Williams syndrome demonstrate a small head circumference. However, the frontal regions and the limbic structures of the temporal lobe, including the uncas, amygdala, and hippocampus, appear to be proportionately spared in patients with Williams syndrome compared with other cerebral structures (Jernigan et al., 1993; Wang and Bellugi, 1993). A postmortem study of a 31-year-old male with WS demonstrated a dramatic reduction in the size of the brain posterior to the rolandic sulcus, almost as if a band constricted the posterior aspect of the brain (Galaburda et al., 1994). The frontal lobes and the anterior portion of the temporal lobes were spared from the reduction in size. The corpus callosum showed a narrowing in the isthmus just anterior to the splenium (Galaburda et al., 1994). Wang et al. (1992) found that the anterior portion of the corpus callosum was preserved in individuals with WS in contrast to individuals with Down syndrome. In addition, the cerebellum, which is dramatically reduced in Down syndrome, is also relatively spared in individuals with Williams syndrome, particularly the neocerebellar area (Bellugi et al., 1999; Wang and Bellugi, 1993). An area in the primary auditory cortex called Heschl's gyrus showed a normal absolute volume which was the same as that of normal control subjects despite evidence of cerebral hypoplasia in other areas of the brain (Hickok et al., 1995). There appears to be a disproportionate development of Heschl's gyrus in Williams syndrome compared with other patient groups. In addition in individuals with Williams syndrome, another auditory area, the planum temporale, also looks similar to that of control patients (Hickok et al., 1995). The patients with Williams syndrome, however, differed from normals in the symmetry of the planum, with the normal leftward asymmetry exaggerated in Williams syndrome compared with controls. This finding is typical of professional musicians, suggesting that patients with WS have the neuroanatomical substrate to do well in music (Hickok et al., 1995; Lenhoff et al., 1997).

The Galaburda et al. (1994) study also demonstrated abnormally oriented pyramidal neurons especially in the visual cortex and the presence of neurons in subcortical white matter, suggesting a migration defect and incomplete connectivity from afferent axons to the abnormally oriented pyramidal neurons. Both of these problems can contribute to the cognitive and behavioral problems associated with WS.

Recent studies of the distribution of elastin fibers in the rat brain have detected neuronal expression of the elastin precursor in the cerebellar Purkinje cells throughout the cerebellar cortex, but it was most robust over the lingula of the anterior cerebellum and over the floccular and para floccular lobes (Sawchenko et al., 1997). The elastin precursor was also seen in the vascular system of the brain and in the neurons of the subfornical organ. Recent neuroanatomical studies of four brains from patients with WS demonstrated an increase in neuronal size, a tendency for decreased cell packing density of neurons, and abnormal orientation of neurons with slight disorganization of layering and columnar organization (Galaburda and Bellugi, 1998). There was no staining for elastin in Purkinje cells in contrast to controls, and three of the four brains showed relative curtailment of the posterior portions of the hemispheres involving mostly the occipital lobes, and also dorsal involvement. This is consistent with the finding that the dorsal stream of visual-spatial processing is more severely involved than the ventral stream (Atkinson et al., 1997; Wang et al., 1995). In addition, Galaburda and Bellugi (1998) found microvascular injury to the cortex consistent with showers of emboli affecting predominantly dorsal posterior portions of the hemispheres. The elastin defect could have contributed to this occurrence because of cardiac pathology.

Molecular Studies

Several pedigrees have now been identified that have only the elastin gene (*ELN*) disrupted without further deletion. All affected members have supravalvular aortic stenosis (SVAS) and some facial features of WS, but they do not have the cognitive profile, the personality, or the hypercalcemia of WS (reviewed by Mervis et al., 1999). This suggests that the *ELN* gene defect is not responsible for the neurocognitive or the behavioral problems in WS.

In a detailed study of two families with a more limited deletion (85 kb and 300 kb) than what is typically seen in WS (>500 kb), the affected members demonstrated a deletion of the *ELN* gene and the LIM-Kinase1 (*LIMK1*) gene, a protein kinase expressed in the brain, which is located 15.4 kb 3′ to the *ELN* gene (Frangiskakis et al., 1996). All of the affected individuals in these two pedigrees had the vascular and facial features of WS, in addition to the visual-spatial deficits typical of the syndrome; however, mental retardation was not present. The *ELN* gene is not expressed in the brain, and the LIMK1 protein is expressed mainly in neurons in human and mice brains, particularly in the basal ganglia, Purkinje cells, and pyramidal neurons (Frangiskakis et al., 1996). The protein tyrosine kinase from *LIMK1* phosphorylates a protein that is required for turnover of actin filaments which are required at the leading edge of a moving cellular process (Tassabehji et al., 1999). Defects in actin turnover could affect axonal guidance during CNS development (Tassabehji et al., 1999). Mice who are deficient in similar protein kinases have demonstrated impairment of long-term potentiation, spatial learning, and hippocampal development (Frangiskakis et al., 1996). Hemizygosity, or one copy, of the *LIMK1* gene is therefore hypothesized to be responsible for the visual-spatial deficits found in WS. A follow-up study of 84 patients with WS and the typical cognitive profile have demonstrated a deletion of both the *ELN* gene and the *LIMK1* genes (Mervis et al., 1997). Individuals without the visual-spatial deficits but with SVAS do not have the *LIMK1* gene deletion (Frangiskakis et al., 1996). A recent report by Tassabehji et al. (1999) evaluated four individuals with small deletions within the WS critical region, including *LIMKl*, but psychological testing of three of them did not demonstrate the typical visual spatial deficits in two of the patients. These findings suggest that the *LIMKl* deletion may not be sufficient alone to explain the visual spatial deficits in WS.

A recent study found that the syntaxin 1A gene (*STX1A*) is within the common WS deletion (Osborne et al., 1997). STX1A is an integral membrane protein found almost exclusively in neurons, and it is essential for neurotransmitter release (Osborne et al., 1997). A reduction of STX1A levels because of hemizygosity could give rise to hyperactivity and other behavior problems associated with WS (Osborne et al., 1997). It is possible that other genes within the deletion region will be found that will be responsible for other aspects of the phenotype of WS, including the hypercalcemia and mental retardation (Ashkenas, 1996).

The diagnosis of Williams syndrome in the past has involved cytogenetic testing, and now a fluorescent in situ hybridization (FISH) probe is available for the *ELN* gene. Williams syndrome is therefore a contiguous gene syndrome with a submicroscopic deletion that is well identified by FISH studies. In the study by Joyce et al. (1996), 96%, or 22 of the 23 patients with a classical Williams syndrome phenotype, had the deletion at 7q11.23. The remaining patient had a unique interstitial deletion on chromosome 11, del (11) (q13.5 q14.2). In a group of patients that had only some features of Williams syndrome phenotype, 2 of

22, or only 9%, had the *ELN* gene deletion. It is therefore recommended that cytogenetic studies be carried out with FISH analysis for the *ELN* gene defect, and, if that is not found, other karyotype abnormalities may also be associated with a Williams syndrome-like phenotype.

TREATMENT

Infancy and Preschool

Reports of feeding difficulties, including swallowing problems, floppiness, food refusal, and even constipation, are common in infants with WS, and they usually begin between 2 and 3 months of age (Martin et al., 1984). More severe problems, including vomiting, which was often projectile, and failure to thrive with a lack of weight gain, were seen in 74% of infants with documented hypercalcemia compared with 44% of infants with WS without hypercalcemia (Martin et al., 1984). Reflux is a common problem in infancy and may require thickened feedings and upright posture after feedings. Persistent problems may require a medical workup to document reflux, such as a barium swallow. Medications to treat reflux, such as metoclopromide or bethanacol or propulside, may be necessary. Hypercalcemia may also exacerbate reflux, and all children with WS should be tested for it.

The hypercalcemia requires treatment when documented, and the treatment involves restriction of calcium and vitamin D in the diet. Since vitamin D is present in all children's vitamins, it is recommended that children with WS should not receive multiple vitamins (Pober et al., 1997). Although hypercalcemia is seen in approximately 15% (Table 8.1), it is usually transient, although it may reoccur even in adolescence or adulthood. It is also recommended that a random spot urine be taken at the time of diagnosis to evaluate hypercalciuria (an elevated urinary calcium). This is assessed by a urine calcium-to-creatinine ratio. Hypercalciuria is defined as follows: infants younger than 7 months, calcium (mg/dl): creatinine (mg/dl) greater than 0.86; 17 to 18 months, greater than 0.60; 10 months to 6 years, greater than 0.42, and adults greater than 0.22 (Pober et al., 1997). If hypercalciuria is documented, repeated spot urines or a 24-hour calcium-to-creatinine ratio and total calcium excretion should be obtained. If the hypercalciuria is persistent, a renal ultrasound for nephrocalcinosis should be obtained, and, if it is present, the patient should be referred to a nephrologist (Pober et al., 1997). Consultation with a nutritionist can also help lower calcium and vitamin D intake when hypercalcemia or persistent hypercalciuria is present.

Usually the hypercalcemia is transient, lasting only a few weeks or months, so monitoring of blood calcium levels is important to avoid hypocalcemia. Sixteen of 76 patients with WS and hypercalcemia became hypocalcemic with treatment, and seven patients developed rickets (Martin et al., 1984). Occasionally a short course of corticosteroids (1 to 4 weeks) is needed for severe hypercalcemia when dietary restrictions do not bring the calcium levels down. Hypercalcemia can cause irritability, muscle cramps, and constipation, and longer-term hypercalcemia can also cause nephrocalcinosis (Gustafson and Traub, 1997; Pober et al., 1997).

Infants with feeding or oral motor coordination problems should be referred for occupational therapy (OT) to help develop sucking, swallowing, and chewing skills (Meyerson and Frank, 1987). As the infant grows, the OT should focus on overall motor coordination, and therapy can enhance the attainment of motor milestones. Sensory integration problems are particularly problematic with auditory and vestibular stimuli and can be addressed in therapy. As the child ages, the fine motor skills should be a focus of therapy. Paper and pencil tasks, utensil use, and tool use are significant problems for most individuals with WS. One-third of patients who were school-aged or in adulthood could not use a knife to spread or to cut because of motor deficits (Harris, 1995).

Progressive joint contractures are frequently seen in Williams syndrome, so a physical therapy (PT) evaluation should also be carried out by 3 years of age, and joint range of motion should be regularly monitored as part of a PT or OT program (Pober et al., 1997).

A detailed cardiology evaluation must be undertaken when the diagnosis of WS is made or if a murmur is heard or cardiac exam is abnormal. The cardiology evaluation should include echocardiography, Doppler flow studies, and four-limb blood pressures at the time of diagnosis (Pober et al., 1997). Some children have severe cardiac pathology, such as a severe stenosis of the proximal aorta, which will require cardiac surgery if the patient is symptomatic. Other children may have an initial negative cardiac workup, but periodic follow-up by cardiology is recommended, since subsequent disease can be documented, including peripheral pulmonic stenosis or hypertension. The risk for hypertension increases significantly with age in WS, and four-limb blood pressures should be followed regularly for this reason (Pober et al., 1997).

Recurrent otitis media infections are common in young children with WS, and, if present, referral to an ENT specialist for consideration of PE tubes is recommended. Normal hearing should be maintained so that a conductive hearing loss does not interfere with language development. Early language development is usually delayed, and language therapy should be considered by 2 years of age.

Preschool and School-Aged Children

An occasional patient may demonstrate hypothyroidism, so routine screening of thyroid function is recommended in patients who are 5 years old or older (Pober et al., 1997).

Language therapy and motor therapy are essential in the preschool period and can be part of a developmental preschool program. Although verbal skills are a strength later in development, early on language delays necessitate therapy which can focus on attending to and comprehending auditory information, concise and accurate responses, and pragmatic aspects of speech, such as turn taking (Meyerson and Frank, 1987). If severe hypernasality is present, evaluation for velopharyngeal insufficiency should be undertaken. If a hoarse voice is present, vocal therapy can focus on reducing abusive behavior to the vocal cords, such as yelling or the imitation of vehicle or animal sounds (Meyerson and Frank, 1987).

Hyperacusis may be apparent even in infancy or the preschool period, and it can lead to irritability or tantrum behavior in this period. Audiologic evaluation which incorporates reflux threshold, loudness increment, and ultra-high-frequency testing can assess the extent of the hyperacusis objectively (Meyerson and Frank, 1987). Environmental modifications can be made to avoid loud noises when the child is present, such as the dishwasher or vacuum cleaner. Ear protectors or ear plugs can be used as needed, and a few cases have been reported of a successful behavioral desensitization program in which the offending noise is taped and played over and over again beginning at a low-intensity level and then increasing the intensity (Meyerson and Frank, 1987).

Intrinsic strengths in music can be stimulated in the preschool and school-aged period with music lessons (see the Resource section at the end of this chapter). In general, patients with WS enjoy music, and many demonstrate talent in musical abilities.

Educational Approaches

As children with WS enter school, they should be evaluated by a special education team because of their cognitive, language, motor, and attentional deficits. Most children can be mainstreamed into the regular classroom with special education supports and individualized attention when necessary. They benefit from both motor and language therapy in school, as previously described. The teacher must be aware of their attentional problems and distractibility. Perhaps their hyperacusis makes them more sensitive to and easily distracted by background noises. Having the patient sit in the front row of the classroom and in close proximity to the teacher so he or she can be easily redirected may be helpful for ADHD symptoms. Structure and positive reinforcement on a daily basis will help with behavior and ADHD symptoms.

Children with WS do best academically in reading and music, but they have the most difficulty in math and handwriting (Grejtak, 1996). In a survey of 112 families who have a child with WS, the majority felt that a phonics approach to reading worked better than a whole-language approach (Grejtak, 1996). The favorite programs were SRA's Reading Mastery and Edmark's Reading Programs (see Appendixes 2 and 3). Reading Mastery is a phonics-based program which also teaches sight words. The Lindamood-Bell program, Visualizing and Verbalizing, can draw on verbal strengths to assist the children in forming visual mental images; this program looks promising for children with WS (Grejtak, 1996). In general, multisensory programs that also utilize a phonics approach have been most successful. Computer software programs to enhance reading are also helpful, and the favorite programs for children with WS are Reader Rabbit, Kid Phonics (Davidson), Mickey's ABC's, Edmark's Story Book Weaver Delux (Grejtak, 1996). Reading and spelling are often strengths for children with WS.

Although their verbal abilities help these children tell elaborate stories, their visual-motor coordination problems interfere with getting this information on paper. Therefore, use of computer technology can be of dramatic benefit to these children, and keyboard skills should be taught early. Computer programs such as Talking Sticky Bear Typing and Talking Fingers enhance keyboard skills, and Co:Writer and Write: Outloud can enhance written language output. To help handwriting skills, Handwriting Without Tears and the Zaner and Bloser Handwriting programs have been found to be helpful by families of children with WS (Grejtak, 1996).

Math is usually a problematic academic area, especially after the second or third grade when abstract math reasoning and more complex visual sequencing of math problems come into play. Using a hands-on approach to math concepts with the help of manipulatives and then calculators has been most successful (Grejtak, 1996). The Touch Math educational program is helpful, but most children need tutoring support in math. Computer software programs, such as Math Blaster, Sticky Bears Math, Math Splash, Talking Sticky Bear Math, and Math Rabbit have also been helpful (see Appendixes 2 and 3).

Children with WS require special education services, but one-third are integrated into a regular classroom for at least 50% of the day and another one-third are in the regular classroom 80 to 90% of the day (Grejtak, 1996). However, adaptations must be made to the materials, homework, and tests so that the child with WS can be successful in the regular classroom. Some examples of adaptation include (Grejtak, 1996):

- use of small group instruction with an aide
- use of a pencil grip (usually recommended by OT)
- use of a large button calculator for math computations
- individual and oral testing
- reducing the number of problems on homework or study sheets
- use of a stamp if child has trouble handwriting name

Table 8.2 provides additional modifications that may be helpful, and additional educational strategies can be found in Rourke (1995) and Anderson and Rourke (1995).

Psychotherapy and Adult Services

Between 40 and 70% of families with WS seek help from a mental health professional. The presenting problem may include ADHD, anxiety, or depression (Pober and Dykens, 1996). Individuals with WS are good candidates for a verbally oriented therapy because of their language skills. They often have strong and immediate transference with the therapist because of their tendency to overfamiliarity (Pober and Dykens, 1996). An important topic to work on in individual or group therapy is appropriate social skills. Their excessive sociability needs to be fine-tuned with

TABLE 8.2. Educational Strategies

Problem area	Strategies
Short attention span Impulsivity Distractibility	Reduce distractions Utilize study carrel or earplugs Reward for attending behavior Positive behavior reinforcements Use high interest areas in curriculum
Hyperacusis	Provide warning before predictable noises Make tape recording of sound and allow child to make it louder or softer Earplugs
Social deficits	Social skills group (make sure this is incorporated into IEP) Assign a buddy Encourage play days at home Pair up child with a partner during learning activities Have the child or parent present on WS to the class
Anxiety Problems with transitions	Use stories or role-play to act out anxious situations Provide a predictable schedule Use picture for daily routine Give warning before transition and use positive reinforcements for completing transition

Adapted from Levine (1998) and Grejtak, (1996).

appropriate listening skills, turn-taking skills, and wariness of strangers (Pober and Dykens, 1996). These patients are frequent targets for abuse and exploitation because of their excessive friendliness. A social-skills-building group can be helpful, either through the school or privately (Begum, 1996; Mundy, 1991).

A recent survey of 70 adults with WS in England found that most families do not receive adequate services for their adult offspring with WS (Udwin et al., 1998). Forty-eight adults (68.6%) were still living at home, and over half of the families related a number of difficulties and concerns, including behavior problems, lack of stimulation, and lack of personal and social independence. Of the 31.4% who left home, most were living in group homes or residential centers, and only three were living independently. In an additional study of this adult population only one patient had independent employment, and the rest were involved with sheltered workshops, voluntary work, or an adult training center (Davies et al., 1997). Emotional and behavioral problems interfered with their work, including anxiety (90%), overfriendliness (100%), distractability (90%), intolerance of others (57%), and anger management (38%) (Davies et al., 1997).

For some individuals, good verbal abilities may mask deficiencies which interfere with job success and interpersonal skills. Intensive job training with the use of a job coach for a prolonged period of time may be necessary. Work on life skills and personal independence should begin in high school or earlier and continue into adult life (Davies et al., 1997).

A multimodality approach to emotional and behavioral problems should include both counseling and psychopharmacology, as described in the next section (Davies et al., 1998).

Psychopharmacology

ADHD symptoms are seen in approximately 84% of children with WS; they usually respond to a multimodality intervention, including modifications at school, as previously described, and medication intervention. Placebo-controlled trials of stimulant medication, specifically methylphenidate (Ritalin), have been carried out in six cases of WS (Bawden et al., 1997; Power et al., 1997). Four of the six children had a positive response to methylphenidate in both behavioral ratings and neuropsychological testing. Some of the children were also noted to be less quarrelsome, impulsive, and moody during the methylphenidate trial period than a placebo period. In two of the cases (aged 7 and 8 years), a 5-mg and a 10-mg dose were compared, and both boys did better with a 10-mg dose (Power et al., 1997). None of the patients experienced a worsening of anxiety or stereotypic behavior on stimulants. Cardiac complications were not mentioned in these reports, although two of the patients did not have cardiac disease (Power et al., 1997).

The side effects of stimulants include cardiovascular stimulation, which might elevate heart rate and blood pressure; these measurements must be watched closely in patients with WS. Hypertension is a contraindication for the use of stimulants (Barkley, 1990). Appetite suppression, which can interfere with weight gain and height growth, should also be followed closely in children with WS, because short stature is already a problem with this syndrome. Higher doses of stimulants may worsen anxiety, which is an issue for many patients. Other stimulants that may be helpful include dextroamphetamine (Dexedrine) and a mixture of four dextro- and levoamphetamine salts (Adderall; Swanson et al., 1998). Both Dexedrine spansules and Adderall tablets are long-acting and can be given in the morning only.

Adderall is composed of d-amphetamine saccharate, d-amphetamine sulfate, d,l-amphetamine sulfate and d,l-amphetamine aspartate, resulting in a 75 : 25 ratio of dextro- and levoisomers of amphetamine (Swanson et al., 1998). Adderall was previously marketed under the brand name Obetral, but in 1994, it was bought by Richwood Pharmaceuticals and marketed for ADHD treatment under the name of Adderall. Only one controlled study has been published documenting the efficacy of Adderall's use in 30 children with ADHD (Swanson et al., 1998). These authors documented a prolonged duration of action with improvement in attention, behavior, and math performance in patients with ADHD on Adderall. Adderall had up to 6.5 hours of effect with the 20-mg dose compared with almost 4 hours of effect for methylphenidate.

Pemoline (Cylert) has recently been associated with rare cases of acute hepatic failure (Berkovitch et al., 1995; Nehra et al., 1990; Pratt and Dubois, 1990), and so the FDA has recently recommended avoiding pemoline as a first-line stimulant medication. A recent case report found that acute hepatic failure associated with pemoline intake had features of autoimmune hepatitis, specifically elevation of antinuclear antibodies (ANA), and the patient responded to prednisone for treatment of autoimmune hepatitis (Hochman et al., 1998). Because of the liver problems, the other stimulants should be tried first for treatment of ADHD in WS before pemoline is considered.

Stimulants do not prolong cardiac conduction nor lead to arrhythmias at higher doses, but tricyclic medications can cause these cardiac complications, and they should be avoided in patients with cardiac disease. Clonidine or guanfacine (Tenex) may also slightly prolong nodal conduction, although arrhythmias are rare (Hagerman et al., 1998). They may be used in patients with WS (after consultation with cardiology) because they lower blood pressure and they also treat hyperactivity, although they do not improve the attentional problems as well as stimulant medications (Hagerman et al., 1998). Gustafson and Traub (1997) reported an 18-year-old male with WS who was successfully treated with a clonidine patch (TTS 2), in addition to nifedipine in sustained release for hypertension.

The use of psychopharmalogic approaches for the treatment of anxiety or depression can be very helpful in WS, although no controlled studies have been carried out. Anecdotal information suggests that patients with either anxiety or depression respond well to a selective serotonin reuptake inhibitor (SSRI) (Pober and Dykens, 1996). SSRIs have been used in both normal and developmentally disabled children and adults for treatment of anxiety and depression (Hagerman et al., 1994; Kiev and Feiger, 1997; Preskorn, 1996; Riddle et al., 1996), and they have been helpful without serious side effects (see chapter 3 for a more detailed discussion of SSRIs).

CASE HISTORY: ROBERT

Robert is a 29-year-old man with Williams syndrome who presented with significant anxiety. His mother had a normal pregnancy but experienced premature rupture of membranes at 39 weeks of gestation. Robert's birth weight was 6 lb. 1 oz., and he was in the nursery for 3 days prior to going home. He ate well but had poor sleeping habits, and his milestones were delayed. He crawled at 21 months of age, and walked at 28 months, but he did not climb stairs until 10 years of age. He never mastered the riding of a tricycle or a bicycle. He was able to dress himself at age 8 but had great difficulties with buttons until he was in his 20s. In the language area, he said words at 2 years and subsequently full sentences before 3. He was always talkative throughout childhood, which facilitated his social interactions. He was also described as restless, hyperactive, and anxious through most of childhood and into adulthood.

Robert was in special education throughout his schooling, and as an adult he has had difficulty in maintaining employment for a sustained period of time.

He has tried jobs on an assembly line and in a laundry room and is currently doing volunteer work at a local train station. He has lived in an apartment by himself, and he is now doing well in a group home.

His mother was concerned about several behavioral problems, including anxiety and obsessive-compulsive behavior, both of which have been long-term difficulties. When he becomes anxious, he calms himself by applying makeup, which he learned to do from his sister. He has modeled his sister's behaviors throughout his life. In addition, he has certain rituals, such as a very specific way of folding his newspaper, and when he is unable to do it, he becomes uncomfortable. He also has problems with picking at sores and scratching his skin.

Cognitive testing 1 year before presentation demonstrated a Full-Scale IQ of 56 with a Verbal IQ of 60 and a Performance IQ of 57 on the WAIS-R. An emotional evaluation demonstrated a need for psychotherapy to increase his trust in peers and to decrease his anxiety level.

On physical examination his head circumference was in the 25th percentile for age. He had a mildly dysmorphic face, which had a triangular shape with a pointed chin, mildly prominent lips, full cheeks, a high, narrow palate, and tooth enamel hypoplasia. His iris pigmentation demonstrated a stellate pattern. He had several areas of scars on his extremities related to previous picking of lesions. Robert had difficulty with motor coordination, including a poor tandem walk, and a mild intention tremor on cerebellar testing. Problems were also seen with rapid alternating movements, and he was unable to coordinate a skip or to stand on one foot for more than 3 seconds. He also had severe visual motor coordination problems, as seen in his design copying and his Draw-A-Person Test. His joints were somewhat stiff. A genital exam demonstrated a small phallus and a testicular volume of 25 ml bilaterally, which is normal. His blood pressure was 150/100. Heart exam was normal, with a regular rhythm without murmur, and abdomen was soft without hepatosplenomegaly.

DNA cytogenetic testing with FISH studies demonstrated a deletion on chromosome 7 at q11.2, consistent with Williams syndrome. Calcium levels were normal, as were kidney function studies, including BUN and creatinine.

In treatment, sertraline (Zoloft) at a dose of 50 mg was given for his anxiety and obsessive-compulsive behavior, and Robert had a good response to this medication. He and his mother felt this medication also improved his hyperacusis. Hippotherapy (horseback riding therapy) has been very helpful for his balance and coordination. Follow-up studies were carried out to evaluate his high blood pressure, including ruling out renal artery stenosis. Ongoing counseling has also been recommended for him.

FUTURE DIRECTIONS

The molecular tapestry is beginning to be deciphered, and three of the genes responsible for components of the phenotype, *ELN*, *LIMK1*, and *STX1A*, have now been identified. Newer genes will be discovered within the deletion at 7q11.23 which will cover other aspects of the phenotype, including hypercalcemia and mental retardation (Ashkenas, 1996; Osborne et al., 1996). An understanding of the function of these new genes and their proteins will lead to new ways to compensate for their lack of function and thus new treatments. The psychiatric problems associated with WS, including anxiety and perhaps depression, should be better delineated so that present psychopharmacological interventions can be more readily used and controlled efficacy studies carried out. The study of the association between sensory modulation problems and anxiety in WS and other disorders discussed in this volume may lead to new approaches in treatment and early intervention. The study of the unique aspects of cognitive function which are controlled by the genes at 7q11.23 will not only be helpful for individuals with WS but will help our global understanding of the mechanisms of brain function and will lead to new educational, medical, and molecular interventions.

ACKNOWLEDGMENTS   Thanks to Ursula Bellugi, Paul Wang, and Cynthia Allman for very thorough reviews of chapter 8 and excellent comments that greatly improved the quality of this chapter. This work was supported in part by MCH grant no. MCJ-089413. Discussions with the Developmental Psychobiology Research group at the University of Colorado Health Science Center were also helpful.

REFERENCES

Anderson, P. E., and Rourke, B. P. (1995) Williams syndrome. In: Syndrome of nonverbal learning disabilities: Neuro-developmental manifestations. Rourke, B. P. (ed.). Guilford, New York, pp. 138–70.

Ashkenas, J. (1996) Williams syndrome starts making sense [Editorial]. American Journal of Human Genetics 59 (4): 756–61.

Atkinson, J., King, J., Braddick, O., Nokes, L., Anker, S., Braddick, F. (1997) A specific deficit of dorsal stream function in Williams syndrome. Neuroreport 8 (8): 1919–22.

Barkley, R. A. (1990) Attention deficit hyperactivity disorder: A handbook for diagnosis and treatment. Guilford, New York.

Bawden, H. N., MacDonald, G. W., Shea, S. (1997) Treatment of children with Williams syndrome with methylphenidate. Journal of Child Neurology 12 (4): 248–52.

Begum, R. W. (1996) Social skills lessons and activities. Center for Applied Research in Education, West Nyack, New York.

Bellugi, U., Wang, P., Jernigan, T. L. (1994) Williams syndrome: An unusual neurocognitive profile. In: Atypical cognitive deficits in developmental disorders. Browman, S. H. and Grafam, J. (eds.). Erlbaum, Hillsdale, NJ, pp. 23–56.

Bellugi, U., Klima, E. S., Wang, P. P. (1996) Cognitive and neural development: Clues from genetically based syndromes. In: The life-span development of individuals: A synthesis of biological and psychological perspectives.

Magnusson, D. (ed.). Cambridge University Press, New York, pp. 223–43.

Bellugi, U., Mills, D., Jernigan, T., Hickok, G., Galaburda, A. (1999) Linking cognition, brain structure, and brain function in Williams syndrome. In: Neurodevelopmental disorders: Contributions to a new framework from the cognitive neurosciences. Tager-Flusberg, H. (ed.). MIT Press, Cambridge, Mass.

Berkovitch, M., Pope, E., Phillips, J., Koren, G. (1995) Pemoline-associated fulminant liver failure: Testing the evidence for causation. Clinical Pharmacology and Therapeutics 57 (6): 696–8.

Beuren, A. J., Schulze, C., Eberle, P., Harmjanz, D., Apitz, J. (1964) The syndrome of supravalvular aortic stenosis, peripheral pulmonary artery stenosis, mental retardation and similar facial appeaarance. American Journal of Cardiology 13: 471–83.

Bird, L. M., Billman, G. F., Lacro, R. V., Spicer, R. L., Jariwala, L. K., Hoyme, H. E., Zamora-Salinas, R., Morris, C., Viskochil, D., Frikke, M. J., Jones, M. C. (1996) Sudden death in Williams syndrome: Report of ten cases. Journal of Pediatrics 129 (6): 926–31.

Black, J. A., and Bonham Carter, R. E. (1963) Association between aortic stenosis and cases of severe infantile hypercalcaemia. Lancet ii: 745–9.

Cassady, C., Bellugi, U., Grafstein, S., Reilly, J., Adolphs, R. (1997) Hypersociability in Williams syndrome: Similarities to bilateral amygdala patients. Poster presented at the International Behavioral Neuroscience Society Annual Meeting, San Diego, Calif.

Chapman, C. A., du Plessis, A., Pober, B. (1995) Neurologic findings in children and adults with Williams syndrome. Journal of Child Neurology 10: 63–65.

Courchesne, E., Bellugi, U., Singer, N. (1995) Infantile autism and Williams syndrome: Social and neural worlds apart. Genetic Counseling 6 (1): 144–5.

Crisco, J. J., Dobbs, J. M., Mulhern, R. K. (1988) Cognitive processing of children with Williams syndrome. Developmental Medicine and Child Neurology 30 (5): 650–6.

Curran, M. E., Atkinson, D. L., Ewart, A. K., Morris, C. A., Leppert, M. F., Keating, M. T. (1993) The elastin gene is disrupted by a translocation associated with supravalvular aortic stenosis. Cell 73 (1): 159–68.

Davies, M., Howlin, P., Udwin, O. (1997) Independence and adaptive behavior in adults with Williams syndrome. American Journal of Medical Genetics 70: 188–95.

Davies, M., Udwin, O., Howlin, P. (1998) Adults with Williams syndrome: A preliminary study of social, emotional and behavioral difficulties. British Journal of Psychiatry 172: 273–6.

Einfeld, S. L., Tonge, B. J., Florio, T. (1997) Behavioral and emotional disturbance in individuals with Williams syndrome. American Journal of Mental Retardation 102 (1): 45–53.

Frangiskakis, J. M., Ewart, A. K., Morris, C. A., Mervis, C. B., Bertrand, J., Robinson, B. F., Klein, B. P., Ensing, G. J., Everett, L. A., Green, E. D., Proschel, C., Gutowski, N. J., Noble, M., Atkinson, D. L., Odelberg, S. J., Keating, M. T. (1996) LIM-kinase1 hemizygosity implicated in impaired visuospatial constructive cognition. Cell 86 (1): 59–69.

Galaburda, A. M., and Bellugi, U. (1998) Brain cytoarchitectonic findings in Williams syndrome. Paper presented at the Cognitive Neuroscience Society, San Francisco, Calif.

Galaburda, A. M., Wang, P. P., Bellugi, U., Rossen, M. (1994) Cytoarchitectonic anomalies in a genetically based disorder: Williams syndrome. Neuroreport 5 (7): 753–7.

Garcia, R. E., Friedman, W. F., Kaback,

M. M., Rowe, R. D. (1964) Idiopathic hypercalcemia and supravalvular aortic stenosis. Documentation of a new syndrome. New England Journal of Medicine 271: 117–20.

Grejtak, N. (1996) Education survey results. Available at the Williams Syndrome Association Web site: http://www.williams-syndrome.org/survey.htm.

Gustafson, R., and Traub, D. (1997) Williams syndrome: A guide to diagnosis and treatment. South Dakota Journal of Medicine 50 (3): 89–91.

Hagerman, R. J., Fulton, M. J., Leaman, A., Riddel, J., Hagerman, K., Sobesky, W. (1994) A survey of fluoxetine therapy in fragile X syndrome. Developmental Brain Dysfunction 7: 155–64.

Hagerman, R. J., Bregman, J. D., Tirosh, E. (1998) Clonidine. In: Psychotropic medication and developmental disabilities: The international consensus handbook. Reiss, S., and Aman, M. G. (eds.). Ohio State University Nisonger Center, Columbus, Ohio, pp. 259–69.

Harris, J. C. (1995) Williams (Williams-Beuren) syndrome. In: Developmental neuropsychiatry: Assessment, diagnosis, and treatment of developmental disorders. Vol. 2. Oxford University Press, New York, pp. 319–32.

Hertzberg, J., Nakisbendi, L., Needleman, H. L., Pober, B. (1994) Williams syndrome—oral presentation of 45 cases. Pediatric Dentistry 16 (4): 262–7.

Hickok, G., Bellugi, U., Jones, W. (1995) Asymmetrical ability [Letter to the editor]. Science 270 (5234): 219–20.

Hochman, J. A., Woodard, S. A., Cohen, M. B. (1998) Exacerbation of autoimmune hepatitis: Another hepatotoxic effect of pemoline therapy. Pediatrics 101 (1): 106–8.

Holmstrom, G., Almond, G., Temple, K., Taylor, D., Baraitser, M. (1990) The iris in Williams syndrome. Archives of Disease in Childhood 65 (9): 987–9.

Hovis, C. L., and Butler, M. G. (1997) Photoanthropometric study of craniofacial traits in individuals with Williams syndrome. Clinical Genetics 51 (6): 379–87.

Howlin, P., Davies, M., Udwin, O. (1998) Cognitive functioning in adults with Williams syndrome. Journal of Child Psychology and Psychiatry 39 (2): 183–9.

Jarrold, C., Baddeley, A. D., Hewes, A. K. (1998) Verbal and nonverbal abilities in the Williams syndrome phenotype: Evidence for diverging developmental trajectories. Journal of Child Psychology and Psychiatry 39 (4): 511–23.

Jernigan, T. L., Bellugi, U., Sowell, E., Doherty, S., Hesselink, J. R. (1993) Cerebral morphologic distinctions between Williams and Down syndromes. Archives of Neurology 50 (2): 186–91.

Joyce, C. A., Zorich, B., Pike, S. J., Barber, J. C., Dennis, N. R. (1996) Williams-Beuren syndrome: Phenotypic variability and deletions of chromosomes 7, 11, and 22 in a series of 52 patients. Journal of Medical Genetics 33 (12): 986–92.

Kiev, A., and Feiger, A. (1997) A double-blind comparison of fluvoxamine and paroxetine in the treatment of depressed outpatients. Journal of Clinical Psychiatry 58: 146–52.

Lai, Z. (1998) Emotional expression and perception in Williams syndrome. Paper presented at the Cognitive Neuroscience Society, San Francisco, Calif.

Lenhoff, H. M., Wang, P. P., Greenberg, F., Bellugi, U. (1997) Williams syndrome and the brain. Scientific American 277 (6): 42–7.

Levine, K. (1998) Williams syndrome: Information for teachers. Williams Syndrome Association, Clawson, MI. (Also available at http://www.williams-syndrome.org/teacher.htm)

Lowery, M. C., Morris, C. A., Ewart, A., Brothman, L. J., Zhu, X. L., Leonard, C. O., Carey, J. C., Keating, M., Brothman, A. R. (1995) Strong correlation of elastin deletions, detected by FISH, with Williams syndrome: Evaluation of 235 patients. American Journal of Human Genetics 57 (1): 49–53.

Marriage, J. (1995) Central hyperacusis in Williams syndrome. [Abstract; Special issue]. Genetic Counseling 6 (1): 152–3.

Martin, N. D., Snodgrass, G. J., Cohen, R. D. (1984) Idiopathic infantile hypercalcaemia—a continuing enigma. Archives of Disease in Childhood 59 (7): 605–13.

Mervis, C., Morris, C., Robinson, B., Klein, B., Bertrand, J., Armstrong, S., Frangiskakis, J., Keating, M. (1997) The deficit in visual-spatial constructive cognition in Williams syndrome is associated with a hemizygous deletion of LIM-Kinase1. Paper presented at the International Conference on Mental Retardation: Genes, Brain and Behavior, Staten Island, NY.

Mervis, C. B., Morris, C. A., Bertrand, J., Robinson, B. F. (1999) Williams syndrome: Findings from an integrated program of research. In Neurodevelopmental disorders: Contributions to a new framework from the cognitive neurosciences. Tager-Flusberg, H. (ed.). MIT Press, Cambridge, Mass.

Meyerson, M. D., and Frank, R. A. (1987) Language, speech and hearing in Williams syndrome: Intervention approaches and research needs. Developmental Medicine and Child Neurology 29 (2): 258–62.

Morris, C. A., Demsey, S. A., Leonard, C. O., Dilts, C., Blackburn, B. L. (1988) Natural history of Williams syndrome: Physical characteristics. Journal of Pediatrics 113 (2): 318–26.

Mundy, J. (1991) Let's talk. Western Psychological Services, Los Angeles.

Nehra, A., Mullick, F., Ishak, K. G., Zimmerman, H. J. (1990) Pemoline-associated hepatic injury. Gastroenterology 99 (5): 1517–9.

Neville, C. E., Mahadevan, M. S., Barcelo, J. M., Korneluk, R. G. (1994) High resolution genetic analysis suggests one ancestral predisposing haplotype for the origin of the myotonic dystrophy mutation. Human Molecular Genetics 3 (1): 45–51.

Osborne, L. R., Martindale, D., Scherer, S. W., Shi, X. M., Huizenga, J., Heng, H. H. Q., Costa, T., Pober, B., Lew, L., Brinkman, J., Rommens, J., Koop, B., Tsui, L. C. (1996) Identification of genes from a 500-kb region at 7q11.23 that is commonly deleted in Williams syndrome patients. Genomics 36 (2): 328–36.

Osborne, L. R., Soder, S., Shi, X. M., Pober, B., Costa, T., Scherer, S. W., Tsui, L. C. (1997) Hemizygous deletion of the syntaxin 1A gene in individuals with Williams syndrome [Letter to the editor]. American Journal of Human Genetics 61 (2): 449–52.

Pankau, R., Partsch, C. J., Gosch, A., Oppermann, H. C., Wessel, A. (1992) Statural growth in Williams-Beuren syndrome. European Journal of Pediatrics 151 (10): 751–5.

Pankau, R., Partsch, C. J., Winter, M., Gosch, A., Wessel, A. (1996) Incidence and spectrum of renal abnormalities in Williams-Beuren syndrome. American Journal of Medical Genetics 63 (1): 301–4.

Perez Jurado, L. A., Peoples, R., Kaplan, P., Hamel, B. C., Francke, U. (1996) Molecular definition of the chromosome 7 deletion in Williams syndrome and parent-of-origin effects on growth. American Journal of Human Genetics 59 (4): 781–92.

Pober, P. R., and Dykens, E. M. (1996) Williams syndrome: An overview of medical, cognitive, and behavioral features. Child and Adolescent Psychiatric Clinics of North America 5: 929–43.

Pober, B., Greenberg, F., Kaplan, P., Lacro, R., Levinson, M., Morris, C., Wang, P. (1997) Medical guidelines for Williams syndrome. (Also available at the Williams Syndrome Association

Web site: http://www.williams-syndrome.org/medical.htm.)

Power, T. J., Blum, N. J., Jones, S. M., Kaplan, P. E. (1997) Brief report: Response to methylphenidate in two children with Williams syndrome. Journal of Autism and Developmental Disorders 27 (1): 79–87.

Pratt, D. S., and Dubois, R. S. (1990) Hepatotoxicity due to pemoline (Cylert): A report of two cases. Journal of Pediatric Gastroenterology and Nutrition 10 (2): 239–41.

Preskorn, S. H. (1996) Clinical pharmacology of selective serotonin reuptake inhibitors. Professional Communications, Caddo, Okla.

Reilly, J., Lima, E. S., Bellugi, U. (1990) Once more with feeling: Affect and language in atypical populations. Development and Psychopathology 2: 367–91.

Reiss, A. L., Feinstein, C., Rosenbaum, K. N., Borengasser-Caruso, M. A., Goldsmith, B. M. (1985) Autism associated with Williams syndrome. Journal of Pediatrics 106 (2): 247–9.

Riddle, M. A., Claghorn, J., Gaffney, G. (1996) A controlled trial of fluvoxamine for OCD in children and adolescents. Biological Psychiatry 39 (7): 568.

Rourke, B. P. (1995) Treatment program for the child with NLD. In Syndrome of nonverbal learning disabilities: Neurodevelopmental manifestations. Rourke, B. P. (ed.). Guilford, New York.

Sawchenko, P., Dargusch, R., Arias, C., Bellugi, U. (1997) Evidence for elastin expression in cerebellar Purkinje cells: Implications for Williams syndrome. Poster presented at the International Behavioral Neuroscience Society Annual Meeting, San Diego, Calif.

Scarborough, H. S., Rescorla, L., Tager-Flusberg, H., Fowler, A., Sudhalter, V. (1991) The relation of utterance length to grammatical complexity in normal and language disordered groups. Applied Psycholinguistics 12: 23–45.

Schulman, S. L., Zderic, S., Kaplan, P. (1996) Increased prevalence of urinary symptoms and voiding dysfunction in Williams syndrome. Journal of Pediatrics 129 (3): 466–9.

Scothorn, D. J., and Butler, M. G. (1997) How common is precocious puberty in patients with Williams syndrome? [Letter to the editor]. Clinical Dysmorphology 6 (1): 91–3.

Singer Harris, N. G., Bellugi, U., Bates, E., Jones, W., Rossen, M. (1997) Contrasting profiles of language development in children with Williams and Down syndromes. Developmental Neuropsychology 13 (3): 345–70.

Swanson, J. M., Wigal, S., Greenhill, L. L., Browne, R., Waslik, B., Lerner, M., Williams, L., Flynn, D., Agler, D., Crowley, K., Fineberg, E., Baren, M., Cantwell, D. P. (1998) Analog classroom assessment of Adderall in children with ADHD. Journal of American Academy of Child and Adolescent Psychiatry 37 (5): 519–26.

Tassabehji, M., Metcalfe, K., Karmiloff-Smith, A., Carette, M. J., Grant, J., Dennis, N., Reardon, W., Splitt, M., Read, A. P. Donnai, D. (1999) Williams syndrome: Use of chromosomal microdeletions as a tool to dissect cognitive and physical phenotypes. American Journal of Human Genetics 64: 118–25.

Tsao, C. Y., and Westman, J. A. (1997) Infantile spasms in two children with Williams syndrome. American Journal of Medical Genetics 71 (1): 54–6.

Udwin, O. (1990) A survey of adults with Williams syndrome and idiopathic infantile hypercalcaemia. Developmental Medicine and Child Neurology 32: 129–41.

Udwin, O., and Yule, W. (1989) Infantile hypercalcaemia and Williams syndrome: Guidelines for parents. Bell Press, London.

Udwin, O., and Yule, W. (1991) A cognitive and behavioural phenotype in Williams syndrome. Journal of Clinical and Experimental Neuropsychology 13 (2): 232–44.

Udwin, O., Yule, W., Martin, N. (1987) Cognitive abilities and behavioural characteristics of children with idiopathic infantile hypercalcaemia. Journal of Child Psychology, Psychiatry and Allied Disciplines 28 (2): 297–309.

Udwin, O., Howlin, P., Davies, M., Mannion, E. (1998) Community care for adults with Williams syndrome: How families cope and the availability of support networks. Journal of Intellectual Disability Research 42 (3): 238–45.

Wang, P. P., and Bellugi, U. (1993) Williams syndrome, Down syndrome, and cognitive neuroscience. American Journal of Diseases of Children 147 (11): 1246–51.

Wang, P. P., Doherty, S., Hesselink, J. R., Bellugi, U. (1992) Callosal morphology concurs with neurobehavioral and neuropathological findings in two neurodevelopmental disorders. Archives of Neurology 49 (4): 407–11.

Wang, P. P., Doherty, S., Rourke, S. B., Bellugi, U. (1995) Unique profile of visuo-perceptual skills in a genetic syndrome. Brain and Cognition 29 (1): 54–65.

Williams, J. C. P., Barratt-Boyes, B. G., Lowe, J. B. (1961) Supravalvular aortic stenosis. Circulation 24: 1311–8.

Winter, M., Pankau, R., Amm, M., Gosch, A., Wessel, A. (1996) The spectrum of ocular features in the Williams-Beuren syndrome. Clinical Genetics 49 (1): 28–31.

RESOURCES

Williams Syndrome Association
P.O. Box 297
Clawson, MI 48017-0297
telephone: (248) 541-3630
fax: (248) 541-3631
http://www.williams-syndrome.org

Williams Syndrome Foundation
University of California
Irvine, CA 92697-2310
telephone: (714) UCI-7259; (714) 824-7259
e-mail: hmlenhof@uci.edu
http://www.wsf.org

American Music Therapy Association, Inc.
8455 Colesville Road, Suite 1000
Silver Spring, MD 20910
telephone: (301) 589-3300
fax: (301) 589-5175

e-mail: info@musictherapy.org
http://www.musictherapy.org

Newsletters

Heart to Heart
Williams Syndrome Association
1312 N. Campbell, Suite 33
Royal Oak, MI 48067

Reading for Families and Teachers

Udwin, O., and Yule, W. (1989) Infantile hypercalcaemia and Williams syndrome: Guidelines for parents. Bell Press, London.

Levine, K. (1994) Williams syndrome: Information for teachers. Williams Syndrome Association, Clawson, MO.

Educational Resources

Handwriting without Tears by Janice Z. Olsen
Available from:
Fred Sammons, Inc.,
Box 32
Brookfield, IL 60513
telephone: (800) 323-7305; (312) 971-0610

Slantboard and Raised Line Paper
K&L Resources, Inc.
P.O. Box 2612
Springfield, VA 22152
telephone: (703) 455-1503
paper: Flaghouse catalog 250 sheets: $42;
(800) 793-7900

Testing and Evaluation Strategies for Children with Williams Syndrome
(Early Intervention to Vocational Options)
Williams Syndrome Association
P.O. Box 297
Clawson, MI 48017-0297
telephone: (248) 541-3630

How to Participate in Your Child's IEP
Coordinating Council for Handicapped Children
20E Jackson Boulevard, Room 900
Chicago, IL
Publication no. 312-939-3513

Videotapes

Thirty-minute videotapes containing the Williams syndrome segments from both the *60 Minutes* and *Chronicle* television shows are available from the Williams Syndrome Association national office. The tape can be released only for home use or educational purposes. A small donation to the Williams Syndrome Association is appreciated to cover production costs. Contact the national office at (248) 541-3630 for details.

Music Education Resources

National Association for Music Therapy, Inc.
8455 Colesville Road, Suite 930
Silver Spring, MD 20910-3392
telephone: (301) 589-3300
fax: (301) 589-5175

Guide to the Selection of Musical Instruments with Respect to Physical Ability and Disability
Developed by the Moss Rehabilitation Hospital Settlement School, Therapeutic Music Program.

Distributed by:
Magnamusic—Baton
10370 Page Industrial Blvd.
St. Louis, MO 63132

Treatment with Music: A Manual for Allied Health Professionals, by Karen J. Miller
Department of Occupational Therapy
College of Health and Human Services
Western Michigan University
Kalamazoo, MI 49008

Available through interlibrary loan or through:
Occupational Therapy Association, Inc.
4720 Montgomery Lane
P.O. Box 31220
Bethesda, MD 20824-1220
telephone: (301) 652-2682
fax: (301) 652-7711

American Association for Music Therapy
P.O. Box 80012
Valley Forge, PA 19484
telephone: (610) 265-4006

Nordoff-Robbins Music Therapy Clinic
New York University
26 Washington Place
New York, NY 10030
telephone: (212) 998-5151
fax: (212) 995-4045

9

Smith-Magenis Syndrome

Smith-Magenis syndrome (SMS) is a mental retardation and multiple congenital anomaly syndrome that was first reported by Ann Smith and Ellen Magenis (Smith et al., 1982, 1986). It is associated with a deletion at chromosome 17p11.2 that is recognized in the majority of patients through high-resolution cytogenetic studies, although fluorescent in situ hybridization (FISH) studies are now available and can detect the deletions that may not be seen in cytogenetic studies. The clinical phenotype is thought to be a contiguous gene syndrome, although it may be possible that only one gene among several which are deleted causes the majority of the clinical features. The deletion occurs on only one chromosome, so haplotype insufficiency in genes that are most likely dosage-sensitive is causing the phenotype. Almost all of the patients have de novo deletions, although there have been two reports of deletions present in the parents (Howard-Peebles et al., 1985; Zori et al., 1993). It is therefore recommended that parental chromosomes be routinely studied, including the use of FISH testing whenever the diagnosis of SMS is made in the child. There is no preferential pattern of deletions in maternal- or paternal-derived chromosomes, so there does not appear to be an imprint effect (Greenberg et al., 1991; Juyal et al., 1995b).

The incidence of this disorder is estimated to be 1/25,000 in the general population, but this may be a low estimate because of poor recognition of this disorder clinically and because FISH testing has only recently been made available for this disorder. At the time of this writing there have been over 100 cases reported in the literature (Smith et al., 1998a).

Neurodevelopmental Disorders: Diagnosis and Treatment, by Randi Jenssen Hagerman. New York: Oxford University Press, 1999. © Oxford University Press, Inc.

CLINICAL PHENOTYPE

The original reports of Smith et al. (1982, 1986) emphasized the presence of brachycephaly, microcephaly, midface hypoplasia, broad nasal bridge, prognathism, low-set and/or posteriorly rotated ears, short broad hands, short stature, scoliosis, speech delay with or without hearing loss, hyperactivity, self-destructive behavior, and moderate to severe mental retardation, which were seen in the majority of patients. Less consistent findings, seen in under 50%, include cardiac disease, cleft palate or cleft lip, genital or renal problems, hoarse or deep voice, and seizures. It is interesting that two of the original nine patients reported by Smith et al. (1986) were treated for a prolonged period of time with methylphenidate for their severe hyperactivity. Subsequent reports have expanded the phenotype and clarified the frequency of several physical and behavioral features described herein and outlined in Table 9.1 (Chen et al., 1996b; Colley et al., 1990; Dykens et al., 1997; Greenberg et al., 1991, 1996; Smith et al., 1998a; Stratton et al., 1986).

Craniofacial

The typical facial features include a broad face with a wide nasal bridge; upslanting palpebral fissures; epicanthal folds; synophrys (the growing together of the two eyebrows); downturned mouth with a cupid's bow shape; ear anomalies, including a small but sometimes prominent ear which is posteriorly rotated; midface hypoplasia; frontal bossing; and prognathism (prominent jaw) with age (Table 9.1; Figure 9.1). Brachycephaly, in combination with the facial dysmorphic features, sometimes suggests Down syndrome, leading to cytogenetic studies and usually the correct diagnosis. Behjati et al. (1997) reported that over half of new patients diagnosed with SMS were originally referred for fragile X testing because of developmental delays, mood lability, or aggression. Although two of the originally described patients had cleft palates and one had a cleft lip, these findings have been less common in subsequent reports, including the survey by Greenberg et al. (1996) in which only 2 of 27 patients had cleft palates, although 2 additional patients had velopharyngeal incompetence. On occasion, the patients with cleft palate have been diagnosed with the Pierre-Robin sequence. Only 5% of cases overall demonstrate cleft lip. Dental problems, including delayed eruption and malocclusion, are not uncommon.

A mild conductive hearing loss was present in 48% of the patients studied by Greenberg et al. (1996). This problem usually occurred in association with recurrent otitis media. In addition, 28% had sensorineural hearing loss, which is of great interest because a gene for hereditary deafness lies within the deleted region in SMS (Friedman et al., 1995; Greenberg et al., 1996).

Neurological and Behavioral Findings

The report by Greenberg et al. (1996) emphasized findings associated with a peripheral neuropathy that were seen in 75% of patients and included one or

TABLE 9.1. Clinical Features in Smith-Magenis Syndrome

Feature	Proportion of patients with feature	Percentage of patients with feature
Craniofacial		
midface hypoplasia	92/99	93
brachycephaly	85/95	89
broad nasal bridge	72/86	84
broad face	43/53	81
abnormal ears	71/96	74
downturned upper lip	48/66	73
synophrys	25/40	62
frontal bossing	51/90	57
prognathia	43/83	52
Skeletal		
short stature/FTT	39/50	78
short broad hands	82/96	85
scoliosis	22/52	42
syndactaly	18/49	37
Neurological or behavioral problems		
hyperactivity	75/90	83
attention seeking	8/10	80
tantrums	7/10	70
anxiety	7/10	70
aggression	7/10	70
self-destructive behavior	63/85	74
sleep disorder	38/55	69
hypotonia	37/69	54
seizures	15/80	19
self-hugging	11/11	100
EEG epileptiform findings without seizures	5/24	21
microcephaly	10/25	40
Opthalmic		
iris anomolies	25/38	66
microcornia	14/38	37
myopia	19/36	53
strabismus	19/38	50
cataracts	3/38	8
retinal detachment	3/38	8
Otolaryngologic		
hoarse voice	53/66	80
sensory neural hearing loss	7/25	28
conductive hearing loss	12/25	48
Visceral		
cardiovascular	20/70	29
renal or urinary tract problems	12/43	28
genital abnormalities	6/15	40
Other Problems		
low T4 levels	8/24	33
low immunoglobulin levels	3/13	23

Data derived from Chen et al. (1996b,c), Finucane et al. (1994), Greenburg et al. (1996), Dykens et al. (1997), Smith et al. (1998a).

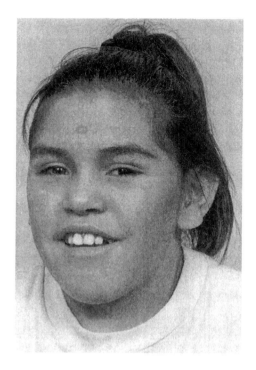

FIGURE 9.1:   A 12-year-old girl with Smith-Magenis syndrome. Note cupid's bow shape of mouth, prominent and posteriorly rotated ears, and mild synophrys.

more of the following: decreased sensitivity to pain or temperature, pes cavus or planus, and decreased deep tendon reflexes. Greenberg et al. (1991) hypothesized that the unusual behavior of onychotillomania, the pulling out of fingernails and toenails, which is common in older patients, and perhaps the behavior of polyembolokoilamania, the insertion of foreign bodies into various body orifices, which is less common, may be secondary to a decreased sensitivity to pain. Nerve conduction studies were found to be normal in all patients except one, who had slightly decreased nerve conduction velocities and muscle wasting in the lower extremities (Greenberg et al., 1991; Greenberg et al., 1996). These authors suggest that the gene *PMP22* which lies just distal to the critical region for SMS is perhaps also deleted in this patient, because deletion of *PMP22* causes hereditary neuropathy with liability to pressure palsy (HNPP) and delayed nerve conduction velocities. The duplicated *PMP22* gene causes Charcot-Marie-Tooth disease type 1A.

Approximately 19% of patients have clinical seizures (Greenberg et al., 1996). There has been no study of the type of seizures that occur, although in one case seizures were precipitated by rage episodes (Smith et al., 1986). Five of 24 patients with SMS had epileptiform findings on the EEG without clinical seizures, but it is unclear whether these findings are associated with behavioral difficulties (Greenberg et al., 1996).

Approximately 70% of patients with SMS have sleep disturbances, including difficulties in falling asleep and frequent night awakenings that lead to exhaustion in the parents (Colley et al., 1990; Smith et al., 1998a, 1998b). Greenberg et al. (1996) carried out sleep studies in 24 patients and found reduced REM sleep in approximately half and reduced sleep time because of frequent awakenings in 29%. Potacki et al. (1997) found elevations in urinary 6-sulphatoxymelatonin (aMT6s), the metabolite of melatonin, during a 24-hour sleep study in five of six patients with SMS. The elevations occurred during the daylight hours, which suggests that the normal pattern of melatonin secretion at night is reversed, such that daytime excretion is high but nighttime secretion is low in patients with SMS. The melatonin deficiency at night could cause the sleep problems in SMS. Smith et al. (1998b) studied sleep behaviors of 39 patients and found that 79% have enuresis, 69% have snoring, 59% use sleep medications, and over half awaken during the night to go to the bathroom or to get a drink. They also found a steady decline in total hours of sleep needed at night and an increased frequency of daytime naps as the patients grow older (Smith et al. 1998b).

Hypotonia has been reported in over half of patients with SMS. It is usually present in infancy, and it is associated with delays in motor milestones. A hoarse voice is seen in approximately 80%, but it is more common as patients age. Only 4 of 12 patients who underwent laryngoscopy were found to have such problems as polyps, nodules, edema, and paralysis of the vocal chords (Greenberg et al., 1996). More significant oral-motor and tracheobronchial problems were seen in 14 patients with SMS who underwent detailed otolaryngologic and speech pathology evaluations (Sonies et al. 1997). Velopharyngeal insufficiency was present in 75%, lingual (tongue) weakness in 71%, severely limited tongue motion in 92%, palatal abnormalities in 64%, and structural vocal fold abnormalities in all but the youngest patients.

Behavior problems are a great difficulty in this disorder. Hyperactivity or ADHD occurs in over 80%, and it is usually associated with aggression, self-destructive behavior, and tantrums. Attention-seeking behavior combined with impulsivity can be a constant problem at home and at school and can interfere with learning and daily activities. Perhaps some of these problems are related to the sleep disturbance and resulting exhaustion during the day, but the behavioral phenotype even after treatment of the sleep problems includes ADHD, mood fluctuations leading to tantrums, and some unusual stereotypic behavior. Dykens et al. (1997) have reported in 9 of 10 patients a characteristic behavior during testing of inserting four fingers of one hand deeply into the mouth (a form of polyembolokoilamania) and then rapidly flipping the pages of a book with the wet fingers. Half of these patients also demonstrated a self-hug, which was originally described by Finucane et al. (1994). The self-hug or spasmodic upper body squeeze usually takes two forms. In one, the arms are crossed over the chest or abdomen with the head tucked into the chest and the upper body is tensed with the arms tightened for only a few seconds. The second form involves clasping the hands at chest level and squeezing the arms against the chest and sides. The authors found this behavior in all 11 patients studied, and they consider it pathognomic for SMS (Finucane et al., 1994). It usually occurs when the patients are excited, and it may often be repetitive or tic-like. The second form is actually very similar to the tensing of the fists that has been described in patients with fragile X syndrome when they are excited, overstimulated, or angry (Hagerman, 1996). This behavior is not problematic, unlike self-injurious or aggressive behavior.

Self-injurious behavior, including head banging, hand biting, wrist biting, or skin picking, occurs in 40 to 100% of patients with SMS (Chen et al. 1996b, Smith et al. 1998a, Dykens and Smith 1998).Dykens and Smith (1998) found that onchotillomania (pulling out fingernails or toenails) occurred in only 29% and inserting objects into body orifices occurred in only 25%. Onchotillomania was positively correlated with age and degree of sleep disturbance. Tantrums, particularly in early childhood, are a problem for 70%, aggression occurs in 70%, and anxiety, which has not been well studied in this disorder, also occurs in 70% (Dykens et al., 1997). Perhaps the anxiety problem is linked to the aggression, as we see in fragile X syndrome; this makes a difference in treatment approaches.

Cognitive Profile

Cognitive abilities range from profound mental retardation to borderline functioning, with the majority in the moderately mentally retarded range, with IQ scores usually between 40 and 50. There is limited evidence that those with a more extensive deletion than what is usually seen in SMS are more severely affected and may even die early in childhood, as seen in one case reported by Smith et al. (1982; 1986). The Verbal and Performance IQ scores on the WISC-III are comparable, and adaptive behavior is also usually consistent with cognitive abilities (Greenberg et al., 1996). Expressive language abilities are worse than receptive language abilities, and Greenberg and colleagues (1996) suggest that some of the behavioral problems are related to the frustrations that these children experience with poor expressive language skills.

Dykens and colleagues (1997) assessed cognitive profiles in 10 patients utilizing the Kaufman Assessment Battery for Children (K-ABC) and found significant weaknesses in Sequential Processing, most likely related to their ADHD symptoms, including impulsivity, hyperactivity, and inattention, although problems in short-term memory and ordering may also contribute to these low scores. Strengths were also seen in Achievement scores and in one-word expressive vocabulary scores. This pattern of strengths and weaknesses has also been reported in patients with fragile X syndrome who experience similar levels of hyperactivity and inattention (reviewed by Bennetto and Pennington 1996).

Neuroimaging and Neuroanatomical Studies

The only detailed neuroanatomical study reported is the case of a child with a severe form of SMS who died at 6 months, after cardiac surgery (Smith et al.,

1986). This baby boy had microcephaly and foreshortened frontal lobes with depletion of neurons frontally in layers 3 and 4. In addition, a small choroid plexus hemangioma was noted in the lateral ventricle. Greenberg et al. (1996) studied 25 patients with CT scanning and found abnormalities in 52%, specifically ventriculomegaly in nine, enlargement of the cisterna magna in two, and partial absence of the cerebellar vermis in one. Although one patient reported by Masuno et al. (1992) had hypoplasia of the cerebellar vermis and pons, these problems appear uncommon in patients with SMS, and routine CNS imaging is not recommended unless there is an additional clinical indication.

Ophthalmological Features

Finucane and colleagues (1993) carried out the first detailed ophthalmological study of patients with SMS. They studied 10 patients and found that all 10 had strabismus and 2 required surgery. They also reported myopia in eight patients, with high myopia in six that led to a progressive degeneration and retinal detachment in three. In two cases retinal detachment occurred after trauma, such as head banging. Cataracts were present in three patients, and abnormalities of the iris, including Brushfield-like spots which were raised nodules of the peripheral iris, midiris stromal ring, and heterochromatic irides, were present in six patients. Greenberg et al. (1996) carried out ophthalmological studies on 27 patients and found that one-third had strabismus or myopia. In addition, 10 patients had microcornea, and 16 had iris dysplasia, including one patient with an iris coloboma. Chen et al. (1996c) evaluated 28 patients with SMS and reported similar findings to the previous studies, including microcornea in 50%, myopia in 42%, and iris anomalies in 68%; but they did not find retinal detachment, perhaps because their patients were generally younger than those reported by Finucane and colleagues. It has been postulated that a gene related to connective tissue integrity may be within the deletion region for SMS, leading to the myopia and progressive retinal changes that culminate in retinal detachment in some patients (Finucane et al., 1993).

Cardiovascular and Renal Features

The overall prevalence of cardiovascular abnormalities in SMS is reported at 29% when combining several reports (Table 9.1). However, Greenberg et al. (1996) carried out echocardiograms on 12 patients and found that 42% were abnormal. The abnormalities included atrial septal defects (ASDs), ventricular septal defects (VSDs), mild mitral or tricuspid regurgitation, and subvalvular aortic stenosis. These authors also reported one patient with a right ventricular conduction defect discovered on EKG.

Greenberg et al. (1996) also carried out renal ultrasonography on 26 patients and found 4 with duplication of the collecting system, 1 with unilateral renal agenesis, and 1 with ectopic kidney. Because of the relatively high frequency of renal and cardiovascular problems, Greenberg and colleagues (1996) recommend routine renal ultrasonography and echocardiography when the diagnosis of SMS is initially made.

Endocrine and Immunological Features

Only one study has been undertaken to assess endocrine and immunological function in patients with SMS. Greenberg et al. (1996) studied thyroid function in 24 patients and found that 7 had thyroxine levels below the normal range, with 2 patients demonstrating an elevated TSH level. None of these patients demonstrated clinical symptoms of hypothyroidism, although all had developmental problems. In addition, 3 of 13 patients demonstrated mildly decreased levels of immunoglobulins, and 1 had mildly elevated IgM levels. These initial studies demonstrate the need for further research to clarify the reason for these findings and the intervention needs. Because occult hypothyroidism can further interfere with development, low thyroid levels require endocrine consultation and treatment as early as possible.

Hypoplasia of the genitalia has been described in SMS for both males and females, and the overall rate of genital abnormalities is 40% including mild degrees of hypoplasia, undescended testes, small penis, and hypoplastic uterus.

Growth and Skeletal Features

Deficits in growth measurements, including height, weight, and head circumference, are common problems in children with SMS. These problems occur even in those patients without heart disease. Approximately 40% have microcephaly, 89% have brachycephaly, and 78% have short stature and/or failure to thrive in infancy (Chen et al., 1996b; Smith et al., 1986; Stratton et al., 1986).

Skeletal abnormalities include scoliosis in 42%, which usually does not require therapy, and a variety of hand abnormalities (Table 9.1). Short, broad hands and fingers (Figure 9.2) are typically seen with partial syndactyly present in one-third of patients. Kondo et al. (1991) also reported on prominent fingertip pads, clinodactyly of the fifth finger, and a single palmar crease in all four of the patients with SMS that they studied. Three patients have been described with polydactyly, and this problem has been reviewed by Yang et al. (1997).

CASE STUDY: LUCY

Lucy is a 12-year-old girl who was diagnosed with Smith-Magenis syndrome when chromosomal testing when she was 11½ years old with FISH studies demonstrated the typical deletion for this disorder at 17p11.2. She was born in Mexico after a normal pregnancy, and her birth weight was 6 lbs. 13 oz. Although she was described as an easy baby, she was significantly delayed in her developmental milestones, and she did not walk until 2 years of age. At the present time, she says only one English word and approximately 10 words in Spanish. She has not had the benefit of intensive language therapy or training in signing. At 2

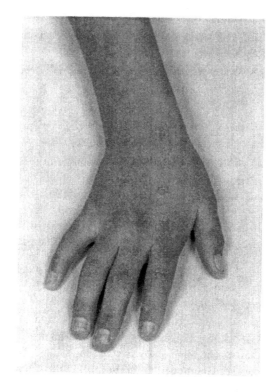

FIGURE 9.2: Short, broad hands and fingers in a
12-year-old girl with Smith-Magenis syndrome.
Note lesions on dorsum of hand and wrist secondary to skin picking and short, irregular nails,
which are often bloody from excessive nail biting
and nail cutting.

years old, after she learned to walk, her behavior changed remarkably, with the
onset of hyperactivity and sleeplessness at night. At her normal bedtime, she
would sleep for only 40 minutes. She would then get up and want to eat for
most of the rest of the night. Her hyperactivity has been severe, and she will
roam the house and often carry out destructive acts, including turning on the
stove or jumping out the window.

At approximately 5 years of age Lucy began self-mutilating behavior, including picking at lesions, poking herself, biting her nails (Figure 9.2), and pulling
her hair out. At approximately 5 years old she also developed some significant
mood swings, with angry episodes and tantrums. These behaviors developed when
her parents said that she was unable to do something that she wanted to do.
When she became angry, she would self-mutilate by poking her skin and biting
her nails. She cuts her nails down with a nail clipper until they bleed. She also

has a habit of putting stones in her ears and up her nose. When she becomes angry, which is usually many times during the day, she will destroy personal property of family members, and she will hit her sisters or other peers. She will not hit her parents but will instead destroy their belongings, for instance, by cutting up their clothes.

Lucy has difficulty in chewing foods, and she tends to either eat foods whole or eat only very soft foods. She is tactilely defensive and will sometimes pull away from touch, but she has a high pain threshold, and she does not appear to experience pain when she hurts herself, as other people do.

She has never had seizures or heart murmurs, but she wets her bed every night and sometimes will urinate in the classroom at school. The parents must lock her bedroom door at night, or else she will run throughout the house and sometimes leave the house in the middle of the night.

The family moved from Mexico to the United States when Lucy was 11½, and a medical evaluation at that time documented her diagnosis. She was started on methylphenidate (Ritalin) at a dose of 10 mg three times a day, and this improved her hyperactivity for the first month or two of use. She was also treated with thioridazine (Mellaril), 25 mg at bedtime, and this helped her sleep through the night until 5 or 6 a.m.

Both of Lucy's parents had normal development, but her maternal grandmother is epileptic. Lucy also has two older sisters who developed normally. An evaluation at her school when she moved to the United States demonstrated an Adaptive Behavior Composite on the Vineland of 25, with Communication Skills at 20, Daily Living Skills at 26, and Socialization at 36. Her behavior at school has involved significant aggression, including kicking, hitting, and biting her teachers and other peers. For this reason she was shifted from her special education classroom into a home schooling program, and since both of her parents work, her oldest sister has been pulled out of school to take care of her at home.

Lucy was evaluated at our child development unit after turning 12 years of age, and at that time her height was below the fifth percentile, with weight at the 15th percentile and head circumference just below the second percentile. Her dysmorphic features included microcephaly; prominent ear pinnae; broad, flat nasal bridge; low hairline anteriorly and posteriorly; short fingers and toes; and closely cropped nails, leading to irritation and inflammation, particularly in the toes. She was hyperactive during the examination and would frequently hug clinic helpers. Limited range of motion was seen in her finger joints and also at her elbow, the latter finding consistent with radial ulnar synostosis. She also had a short neck with limited range of motion at the neck, but she did not demonstrate scoliosis. She had a hoarse voice and was only able to say approximately 10 words.

Her treatment program included increasing her methylphenidate to 20 mg three times a day and subsequently shifting the thioridazine to melatonin at a 3-mg dose in the evening. She was later tried on fluvoxamine (Luvox) at a dose of 50 mg at bedtime to improve her aggression and irritability, but this was not helpful. She was then tried on risperidone (Risperdal), a new atypical antipsychotic, for treatment of her aggression and hyperactivity, and this has helped remarkably at a dose of 1 mg twice a day. Laboratory work included thyroid studies, which were normal. Her immunoglobulin studies showed a mild elevation of IgG levels. She was referred to a psychologist for a behavior program at school. Subsequent evaluations will include an echocardiogram with cardiology consultation, renal ultrasound studies, an augmentative communication evaluation, PT/OT assessment, and an ophthalmology evaluation.

MOLECULAR STUDIES

The deletion associated with SMS can vary in size from 1.5 Mb to 9 Mb, but they typically are approximately 5 Mb in size (Juyal et al., 1996). In patients with typical SMS, the deletion is almost always seen with high-resolution chromosomal studies. However, in patients with a milder clinical phenotype, the cytogenetic studies may look normal or show a mosaic pattern (Juyal et al., 1996). Fluorescent in situ hybridization (FISH) studies are then needed to clarify the presence of the deletion. In two cases, an apparent mosaic pattern by cytogenetic studies was shown to have the deletion in 100% of the cells studied (Juyal et al., 1995a, 1995b). There are only two cases reported with a mosaic pattern in blood confirmed by FISH or additional molecular studies. One case was a mother who had mild physical features, including a broad face, short hands and fingers, clinodactyly, pes cavus, and a history of feeding problems at birth, head banging, temper tantrums, and learning problems in school that required a tutor. The deletion was documented by cytogenetic and molecular studies in 55% of her lymphocytes, and it was also seen in 100% of the lymphocytes of her daughter (Zori et al., 1993). The second case was a patient with the typical SMS phenotype, and the deletion was documented in 63% of his lymphocytes (Juyal et al., 1996).

More severe clinical involvement may be seen with a large deletion that removes more genes than are typically removed in cases of SMS (Smith et al., 1986). It is also possible for a severe phenotype to be influenced by a mutation in the nondeleted chromosome for a recessive allele that is unmasked because of the presence of the deletion. Such a situation is hypothesized for the severe case of SMS reported by Yang et al. (1997).

The reason for deletions in this area is not yet known. However, structural changes in the DNA can predispose to deletions through abnormal pairing and unequal crossing over. These areas of the DNA are considered hot spots because of breakage and rearrangements, leading to deletions and translocations. Wilgenbus and colleagues (1997) have carried out detailed molecular studies of the 17p11 region and have found low abundant repetitive sequences in this region which may be the cause of the frequent deletions.

Prenatal diagnosis with high-resolution cytogenetic studies or FISH studies are clinically possible but have been documented in only one case (Fan and Farrell, 1994). This is because most of the cases of SMS are de novo or new deletions, so it is rare that a mother would come in requesting prenatal diagnosis for SMS. The one case identified was picked up on a routine amniocentesis for low maternal serum alpha-fetoprotein screening; the patient was just under 35 years of age. Fan and Farrell (1994) recommend using a resolution level of at least 500 bands so this deletion can be identified routinely in amniocentesis.

Only a few genes have been found to be consistently deleted in patients with SMS so far. The more interesting deleted genes include (a) the human homologue (FLII) of the *Drosophila melanogaster* flightless −1 gene, which is involved in actin binding and important in cellular functions such as motility, cell division, and chemotaxis and has a leucine-rich region that is important in protein–protein interactions such as cell adhesion and cell recognition; (b) the human microfibril-associated protein (MFAP4) gene that codes for a calcium-dependent adhesive protein associated with elastin-microfibrils and that may be important for the connective tissue aspects of SMS; and (c) the cytosolic serine hydroxymethyltransferase (cSHMT) gene (Chen et al., 1996a; Elsea et al., 1995). SHMT is an enzyme that cleaves serine to produce glycine and one carbon units in the brain. Reduced SHMT levels lead to excess serine levels, which may in turn enhance N-methyl-D-asparate (NMDA) receptor-produced neurotoxicity (Elsea et al., 1995). A 50% reduction of SHMT levels has been documented in the three patients with SMS who were studied by Elsea et al. (1995). SHMT is also important for folate-dependent one carbon transfers, and reduced levels of folate have been found in one patient with SMS (Elsea et al., 1995). Decreased SHMT levels can also lead to low levels of adenosine, which is a neuromodulator of dopamine and glutamate; adenosine also acts as a neuroprotective agent (Elsea et al., 1995). The secondary effects on the dopamine system may relate to the attentional and hyperactivity problems in SMS. In addition, the possible neurotoxicity produced by low levels of SHMT may cause additional behavior problems such as head banging. A similar neurotoxic process has been documented in the brains of some psychotic patients who have lowered levels of SHMT (Elsea et al., 1995). Elsea and colleagues (1995) have suggested that new antipsychotic agents, such as glycine, and NMDA antagonists or even folic acid may be helpful in treatment of patients with SMS.

Two additional genes of interest have been mapped to the SMS region, including the adenosine A2b receptor subtype gene (ADORA2B) and a gene for one form of nonsyndromal recessive deafness (DFNB3) (Chen et al., 1996a). The adenosine A2b receptor is widespread in the CNS, and it is associated with stimulation of adenylate cyclase activity and cAMP levels, which are important for many neurotransmitter systems. A mutation in the DFNB3 gene could be unmasked by the deletion in SMS and could be responsible for the sensorineural hearing loss present in a limited number of patients with SMS (Table 9.1) (Chen et al., 1996a). Last, a recent report mapped a human gene, RIGUI, to 17p12, which is the mammalian equivalent to the *Drosophila* period gene (Sun et al.,

1997). Although this gene may be distal to the SMS critical region, it may be important in the sleep disturbance found in SMS.

TREATMENT

Infancy and Early Childhood

Although a small number of patients show failure to thrive in infancy because of oral-motor coordination problems and a poor suck, many patients are described as normal infants who are easy to care for and who gain weight well, even to the point of developing redundant fat folds that have been described as resembling the Michelin man (Smith et al., 1998a). Hypotonia is common, and most patients cry very little (Smith et al. 1998a). The excessive wakefulness may not develop during the first year, and parents have reported the need to wake up their child to feed (Smith et al., 1998a).

Greenberg et al. (1996) recommend studying thyroid function and immunoglobulin levels at the time of diagnosis because of the limited number of patients who have had deficiencies. Blood work should also include parental chromosomes and FISH studies to rule out an inversion or deletion in one of the parents. Because of the malformations in patients with SMS, renal ultrasonography, echocardiogram with a cardiology consultation, a detailed ophthalmological examination, spine films for scoliosis, audiometric testing, and an otolaryngologic assessment for velopharyngeal incompetence or other oral-motor problems are recommended. Appropriate follow-up and treatment are needed for any of the abnormalities found. For instance, thyroid replacement may be indicated if the thyroid levels are low, and intensive follow-up by cardiology and even surgery are sometimes necessary for complex cardiac malformations. Annual ophthalmological evaluations are recommended because the myopia is usually progressive and retinal detachment may occur.

Seizures are not infrequent in SMS, and an EEG is indicated when the behavior suggests seizures or when severe tantrums or aggression are present. Sometimes these latter two behaviors are associated with occult seizure activity or with spike and wave discharges on the EEG without clinical seizure activity. Greenberg et al. (1996) have reported that carbamazepine (Tegretol), which is an anticonvulsant, is often helpful for severe behavioral problems, although the effect may sometimes be transient. Carbamazepine is more commonly used in the school-aged child, so it is described in more detail in the next section.

Sleep disturbances, including frequent waking, commonly develop in the second to fourth years of life and usually require intervention. Although behavioral or environmental manipulations—such as positive reinforcers for not getting out of bed, shutting the blinds and eliminating excess noises, and use of a music box to promote self-calming when the child wakes up—may help, medical intervention is often necessary. Anecdotal reports suggest that melatonin, the normal sleep-promoting hormone, may be helpful for wakefulness, which is consistent with early reports demonstrating abnormalities in the melatonin-secretion patterns in patients with SMS (Smith et al., 1998b). Although no controlled studies exist for patients with SMS, a large experience has developed in children with developmental disabilities who have sleep disturbances. Over 80% respond to melatonin treatment (Jan and O'Donnell, 1996). Long-term treatment (experience up to 6 years so far) has been safe without significant side effects (Jan and O'Donnell, 1996; Palm et al., 1997). The typical dose is 1 to 3 mg by mouth at bedtime in the young child and 3 to 6 mg in the older child or adolescent. The use of a selective serotonin reuptake inhibitor (SSRI) has also been reported to be helpful for sleep disturbances and behavioral outbursts in three patients with SMS (Smith et al., 1998b).

Speech and language delays are seen in all patients, and they require early intervention by a speech and language pathologist, in addition to careful follow-up of hearing abilities, since recurrent otitis media is common. The placement of PE tubes may be necessary to normalize hearing, or, in the case of a sensorineural hearing loss, hearing aids may be necessary. Velopharyngeal incompetence is not uncommon, so evaluation by a cleft palate team or an ENT specialist and cinefluoroscopy studies of palatal function may be necessary.

Severe delays in expressive language may occur and necessitate the use of signing and a total communication approach in the educational setting for the preschool period. An intensive program in signing seems to facilitate later language development (Ann C. M. Smith, personal communication 1998). Motor delays are also common and can be treated with occupational therapy in the preschool period.

The School-Aged Children

Behavioral difficulties have blossomed by this time in the majority of patients with SMS. Their great need for individualized attention causes problems in the classroom and at home, and when attention is not received or when transitions occur, they often escalate their behavior to a tantrum or to aggressive or self-injurious behavior (Smith et al., 1998a). Table 9.2 includes both the positive and the negative aspects of the behavior of children with SMS that affect learning, from the perspective of a special education teacher who has worked with many children with this disorder (Haas-Givler, 1994).

Haas-Givler and Finucane (1995) have recommended a self-contained placement with no more than five to seven students so that a calm, structured setting can be maintained and so that excessive competition for the teacher's attention does not occur. Inclusion into the regular classroom is usually not possible for patients typically affected with SMS because of easy overstimulation, behavioral outbursts, out-of-seat activity, and excessive drive for the teacher's attention. Higher-functioning children with SMS may do well in an inclusion setting with an aide who focuses on their needs. Further research into sensory integration problems that lead to overstimulation in this syndrome and into the efficacy of sensory integration therapy from an OT is needed.

TABLE 9.2. Behaviors That Positively and Negatively Affect Learning

Attributes that positively affect learning
  Engaging and endearing personality
    usually patients have good eye contact and smile and hug people frequently
  Enjoy interpersonal interactions
    appreciate attention from the teacher and use appropriate social expressions such as "please"
    and "thank you"
  Responsive to structure and routine
    follow classroom routine and react positively to consistency in a stable environment
  Motivated by many reinforcers
    positive behavior reinforcement with the use of stickers, food, individual time with the
    teacher, or favorite activities works well
  Eager to please
    will usually try to please the teacher and are usually positive in verbal and facial expressions
  Enjoy communication
    eager to communicate either verbally, gesturally with sign language, or visually with a picture
    board; enjoy many activities such as music, songs, water play, puzzles, and games
  Fascinated with electronics
    enjoy working with calculators, computers, and other machines
  Well-developed sense of humor
    enjoy joking and laugh at appropriate times
  Predictability of tantrums and aggression
    easily overstimulated due to changes in routine or emotional upset. These behaviors can often
    be redirected if the staff or parent intervene before the child becomes too upset.

Attributes that negatively affect learning
  Attention seeking
    often demand excessive time from the teacher with one-to-one attention
  Aggression toward others
    may demonstrate aggression to other students who compete for their teacher's attention and
    when emotionally upset
  Frequent tantrum behavior
    tantrums may include falling to the ground, refusing to walk, or hitting other children
  Self-injurious behavior
    problems with picking at nails and skin, head banging, and other behaviors that interfere with
    learning
  Poor impulse control
    frequently act impulsively, such as jumping out of the seat, grabbing things without asking, or
    demonstrating aggressive behavior
  Negative reaction to changes in routine.
    children must be prepared for changes in activity
  Attention deficit hyperactivity disorder
    attentional problems with or without hyperactivity occur in the majority of patients
  Perseveration
    frequent repetition of questions can interfere with the classroom routine
  Sleep disturbance
    may fall asleep in the classroom because of nighttime difficulties

Adapted from Haas-Givler (1994).

Additional educational strategies that may be helpful to children with SMS include the use of reinforcers and motivators such as stickers, individual teacher time, or a favorite activity. Children can become very motivated to learn or to keep their behavior problems under control if a reward is given after finishing an activity or during a transition period. Visual reminders also help them process sequential information in an academic task or in a daily schedule. Groups of pictures can be used to outline a multistep task, such as preparing a meal or carrying out a math problem. The daily schedule of events in the classroom can be displayed visually so that the child can refer to it independently during the day instead of persistently asking the teacher what the next activity is (Haas-Givler and Finucane, 1995). The teacher and the parent should become aware of what usually precipitates a tantrum and try to intervene early to deescalate an outburst when early signs appear. For instance, taking the child aside and talking in a calm voice or telling a favorite story that the child has to calm down to hear may defuse the situation (Haas-Givler and Finucane, 1995). If a tantrum develops in the classroom, it is best to remove the child from the class so that he or she gets the least attention possible and can calm down in an uninteresting time-out room. Many children with SMS do not want to miss the activities of the class or time with their teacher, so they will put extra effort into keeping their tantrums under control when such a behavior program is initiated (Haas-Givler and Finucane, 1995).

Medication use in the school-aged child is usually targeted to improve attentional problems with or without hyperactivity (ADHD) and mood swings that lead to tantrums or aggression. Stimulants such as methylphenidate (Ritalin), dextroamphetamine (Dexedrine), a levoamphetamine and dextroamphetamine mixture (Adderall), or pemoline (Cylert) can be used for ADHD symptoms. A. J. Allen (personal communication) has found that stimulants, particularly Adderall, are helpful for treatment of ADHD symptoms in approximately one-third of patients. Clonidine, a high blood pressure medication, may also turn out to be helpful in children with SMS because it usually improves hyperactivity and has an overall calming effect which decreases overstimulation and tantrums (Hagerman et al., 1998). One of the main side effects of clonidine is sedation, but this may be helpful for the sleeping difficulties; clonidine given before bedtime usually causes drowsiness and subsequent sleep. On rare occasions clonidine may cause wakefulness at night after the sleeping effect has worn off, but in these cases guanfacine (Tenex), which is a long-acting preparation that is similar to clonidine, can be used at bedtime. When clonidine is given in the mornings, it is usually necessary to start with a low dose, because drowsiness can occur in the daytime. An EKG should be done at baseline and in follow-up for patients on clonidine because rare cases of arrythmia have been reported with clonidine use, and occult heart disease or conduction problems may occur in patients with SMS. Sometimes aggression in children with developmental disabilities may improve with clonidine or with the stimulants (Hagerman et al., 1998).

Mood lability or tantrums or aggression that do not improve with stimulants or clonidine usually require a different approach pharmacologically. Greenberg et al. (1996) have suggested that carbamazepine (Tegretol) or valproic acid should be tried initially for these problems. Although they are anticonvulsants, they are also effective mood stabilizers with efficacy similar to lithium. They have significant side effects, however, and careful monitoring of blood levels to maintain a therapeutic range is essential. They may also irritate the liver, drop the white blood cell count or platelets, and cause electrolyte problems, so follow-up of blood chemistries is necessary. A. J. Allen (personal communication 1997) has found carbamazepine to be helpful in approximately one-third of patients with SMS. Newer anecdotal reports suggest that the SSRI agents that boost the serotonin level are helpful for aggression and mood lability in children with SMS (Smith et al., 1998a; Smith and Gropman, 1999). These agents, such as fluoxetine (Prozac), sertraline (Zoloft), paroxetine (Paxil), and fluvoxamine (Luvox), are helpful in decreasing anxiety that may be precipitating aggression. They also help with decreasing obsessive-compulsive behavior, improving mood, and usually stabilizing mood swings. However, on occasion an increase in hyperactivity secondary to an activation effect may occur. The activation may escalate to symptoms of mania, including an increase in sleep problems. When such symptoms occur, the SSRI should be tapered and discontinued. If the mania persists, then a mood stabilizer should be utilized.

Crumley (1998) recently reported an unusual case of a 12-year-old girl with SMS with a nonverbal IQ in the normal range. Her severe hyperactivity responded well to methylphenidate and dextroamphetamine, and her insomnia responded well to trazodone, an antidepressant with significant sedation as a side effect. Her mood lability, anger, and aggression responded well to lithium.

If the medications described here are not helpful for treatment of aggression and hyperactivity, then a low dose of a new atypical antipsychotic, risperidone, which has a lower risk of extrapyramidal symptoms and tardive dyskinesia, may help (Kapur and Remington, 1996). Although controlled studies of the efficacy of risperidone have not been carried out in SMS, risperidone has been helpful for treatment of aggression in children and adolescents with psychiatric problems or pervasive developmental disorder and mental retardation (Fisman et al., 1996; Khan, 1997; Simeon et al., 1995). We have seen improvement in aggression and mood lability with the use of risperidone in the case of SMS described here (see the preceding case history). Risperidone was used instead of carbamazepine because the latter would require more frequent blood tests than risperidone, which the family could not do because of financial limitations.

Augmentative and Alternative Communication

Many children with SMS are nonverbal or have very poor verbal abilities, which means augmentative and alternative communication (AAC) strategies may be helpful. AAC strategies refer to a variety of techniques or aids, including gestures, signing, picture boards, or computers, which may be helpful in enhancing communication. With the nonverbal or low verbal child, these strategies should be started as soon as possible in the preschool period (Silverman, 1995). They enhance language development and verbal speech, so they do not substitute for oral language but help oral language to develop. As oral language develops, the AAC strategies can be faded out. Children who are nonverbal or who have low verbal abilities should be referred to an AAC specialist or a speech and language therapist who has expertise in AAC strategies. The therapist will determine which strategies will be most useful for the child, and these strategies should be combined with speech and language therapy. Some of the strategies that can be utilized are described here.

Hand signing or gestures are the most portable AAC strategy, but they will be understood only by the communication partners who know the signs. Signing may also be difficult for the child with severe motor coordination problems or dyspraxia. American Sign Language (ASL) evolved from French Sign Language, and it is the most common signing system used in the states. Most bookstores have signing books for beginners. For those who want more detailed information, the Gallaudet University bookstore is a good resource. The American Sign Language Dictionary is on CD-ROM and has over 2,000 words signed on video clips, as well as traditional sign illustrations (Sternberg, 1994). The preschool teacher can introduce a few signs each week that can be taught to all of the students and staff and then can be sent home with illustrations or in a video form so that they can be learned by family and friends (Weitz et al., 1997). The reverse process can occur for signs that are initially learned at home, so that signs from home and school can be practiced in all environments.

A simple aided system is a picture communication board that can be easily understood by everyone in all environments without the specific training that is needed for signing. The Picture Exchange Communication System is one training approach that has worked with severely retarded or autistic individuals (Weitz et al., 1997). It helps children initiate communication because they receive a concrete reinforcement when they point to a picture. The therapist can start with a set of pictures of the child's favorite objects and then can progress to food items and other topics. This program teaches the child how to use a picture or symbol to obtain a desired object (Weitz et al., 1997). The therapist or parent can subsequently build language in a natural environment by modeling ways to combine symbols related to topics of the child's interests. For instance, when the child is eating and wants more, he or she may point to a picture of cookies; the therapist can then point to a picture of *more + cookies* or expand the content by pointing to a picture of *hungry + more + cookies* (Weitz et al., 1997). Easily portable communication boards, including wallet systems and miniboards, have been developed.

High-technology examples of AAC are the voice output communication aids (VOCAs). They include systems such as the Alpha Talker and DynaVox, which have an organized storage of vocabularies that can be accessed for different situations. These devices are often unwieldy to carry around, although lightweight, miniaturized systems are now being developed.

FUTURE THERAPIES

In the future, gene replacement therapy may become a reality, although it is likely that multiple gene deficiencies lead to the phenotype of SMS. For the near future, controlled medication studies are needed to clarify efficacy, and newer medications should be tried because of the molecular advances that suggest dysfunction of certain cellular processes. For instance, Elsea et al. (1995) suggest that new antipsychotic agents, specifically glycine and NMDA antagonists, may be helpful for patients with SMS. In addition, a folic acid trial should be undertaken with patients with SMS because of deficiency of the SHMT gene (Elsea et al., 1995). The field of AAC and computer enhancement of learning is ever expanding, and new instrumentation will be available yearly to improve education and vocational opportunities for patients with SMS.

ACKNOWLEDGMENTS   I thank Ann C. M. Smith and A. J. Allen for their comments and useful information on chapter 9. This work was partially supported by a grant from MCH no. MCJ-089413. Discussions with the Developmental Psychobiology Research Group (DPRG) at the University of Colorado Health Sciences Center and with Tracy Kovach, Clinical Director of the Assistive Technology Clinic at the Children's Hospital in Denver, significantly enhanced this chapter, and I thank them.

REFERENCES

Behjati, F., Mullarkey, M., Bergbaum, A., Berry, A. C., Docherty, Z. (1997) Chromosome deletion 17p11.2 (Smith-Magenis syndrome) in seven new patients, four of whom had been referred for fragile-X investigation. Clinical Genetics 51 (1): 71–4.

Bennetto, L., and Pennington, B. F. (1996) The neuropsychology of fragile X syndrome. In: Fragile X syndrome: Diagnosis, treatment, and research. Hagerman, R. J., and Cronister, A. (eds.). 2nd ed. Johns Hopkins University Press, Baltimore, pp. 210–48.

Chen, C. H., Lee, Y. R., Liu, M. Y., Wei, F. C., Koong, F. J., Hwu, H. G., Hsiao, K. J. (1996a) Identification of a BglI polymorphism of catechol-O-methyltransferase (COMT) gene, and associ-ation study with schizophrenia. American Journal of Medical Genetics 67 (6): 556–9.

Chen, K.-S., Potocki, L., Lupski, J. R. (1996b) The Smith-Magenis syndrome [del(17)p11.2]: Clinical review and molecular advances. Mental Retardation and Developmental Disabilities Research Reviews 2 (3): 122–9.

Chen, R. M., Lupski, J. R., Greenberg, F., Lewis, R. A. (1996c) Ophthalmic manifestations of Smith-Magenis syndrome. Ophthalmology 103 (7): 1084–91.

Colley, A. F., Leversha, M. A., Voullaire, L. E., Rogers, J. G. (1990) Five cases demonstrating the distinctive behavioural features of chromosome deletion 17(p11.2 p11.2) (Smith-Magenis syndrome). Journal of Paediatric Child Health 26: 17–21.

Crumley, F. E. (1998). Smith-Magenis syndrome. Journal of the American Academy of Child and Adolescent Psychiatry 37 (11): 1131–2.

Dykens, E. M., and Smith, A. C. M. (1998) Distinctiveness and correlates of maladaptive behavior in children and adolescents with Smith-Magenis syndrome. Journal of Intellectual Disability Research. 42 (6): 481–9.

Dykens, E. M., Finucane, B. M., Gayley, C. (1997) Brief report: Cognitive and behavioral profiles in persons with Smith-Magenis syndrome. Journal of Autism and Developmental Disorders 27 (2): 203–11.

Elsea, S. H., Juyal, R. C., Jiralerspong, S., Finucane, B. M., Pandolfo, M., Greenberg, F., Baldini, A., Stover, P., Patel, P. I. (1995) Haploinsufficiency of cytosolic serine hydroxymethyltransferase in the Smith-Magenis syndrome. American Journal of Human Genetics 57 (6): 1342–50.

Fan, Y. S., and Farrell, S. A. (1994) Prenatal diagnosis of interstitial deletion of 17(p11.2p11.2) (Smith-Magenis syndrome) [Letter to the editor]. American Journal of Medical Genetics 49 (2): 253–4.

Finucane, B. M., Jaeger, E. R., Kurtz, M. B., Weinstein, M., Scott, C. I., Jr. (1993) Eye abnormalities in the Smith-Magenis contiguous gene deletion syndrome. American Journal of Medical Genetics 45 (4): 443–6.

Finucane, B. M., Konar, D., Haas-Givler, B., Kurtz, M. B., Scott, C. I., Jr. (1994) The spasmodic upper-body squeeze: A characteristic behavior in Smith-Magenis syndrome. Developmental Medicine and Child Neurology 36 (1): 78–83.

Fisman, S., Steele, M., Short, J., Byrne, T., Lavallee, C. (1996) Case study: Anorexia nervosa and autistic disorder in an adolescent girl. Journal of the American Academy of Child and Adolescent Psychiatry 35 (7): 937–40.

Friedman, T. B., Liang, Y., Weber, J. L., Hinnant, J. T., Barber, T. D., Winata, S., Arhya, I. (1995) A gene for congenital, recessive deafness DFNB3 maps to the pericentromeric region of chromosome 17. Nature Genetics 9: 86–91.

Greenberg, F., Guzzetta, V., Montes de Oca-Luna, R., Magenis, R. E., Smith, A. C., Richter, S. F., Kondo, I., Dobyns, W. B., Patel, P. I., Lupski, J. R. (1991) Molecular analysis of the Smith-Magenis syndrome: A possible contiguous-gene syndrome associated with del(17)(p11.2). American Journal of Human Genetics 49 (6): 1207–18.

Greenberg, F., Lewis, R. A., Potocki, L., Glaze, D., Parke, J., Killian, J., Murphy, M. A., Williamson, D., Brown, F., Dutton, R., McCluggage, C., Friedman, E., Sulek, M., Lupski, J. R. (1996) Multi-disciplinary clinical study of Smith-Magenis syndrome (deletion 17p11.2). American Journal of Medical Genetics 62 (3): 247–54.

Haas-Givler, B. (1994) Educational implications and behavioral concerns of SMS: From the teacher's perspective. Spectrum 1: 3–4.

Haas-Givler, B., and Finucane, B. (1995) What's a teacher to do: Classroom strategies that enhance learning for children with SMS. Spectrum 2: 1–6.

Hagerman, R. J. (1996) Physical and behavioral phenotype. In: Fragile X syndrome: Diagnosis, treatment, and research. Hagerman, R. J., and Cronister, A. (eds.). 2nd ed. Johns Hopkins University Press, Baltimore, pp. 3–87.

Hagerman, R. J., Bregman, J. D., Tirosh, E. (1998) Clonidine. In: Psychotropic medication and developmental disabilities: The international consensus handbook. Reiss, S., and Aman, M. G. (eds.). Ohio State University Nisonger Center, Columbus, Ohio, pp. 259–69.

Howard-Peebles, P. H., Friedman, J. M., Harrod, M. J. E., Brookshire, G. S., Lockwood, J. E. (1985) A stable supernumerary chromosome derived from a deleted segment of 17p. American Journal of Human Genetics 37: A97.

Jan, J. E., and O'Donnell, M. E. (1996) Use of melatonin in the treatment of paediatric sleep disorders. Journal of Pineal Research 21: 193–9.

Juyal, R. C., Finucane, B., Shaffer, L. G., Lupski, J. R., Greenberg, F., Scott, C. I., Baldini, A., Patel, P. I. (1995a) Apparent mosaicism for del(17)(p11.2) ruled out by fluorescence in situ hybridization in a Smith-Magenis syndrome patient [Letter to the editor; Comment]. American Journal of Medical Genetics 59 (3): 406–7.

Juyal, R. C., Greenberg, F., Mengden, G. A., Lupski, J. R., Trask, B. J., van den Engh, G., Lindsay, E. A., Christy, H., Chen, K. S., Baldini, A., et al. (1995b) Smith-Magenis syndrome deletion: A case with equivocal cytogenetic findings resolved by fluorescence in situ hybridization. American Journal of Medical Genetics 58 (3): 286–91.

Juyal, R. C., Figuera, L. E., Hauge, X., Elsea, S. H., Lupski, J. R., Greenberg, F., Baldini, A., Patel, P. I. (1996) Molecular analyses of 17p11.2 deletions in 62 Smith-Magenis syndrome patients. American Journal of Human Genetics 58 (5): 998–1007.

Kapur, S., and Remington, G. (1996) Serotonin-dopamine interaction and its relevance to schizophrenia. American Journal of Psychiatry 153: 466–76.

Khan, B. U. (1997) Brief report: Risperidone for severely disturbed behavior and tardive dyskinesia in developmentally disabled adults. Journal of Autism and Developmental Disorders 27 (4): 479–89.

Kondo, I., Matsuura, S., Kuwajima, K., Tokashiki, M., Izumikawa, Y., Naritomi, K., Niikawa, N., Kajii, T. (1991) Diagnostic hand anomalies in Smith-

Magenis syndrome: Four new patients with del (17)(p11.2p11.2). American Journal of Medical Genetics 41 (2): 225–9.

Masuno, M., Asano, J., Arai, M., Kuwahara, T., Orii, T. (1992) Interstitial deletion of 17p11.2 with brain abnormalities. Clinical Genetics 41: 278–80.

Palm, L., Blennow, G., Wetterberg, L. (1997) Long-term melatonin treatment in blind children and young adults with circadian sleep-wake disturbances. Developmental Medicine and Child Neurology 39: 319–25.

Potacki, L., Reiter, R. J., Glaze, D., Lupski, J. R. (1997) Twenty-four hour urinary excretion of 6-sulphatoxymelatonin in Smith-Magenis syndrome. American College of Medical Genetics Conference, abstract no. A31.

Silverman, F. (1995) Communication for the speechless. Allyn & Bacon, Boston.

Simeon, J. G., Carrey, N. J., Wiggins, D. M., Milin, R. P., Hosenbocus, S. N. (1995) Risperidone effects in treatment-resistant adolescents: Preliminary case reports. Journal of Child and Adolescent Psychopharmacology 5 (1): 69–79.

Smith, A. C. M., and Gropman, A. (1999) Smith-Magenis syndrome. In: Clinical management of common genetic syndromes. Cassidy, S., and Allanson, J. (eds.). Wiley, New York.

Smith, A. C. M., McGavran, L., Walkstein, G. (1982) Deletion of the 17 short arm in two patients with facial clefts. American Journal of Human Genetics 34 (suppl.): A410.

Smith, A. C. M., McGavran, L., Robinson, J., Waldstein, G., Macfarlane, J., Zonona, J., Reiss, J., Lahr, M., Allen, L., Magenis, E. (1986) Interstitial deletion of (17)(p11.2p11.2) in nine patients. American Journal of Medical Genetics 24 (3): 393–414.

Smith, A. C. M., Dykens, E., Greenberg, F. (1998a) The behavioral phenotype of Smith-Magenis syndrome (del

17p11.2). American Journal of Medical Genetics (Neuropsychiatric Genetics) 81: 179–85.

Smith, A. C. M., Dykens, E., Greenberg, F. (1998b) Sleep disturbance in Smith-Magenis syndrome (del 17p11.2). American Journal of Medical Genetics (Neuropsychiatric Genetics) 81: 186–91.

Sonies, B. C., Solomon, B., Ondrey, F., McCullagh, L., Greenberg, F., Smith, A. C. M. (1997) Oral-motor and otolaryngologic findings in 14 patients with Smith-Magenis syndrome (17p11.2): Results of an interdisciplinary study. American Journal of Human Genetics 61 (Suppl. 4), abstract no. 13pA5.

Sternberg, M. (1994) The American Sign Language Dictionary on CD-ROM. Harper Collins Interactive.

Stratton, R. F., Dobyns, W. B., Greenberg, F., DeSana, J. B., Moore, C., Fidone, G., Runge, G. H., Feldman, P., Sekhon, G. S., Pauli, R. M., et al. (1986) Interstitial deletion of (17)(p11.2p11.2): Report of six additional patients with a new chromosome deletion syndrome. American Journal of Medical Genetics 24 (3): 421–32.

Sun, Z. S., Albrecht, U., Zhuchenko, O., Bailey, J., Eichele, G., Lee, C. C. (1997) RIGUI, a putative mammalian ortholog of the Drosophila period gene. Cell 90 (6): 1003–1011.

Weitz, C., Dexter, M., Moore, J. (1997) AAC and children with developmental disabilities. In: The handbook of augmentative and alternative communication. Glennen, S. L., and DeCoste, D. C. (eds.). Singular, San Diego, pp. 395–431.

Wilgenbus, K. K., Seranski, P., Brown, A., Leuchs, B., Mincheva, A., Lichter, P., Poustka, A. (1997) Molecular characterization of a genetically unstable region containing the SMS critical area and a breakpoint cluster for human PNETs. Genomics 42 (1): 1–10.

Yang, S. P., Bidichandani, S. I., Figuera, L. E., Juyal, R. C., Saxon, P. J., Baldini, A., Patel, P. I. (1997) Molecular analysis of deletion (17)(p11.2p11.2) in a family segregating a 17p paracentric inversion: Implications for carriers of paracentric inversions. American Journal of Human Genetics 60 (5): 1184–93.

Zori, R. T., Lupski, J. R., Heju, Z., Greenberg, F., Killian, J. M., Gray, B. A., Driscoll, D. J., Patel, P. I., Zackowski, J. L. (1993) Clinical, cytogenetic, and molecular evidence for an infant with Smith-Magenis syndrome born from a mother having a mosaic 17p11.2p12 deletion. American Journal of Medical Genetics 47 (4): 504–11.

RESOURCES

Professional Organizations

PRISMS — Parents and Researchers Interested in Smith-Magenis Syndrome
11875 Fawn Ridge Lane
Reston, VA 20194
fax: (703) 709-0538
e-mail: acmsmith@nhgri.nih.gov

This is a national organization that publishes a newsletter, *Spectrum*, on a twice-a-year basis. Their newsletter has practical information regarding treatment issues and learning issues for children and adults with Smith-Magenis syndrome. They also have a program to link up patients in the same area. The president is Margaret Miller and the chairman of the

Professional Advisory Committee is Ann C. M. Smith.

March of Dimes Birth Defects Foundation
National Headquarters
1275 Mamaroneck Avenue
White Plains, NY 10605
telephone: (888) MO-DIMES; (206) 624-1373

This national organization funds research and also disseminates educational materials.

Association for Retarded Citizens of the United States (ARC)
National Headquarters
2501 Avenue J
Arlington, TX 76006
telephone: (817) 261-6003

This is an association in support of citizens with mental retardation.

The National Organization for Rare Disorders (NORD)
National Headquarters
P.O. Box 8923

New Fairfield, CT 06812-8923
telephone: (800) 999-6673; (203) 746-6518
fax: (203) 746-6481
http://www.pcnet.com/~orphan

NORD is committed to the identification, treatment, and cure of rare disorders through programs of education, advocacy, research, and service.

Alliance of Genetic Support Groups
4301 Connecticut Avenue, NW, Suite 404
Washington, DC 20008-2304
telephone: (800) 336-GENE

General Reading

Haas-Givler, B. (1994) Educational implications and behavioral concerns of SMS: From the teacher's perspective. Spectrum 1: 3–4.

Haas-Givler, B., and Finucane, B. (1995) What's a teacher to do: Classroom strategies that enhance learning for children with SMS. Spectrum 2: 1–6.

Attention Deficit Hyperactivity Disorder

READINGS FOR PARENTS AND TEACHERS

Barkley, R. A. (1998) Attention-deficit hyperactivity disorder: A clinical workbook. 2nd Ed. New York: Guilford Press.

Barkley, R. A. (1998) Your defiant child: 8 steps to better behavior. New York: Guilford Press.

Barkley, R. A. (1995) Taking charge of ADHD: The complete, authoritative guide for parents. New York: Guilford Press.

Barkley, R. A. (1997) ADHD and the nature of self control. New York: Guilford Press.

Barkley, R. A. (1997) Defiant children: A clinician's manual for assessment and parent training. 2nd Ed. New York: Guilford Press.

Braswell, L., Bloomquist, M., Pederson, S. (1991) ADHD: A guide to understanding and helping children with attention deficit hyperactivity disorder in school settings. Minneapolis: University of Minnesota (Available from Department of Professional Development and Conference Services, Continuing Education and Extension, 315 Pillsbury Drive S.E., Minneapolis, MN 55455, (612) 625-3504).

Camp, B., and Bash, M. A. (1981) Think aloud: Increasing social and cognitive skills—a problem solving program for children. Champaign, IL: Research Press.

Clark, L. (1989) The time-out solution: A parent's guide for handling everyday behavior problems. Chicago: Contemporary Books. Much detail on using time-out but also other punishments and positive ways of increasing appropriate behavior. Includes examples, checklists, and tear-out reminder sheets.

Fowler, M. C. (1990) Maybe you know my kid: A parent's guide to identifying, understanding and helping your child with attention deficit hyperactive disorder. New York: Carol.

Garber, S. W., Garber, M. D., Spizman, R. F. (1990) If your child is hyperactive, inattentive, impulsive, distractible . . . helping the ADD (attention deficit disorder) hyperactive child. New York: Villard Books. A practical program for changing behavior with or without medication.

Goldstein, S. (1995) Understanding and managing children's classroom behavior. Wiley.

Goldstein, S., and Goldstein, M. (1987) A teacher's guide: Attention deficit hyperactivity disorder in children. Salt Lake City, UT: Neurology, Learning and Behavior Center.

Hallowell, E., and Ratey, J. (1994) Driven to distraction: Recognizing and coping with attention deficit disorder from childhood through adulthood. New York: Pantheon Books.

Hallowell, E. M., and Ratey, J. J. (1994) Answers to distraction. New York: Pantheon Books.

Ingersoll, B. (1988) Your hyperactive child: A parent's guide to coping with attention deficit disorder. New York: Doubleday. A comprehensive book with many examples. Includes brief guidelines for teachers and an appendix with behavioral management programs for classroom use.

Ingersoll, B., and Goldstein, S. (1993) Attention deficit disorder and learning disabilities: Realities, myths and controversial treatments. New York: Doubleday Main Street Books. An up-to-date review by two psychologists focusing on causes and treatment. Good coverage of common myths and unfounded claims.

Kelly, K., and Ramundo, P. (1996) You mean I'm not lazy, stupid, or crazy?! New York: Fireside Books.

Levine, M. (1994) Educational care: A system for understanding and helping children with learning problems at home and in school. New York: Simon & Schuster.

Nadeau, K. (1994) Survival guide for college students with ADD or LD. New York: Magination Press.

Nadeau, K. G. (1995) A comprehensive guide to attention deficit disorder in adults: Research, diagnosis, and treatment. New York: Brunner/Mazel.

Pierangelo, R. (1994) A survival kit for the special education teacher. Education Publishing Service.

READINGS FOR PATIENTS

Gehert, J. (1992) Eagle eyes: A child's view of ADD. Fairport, NY: Verbal Images Press.

Gordon, M. (1991) Jumpin' Johnny get back to work! A child's guide to ADHD/hyperactivity. DeWitt, NY: GSI.

Gordon, M. (1992) My brother's a world class pain . . . A sibling's guide to ADHD/hyperactivity. DeWitt, NY: GSI.

Gordon, M. (1993) I would if I could: A teenager's guide to ADHD/hyperactivity. DeWitt, NY: GSI.

Kelly, K., and Ramundo, P. (1996) You mean I'm not lazy, stupid, or crazy?! New York: Fireside Books.

Levin, M. (1989) Keeping ahead in school. Cambridge, MA: Educational Publishing Services.

Levin, M. (1992) All kinds of minds. Cambridge, MA: Educational Publishing Services.

Moss, D. (1988) Shelly the hyperactive turtle. Rockville, MD. Woodbine House.

Parker, R. N. (1992) Making the grade: An adolescent's struggle with ADD. Plantation, FL: Impact Publications.

Quinn, P., and Stern, J. (1992) Putting on the brakes: Young people's guide to understanding attention deficit hyperactivity disorder (ADHD). New York: Magination Press.

ORGANIZATIONS

ADDAG (Attention Deficit Disorder Advocacy Group)
A Colorado support group for families affected by ADD.
8091 South Ireland Way
Aurora, CO 80016
(303) 690-7548

CHADD (Children with Attention Deficit Disorder)
A national organization that provides information and support related to ADD.
499 Northwest 70th Avenue, Suite 308
Plantation FL 33317
(305) 587-3700

NEWSLETTERS

Attention!
The Magazine of Children and Adults with Attention Deficit Disorders
449 N.W. 70th Avenue, Suite 208
Plantation, FL 33317

The ADHD Report
Guilford Press
72 Spring Street
New York, NY 10012

Challenge
The First National Newsletter on Attention Deficit (Hyperactivity) Disorder
P.O. Box 2001
West Newbury, MA 01985

TEXTS FOR PHARMACOTHERAPY IN CHILDREN AND ADOLESCENTS

Green, W. H. (1995) Child and adolescent clinical psychopharmacology. Baltimore: Williams and Wilkins.
Greenhill, L. L., and Osman, B. B. (1991) Ritalin: Theory and patient management. New York: Liebert.
Kutcher, S. P. (1997) Child and adolescent psychopharmacology. Philadelphia: Saunders.

Riddle, M. A. (1995) Pediatric psychopharmacology I. Child Adolescent Psychiatry Clinics of North America 4:1–260.

Riddle, M. A. (1995) Pediatric psychopharmacology II. Child Adolescent Psychiatry Clinics of North America 4:261–520.

Rosenberg, D. R., Holttum, J., Gershon, S. I. (1994) Textbook of pharmacotherapy for child and adolescent psychiatric disorders. New York: Brunner/Mazel.

Werry, J. S., and Aman, M. G. (1993) Practitioner's guide to psychoactive drugs for children and adolescents. New York: Plenum.

Wiener, J. M. (1996) Diagnosis and psychopharmacology of childhood and adolescent disorders. New York: Wiley.

PRODUCTS

A.D.D. Warehouse
For a complete listing of products, call for a free catalog—Books, tapes, videos
Assessment Products, Behavioral Programs
Attention Training, Social Skills Training
telephone: (800) 233-9273 (toll free); (305) 792-8944
fax: (305) 792-8545

PHARMACEUTICAL COMPANIES WITH PATIENT ASSISTANCE PROGRAMS FOR MEDICATIONS

Abbot Laboratories/Ross Laboratories   (202) 637-6889; (800) 922-3255
Aldoria Laboratories, Inc.   (614) 764-8100
Allergan Prescription Pharmaceuticals   (800) 347-4500
Amgen, Inc.   (800) 272-9376
Boehringer Inglehelm   (203) 798-4131
Bristol-Meyers Squibb (Prolixin)   (800) 736-0003
Burroughs-Wellcome   (919) 248-4418; (800) 722-9292
Ciba-Geigy   (908) 277-5849
Genetech Inc.   (800) 879-4747
Glaxo, Inc.   (800) 452-9677
Hoescht-Rossel   (800) 776-4563
Hoffman-LaRouche, Inc.   (800) 526-6367
CI/Stuart   (302) 886-2231
Immunex Corporation   (206) 587-0430
Johnson and Johnson, Ortho Biotechnology   (908) 704-5232; (800) 447-3437
Johnson and Johnson (Risperdal), Janssen Pharmaceuticals   (800) 652-6227
Eli Lilly and Company (Prozac)   (317) 276-2950
Marion Merrel Dow   (816) 966-4250
Merck Sharp Dohme   (215) 540-2000
Parke-Davis   (201) 540-2000
Pfizer Pharmaceuticals (Zoloft)   (800) 869-9979
Sandoz Pharmaceuticals (Clozaril)   (800) 937-6673
Sanoft Winthrop   (212) 907-2000

Schering-Plough   (800) 822-7000
G. D. Searle & Co.   (800) 542-2526
Smithkline Beecham (all programs)   (215) 751-5760
Smithkline Beecham (Eminase, Triostat, and Paxil)   (800) 866-6273
Syntex Laboratories   (800) 822-8255
Wyeth-Ayerst Laboratories (Effexor)   (800) 568-9938
Risperidal Patient Assistance Program
4828 Parkway Plaza Boulevard #220
Charlotte, NC 28217-1969
(800) 652-6227; fax: (704) 357-0036

Computer Information and Technology Centers

RECOMMENDED SOFTWARE, CURRICULUM PACKAGES, AND VIDEO ASSISTANCE

Attainment Company: For children and adults with special needs
P.O. Box 930160
Verona, WI 53593-0160
For a free catalog, telephone (800) 327-4269 (toll free)
fax: (800) 942-3865
http://www.attainment-inc.com

Survival Words $195
> CD-ROM interactive. Survival Words covers the key elements of independence. Includes the most important signs from Information, Safety, Public Transportation, and Community Signs. Includes 80 words on one CD-ROM (Win/MAC), an administration manual, and a reproducible student workbook.

Picture Prompt System $327
> The Picture Prompt system provides a library of reproducible illustrations that make teaching daily living tasks easier. Includes Picture Prompt Cards, Stickers, Illustrated Guide Package, Home Cooking Picture Cookbook, the Looking Good and Keeping House Step Pages

School to Work Package $199
> For students with disabilities, the segue from school to real life is not easy and often not successful. The School to Work Package includes: Everyone Can Work video, It's All Part of the Job video, Community Success—an illustrated encyclopedia of community-based activities and corresponding social skills, and Transition Plans.

Attainment's Big Bundle CD-ROM $529
> Attainment's most comprehensive software package. Includes everything from math, spelling, and language to life skills, basic concepts, and money skills. Software includes Picture Cue Dictionary, Looking For Words, Dollars and Cents, Show Me Math, Show Me Spelling, Basic Concepts, and Wordwise.

Picture Cue Dictionary CD-ROM $189
> Five interactive programs help students perform everyday activities independently. Includes Looking Good, Keeping House, Select-A-Meal, Shopping Smart, and Plan Your Day.

Plan Your Day Curriculum $99
> Students can learn how to follow a schedule, even if they can't tell time or remember the date. Plan Your Day Curriculum includes an instructor's guide plus hands-on student resources.

Learn about Life Curriculum $129
> Learn About Life is an illustrated sexual education and social skills program covering puberty, dating, pregnancy, STDs, and more. Candid, realistic, and original graphics and simple text help below-level readers understand important sexual issues. Includes Your Body, Your Mind; Having a Baby; Being a Woman; Being a Man; Be Smart, Be Safe; and Relationships.

It's All Part of the Job Video $59
> One-of-a-kind video features real-life workers with developmental disabilities and their employers. Focuses on social skills needed to succeed on the job in an entertaining and motivational manner. Great for supported employment, work-skill training programs, or to show parents or employers.

Self-Advocacy Package $199
> The Self-Advocacy Package gives you everything you need to facilitate a workshop for a group of adolescents or adults with developmental disabilities. It builds advocacy and self-determination skills by involving participants in the disability rights movement.

Money Math Program $135
> Teaches real-life shopping skills using sales flyers and reproducible worksheets. Includes Money Math Grocery Store, Drug Store and Super Store.

Edmark Reading Programs $475
> A step-by-step program that teaches students with developmental disabilities to read. With two levels, students learn to recognize whole words, match them to pictures, and read them in sentences following a structured lesson plan.

Show Me Math $99
> A CD-ROM interactive, instructive program where students learn in three different critical areas, addition/subtraction, multiplication, and division.

Show Me Reading $129
A CD-ROM interactive, instructive program which allows students to succeed at spelling while learning up to 600 words independently.

Berta Max Educational Software Center
P.O. Box 31849
Seattle, WA 98103

Berta Max Read Alongs $25
A series of emergent and early reading books on the computer. Text is predictable, with rhyme and repetition. Graphics are good, and text is underlined as it is read by the speech synthesizer. Stories include ABC, counting, and Feet (Apple).

Big Top Productions
(800) 900-PLAY

Hello Kitty Big Fun Deluxe $40
Coloring book, piano, animal sounds, storybook, and counting. CD-ROM.

Bright Star
P.O. Box 485
Coarsegold, CA 93614
(800) 743-7725

Dream Team Series $15–25 each
Combination of visual and auditory feedback in interactive programs designed to teach early learning through middle elementary concepts. Some available in CD-ROM format. (MAC/IBM)

Alphabet Blocks
Beginning Reading
Early Math
Kid's Typing
Basic Spelling
Advanced Spelling

Brøderbund
17 Paul Drive
San Rafael, CA 94903
(800) 521-6263

Playworld BUNDLE $90
The Backyard
Playroom
The Tree House

Living Books Series $35–45 each

The Living Books series combines sound and animation to bring children's literature to life. The story can be read aloud, and virtually every object on the page can be manipulated in some way. CD-ROM.

Arthur's Teacher Trouble
Arthur's Birthday
Berenstein Bears Get in a Fight
Dr. Seuss ABC
Green Eggs and Ham
Harry and the Haunted House
Just Grandma and Me
Little Monster at School
The New Kid on the Block
Ruff's Bone
Sheila Rae, The Brave
The Tortoise and The Hare

Amazing Writing Machine $40

Journals, poetry, essays, stories, and more. Includes feature to support building stories from a template. CD-ROM.

Kid Pix Studio $30–40

This is an excellent graphics and drawing program. Children can write by stamping letters, select stamps to put in their pictures, and draw in color. The alphabet talks, and sound effects can be added to pictures. Also integrates features of Kid Pix Companion. (MAC/IBM).

Math Workshop $30–40

Highly interactive problem-solving software. Arithmetic and visual perceptual skills are addressed through seven different activities. Multiple skill levels are available. (MAC/IBM).

Print Shop or Print Shop Deluxe $36

This is an easy-to-use program which allows the user to make signs, banners, and letters. It is an excellent tool for motivational writing and creative activities. (MAC/IBM).

Where in—Is Carmen Sandiego Series $35 each

Reading, attention to detail, discrimination between significant and insignificant facts, note taking, and a variety of other skills are used to catch a crook who flees to different parts of the world.

Computer Options for the Exceptional
49 Overlook Road
Poughkeepsie, NY 12603
(914) 452-1850

Grocery Shop $30
Works on word recognition for grocery and related words. Uses words and photographs to stimulate going to the grocery store to shop for specific list items.

Order at McDonald's $30
Recognition of McDonald's menu words.

Read Community Signs $30
This activity presents four common community signs at once. The user is given an auditory prompt to find a given sign from the four choices.

Read Functional Words $30
Sight word recognition of 45 functional words is taught.

Identify Money $30
Money recognition, making the correct sum, identifying money by its name and amount.

Read a Clock $30
25 situations are presented with auditory prompts indicating the corresponding time. The user needs to match the auditory prompts with the pictures of the appropriate clock.

Creative Wonders
(800) KID-XPRT

Early Learning $35
Sesame Street: Get Set to Learn
Elmo's Preschool
Sesame Street: Let's Make a Word

School House Rock Series $35–40
Grammar Rock
Science Rock
America Rock
Math Rock

Davidson
(800) 567-4321

Kids Can Read—five titles in a bundle $40
A collection of popular books converted to CD-ROM technology. The program will read the story, pronounce words individually, and even give definitions of words. It also creates a list of words which the reader needs to practice. Can read in Spanish or English. CD-ROM

Kid Phonics 1 $40
Kid Phonics 2 $40

Kid Keys $35
   Talking animated typing program. Three activities to familiarize young children with
   keyboard functions. (IBM/MAC)

Math Blaster Series $35 each
   Addition, subtraction, multiplication, and division concepts are taught in a fun ar-
   cade game format. Further into the series, concepts in the areas of geometry and algebra are explored on disks. (MAC/IBM)

   Math Blaster Mystery
   Math Blaster: In Search of Spot
   What's My Angle?
   Alge-Blaster 3

Money Town (grades K–3)   MAC/WIN CD $30.95
   Children will learn about earning, saving, making change, coin recognition, and
   much more.

Don Johnston Developmental Equipment, Inc.
P.O. Box 1000 N. Rand Road, Bldg. 115
Wauconda, IL 60084
(800) 999-4660

Big Calc $29
   Large calculator program that has many features for manipulating numbers as well as
   the layout of the keypad. Has auditory feedback capabilities. (MAC)

Blocks in Motion $79 starter kit
   Building blocks for the computer. New sets of bricks can be purchased for $25 each.

Co:Writer $350
   A word prediction program which "guesses" the word which is to be typed based on
   the first few letters. It collects new words as you use them and adds them to the lists
   of possibilities. This program makes writing much faster.

Gateway Stories I and II $125
Gateway Authoring System $90
   Allows the reader to independently select, hear, and turn pages with a switch or
   mouse click. The authoring program allows you to insert graphics and text onto
   blank pages.

Eensy and Friends $65
   Characters involved in cause/effect games that involve counting, dressing, and prepo-
   sitions.

Write: Outloud $99
   All of the power of a fully functional word processor, including a spell checker, with
   the added feature of speech. The speech output options are flexible enough to meet

every user's needs. There is visual ribbon, which makes changing settings as easy as pointing and clicking.

Edmark Corporation
P.O. Box 3218
Redmond, WA 98073-3218

Imagination Express Series $30 each
    Castle
    Time Trip, USA
    Pyramids
    Ocean
    Neighborhood
    Rain Forest
    Creative Writing programs. CD-ROM

Kid's Desk $59
    A program which allows for single click access to individual applications. The system and other parts of the computer can be locked to avoid inadvertent loss. (IBM/MAC)

Learning House Programs $30–40 each
    Learn about a variety of concepts through interactive games and exploration. (IBM/MAC)

    Bailey's Book House
    Millie's Math House
    Sammy's Science House
    Stanley's Sticker Stories
    Trudy's Time and Place House

Mighty Math Series $60 each
    Interactive math programs in different levels. CD-ROM

    Carnival Countdown
    Zoo Zillions
    Number Heroes
    Calculating Crew
    Cosmic Geometry
    Astro Algebra

Thinkin' Things 1 $40
Thinkin' Things 2 $40
Thinkin' Things 3 $40
    Builds critical thinking skills and creativity. Musical patterns, logical comparison, and deductive reasoning addressed. (MAC/IBM) CD-ROM

Story Book Weaver Delux (grades 1–6) $26
    Students can create stories using hundreds of graphics in any combination

Strategy Games of the World $45
Includes Mancala, Nine Men's Morris, and GO. Can play against computer or another person. CD-ROM

Hartley/Jostens Learning
9920 Pacific Heights Boulevard, Suite 500
San Diego, CA 92121
(800) 247-1380
http://www.jlc.com

Math Skills Collection (grades 4–6)   MAC/WIN CD $64.95
This collection includes whole numbers and fractions, decimals and percents, measurements and representation of data and shapes and figures.

Clock (grades 1–5)   MAC/WIN CD $27.95
Teaches the relationship between digital time and analog time by means of a graphic clock.

Information Services, Inc.
28 Green Street
Newbury, MA 01951
(800) 659-3399

WriteAway $199
This word prediction program "guesses" the next word being typed based on the first few letters. It has the ability to collect new words and add them to its dictionary. This program may greatly increase typing speed. This program is **not** transparent and must be used only with the accompanying word processor. (DOS/Windows)

IntelliTools
55 Leveroni Court, Suite 9
Novato, CA 94949
(800) 899-6687

Click It! $99.95
Software allows programming of any computer input. Allows for more than one switch to be used differentially within any software program.

IntelliTalk $50
A talking word processor which can speak letters, words, sentences, or any combination (MAC, IBM, Apple).

IntelliPics $40
This software allows the user to design software simply and creatively to be used with a mouse or the IntelliKeys, when an overlay is created using Overlay Maker. Specific concepts can be addressed in a fun, interactive way. (MAC)

Overlay Maker $80

This is a program which allows for the IntelliKeys to be programmed to meet an individual's needs.

Knowledge Adventure, Inc.
1311 Grand Central Avenue
Glendale, CA 91201
(800) 542-4240

Jump Start Learning System $20–40 each

A grade-based software series that targets various skills at each grade level.

Toddlers: computer mouse skills, letters and numbers, vocabulary, and music
Preschool: comprehension, phonics, mouse skills, letters and numbers, vocabulary, and music
Pre-K: letter order, quantities, problem solving, decision making, social roles, phonics, counting, vocabulary, and music
Kindergarten: letter combinations, reading and sentences, similarities and differences, sequencing, counting, art, time concepts, comprehension, listening skills, vocabulary, and music
1st Grade: spelling, literature, math, science, geography, phonics, reading, similarities and differences, sequencing, art, vocabulary, and music
2nd Grade: basic grammar, math, social studies, science, geography, vocabulary, writing, spelling, literature, reading, art, sequencing, comprehension, and phonics review
3rd Grade: history, science, geography, spelling, grammar, sentence structure, math, art, music, and astronomy
4th Grade: history, science, geography, parts of speech, spelling, grammar, story creation, math, art history, and music
5th Grade: history, logic, problem solving, deductive reasoning, map skills, science, geography, grammar, math skills (including geometry), and art history

Laureate Learning Systems, Inc.
110 E. Spring Street
Winooski, VT 05404-1837
(800) 562-6801

The purpose of this software series is to introduce the concepts of cause and effect, switch use, visual tracking, discrete pointing, and turn taking.

Creature Antics $75 each
Creature Capers
Creature Features
Creature Chorus

First Words Series $200 each

This series is part of an entire language development program. It can be accessed in a variety of ways, including touch window and single switch. There is a Lesson Editor, which allows for customization of the software. Most pieces of software from this company can be run on a Macintosh with an Apple IIe emulator, and they are currently developing more Macintosh-specific software.

Lawrence Productions
1800 S. 35th Street
Galesburg, MI 49053-9687
(800) 421-4157

These programs allow children to explore different environments on the computer. Children decide what McGee will play with and explore (Apple II available individually, MAC, IBM)

McGee Series $32 each
McGee
McGee at Fun Fair
McGee Visits Katie's Farm

The Learning Company
6493 Kaiser Drive
Freemont, CA 94555
(800) 852-2255

Ancient Empires! $?? each
Treasure Mountain!
Time Riders in American History
Gizmos and Gadgets
Operation Neptune
Midnight Rescue
Spell Bound
  Adventure games that use reading, math, science, comprehension, and critical thinking skills. (IBM, Macintosh)

Reader/Writer Rabbit Series $40–50 each
  Each piece of software works on different reading and writing skills, from letter recognition to word attack strategies. (IBM/MAC)

Interactive Reading Journey $100
  Combines open-ended reading exploration with structured practice. Wide variety of concepts addressed. CD-ROM

Math Rabbit Series $40 each
  Each piece of software works on different math skills, from number recognition to problem solving and arithmetic. (IBM/MAC)

Interactive Math Journey $90
   Combines open-ended math exploration with structured practice. Wide variety of concepts addressed. CD-ROM

The Writing Center (MAC) $55 each
The Bilingual Writing Center (MAC)
The Student's Writing Center (IBM)
The Children's Writing and Publishing Center (Apple)
The Children's Writing and Publishing Center, Spanish Edition (Apple)
   All of the features of the Children's Writing and Publishing Center and much more. It includes a spell checker, thesaurus, and graphics. You can also import graphics from other programs. It will print in color or black and white. This is an easy-to-use and versatile word processing program.

Super Solvers Gizmos and Gadgets (grades 3–6)   MAC/WIN CD $29.95
   Students learn the basic principles of physical science though observation and experimentation. Students build an understanding of force, magnetism, electricity, gears, balance, energy sources, and simple machines.

MacWarehouse
P.O. Box 3013
1720 Oak Street
Lakewood, NJ 08701-3013
(800) 255-6227

OmniPage 3.0 $459
   Optical Character Recognition software which allows for scanned data to be treated as text files. Imperative if the goal is to work with the information scanned in a word processing format.

Madenta Communications
Box 25 Advanced Technology Centre
9650 20 Avenue
Edmonton, Alberta
Canada
(800) 661-8406

Screen Doors $365
   This is a word prediction, on-screen keyboard, and telephone program. The word prediction portion "guesses" the next word being typed based on the first few letters. It has the ability to collect new words and add them to its dictionary. This program greatly increases typing speed. The on-screen keyboard allows for typing using only a mouse or mouse emulator. The telephone feature allows for environmental control of the telephone through the computer and a modem. This program is "transparent" in that it can be used with any word processing program. Pieces of the program can be purchased as needed. (MAC)

Telepathic $250

This word prediction program "guess" the next word being typed based on the first few letters. It has the ability to collect new words and add them to its dictionary. This program may greatly increase typing speed. This program is "transparent" in that it can be used with any word processing program. (MAC)

Mayer-Johnson Co.
P.O. Box 1579
Solana Beach, CA 92075-7579
telephone: (619) 550-0084
fax: (619) 550-0449
e-mail: mayerj@aol.com
http://www.mayer-johnson.com

Boardmaker $399

An incredibly flexible and powerful communication display maker. Boardmaker is a graphics database containing over 3,000 picture communication symbols in bitmap clip art form. Available for both MAC and PC and comes in nine different languages. Also available in a text-based book form.

The Picture Exchange Communication System (PECS) $39

PECS is a popular and well-respected AAC training system designed for use with children with autism and related developmental disabilities. Children are taught to approach and give a picture of a desired item to a communicative partner in exchange for that item.

MECC
3490 Lexington Avenue N.
St. Paul, MN 55126
(800) 228-3504

MECC produces numerous pieces of academic software, with subjects ranging from science to problem solving to telling time. These programs can often be used to integrate with classroom curriculum goals.

Storybook Weaver Deluxe $55

Create a storybook with a picture library and fun fonts.

Trail Programs $60 each

Trail games incorporate multiple skills, including planning and problem solving.
CD-ROM

Oregon Trail
Amazon Trail
Africa Trail
Maya Quest

Microsystems Software, Inc.
600 Worcester Road
Framingham, MA 01701-5342
(800) 828-2600

HandiWORD $290
This word prediction program "guesses" the next word being typed based on the first few letters. It has the ability to collect new words and add them to its dictionary. This program may greatly increase typing speed. This program is "transparent" in that it can be used with any word processing program. (DOS/Windows)

Optimum Resources, Inc.
10 Station Place
Norfolk, CT 060058

Stickybears Math Splash (grades K–5) $35.95
Targets skills in addition, subtraction, multiplication, and division.

Orange Cherry Talking Schoolhouse
P.O. Box 390
Pound Ridge, NY 10576-0390

Many of the programs in this series are available bundled together on a CD-ROM for Macintosh.

Talking Alpha Chimp $40
Alphabet skills and early numbers are taught by Harry the Chimp. Three programs are included: Alphabet Board, Number Tree, and Alphabet Story. (IIgs/IBM)

Jungle Safari $40
Take a safari and learn about animals and their habitats. Prereaders can explore the animals, bypassing the reading sections. Motivating text for beginning and advanced readers. (IIgs)

Talking First Words $40
Introduction to word classes, such as nouns, verbs, and word families. Children complete sentences, solve riddles, and fill in missing letters. (IIgs/IBM)

Talking Addition and Subtraction $40
Beginning math problems are introduced, including number sets, picture problems, and a number line. Immediate feedback is provided for all input. (IIgs/IBM)

Talking Clock $40
Time-telling skills are taught in hours, minutes, and seconds. (IIgs/IBM)

Basic Math Skills (grades preK–3)   MAC/WIN CD $41.95
Program teaches numbers, their values, number words, addition and subtraction, and sets and sequences.

Using Money and Making Change (grades 2–4)   MAC/WIN CD $34.95
A real human voice identifies coins and bills and describes their various values and equivalents. Students run a small business in which they must buy all the ingredients to make and sell cookies. Students are taught to count money, make change, and total their profits.

Slater Software
351 Badger Ln.
Guffey, CO 80820
(719) 479-2255
fax: (719) 479-2254
e-mail: jimslater@earthlink.net
http://home.earthlink.net/~jimslater

Picture It   MAC/WIN $250
A program that automatically adds pictures to the text you type.

Picture It Jr.   MAC/WIN $65
As students type in a word, the computer matches the picture and reads the word. They get immediate visual and auditory feedback for their writing.

PixReader   MAC/WIN $65
Allows students to hear the materials spoken that have been created in Picture It. The computer reads the documents and the students can follow the highlighted words.

PixWriter   MAC/WIN $65
Chooses pictures to write text and hear speech. Great for emergent and developing readers and writers.

Tom Snyder Productions
90 Sherman Street
Cambridge, MA 02140
(617) 876-4433

Flodd the Bad Guy $40–50 each
Jack and the Beanstalk
These programs are interactive storybooks. Children read the story, turn the page, and choose where the story goes. (IBM/MAC)

Toucan Software
21000 Nordhoff Street
Chatsworth, CA 91311
(800) 247-4641

Children create their own stories following familiar story lines and formats. Each program includes graphics and text generation. (IBM/MAC)

Creative Writing Series $50–60 each
Big Book Maker: Fairy Tales and Nursery Rhymes
Big Book Maker: Tall Tales and American Folk Heroes
Monsters and Make Believe
Comic Book Maker
Story Starters: Social Studies, Science
Dinosaur Days Plus
Robot Writer

Walt Disney Computer Software Inc.
500 S. Buena Vista Street
Burbank, CA 91521

Mickey's ABC's, A Day at the Fair $27.95
Mickey's 123's, The Big Surprise Party $27.95
Mickey's Colors and Shapes, The Dazzling Magic Show $27.95
Mickey's Jigsaw $34.95
Beauty and the Beast Print Kit $13.95
Aladdin Print Kit $13.95
  Variety of programs which work on different skill areas. They all have popular Disney characters, high quality graphics, and auditory feedback. (IBM)

Weekly Reader Software
Optimum Resources, Inc.
10 Station Place
Norfolk, CT 06058

This is a fun series of software programs introducing a variety of concepts to children. These included ABC's, Numbers, Shapes, and Opposites, among others. (IBM/MAC)

Talking Sticky Bear Series $25–35 each
    Numbers
    Math
    Word Problems
    ABC's
    Typing
    Reading
    Opposites

William K. Bradford Publishing
310 School Street
Acton, MA 01720

These programs are classic and familiar stories (e.g., Princess and the Pea, The Three Little Pigs, Lima Bean Dream, etc.) that allow the children to read the story, create their own stories, and a variety of other activities related to the story. The graphics on the screen move with a mouse, so children can interact with the story as they read it. (Apple)

Explore-a-Classic $40–50 each
Explore-a-Folktale
Explore-a-Science
Explore-a-Story

Other CD-ROM Disks

MacMillan Dictionary for Children $30
   Includes almost 12,000 word entries, 1,000 illustrations, and 40 sound effects. You can hear a spoken version of any word by clicking on its pronunciation.

Grolier's or Compton's Encyclopedia $240
   Over 33,000 articles featuring audio capabilities, hundreds of maps, and thousands of pictures.

Games

Shanghai   visual/perceptual
Tetris   visual/perceptual
Lemmings (Psygnosis)   problem solving
Columns   visual/perceptual
Jeopardy   knowledge base
Wheel of Fortune   decoding skills/knowledge base
Mr. Potato Head   Playskool
Candy Land Adventure   Playskool

The Think Aloud Program
By Bonnie Camp. Available from the A.D.D. Warehouse
(800) 233-9273

Camp, B., and Bash, M. A. (1981), Think aloud: Increasing social and cognitive skills—A problem-solving program for children. Champaign: Research Press.

TECHNOLOGY RESOURCE CENTERS

Nebraska Assistive Technology Project
(402) 471-0735

This organization can provide families with information regarding technology outreach centers, such as computer labs that may be available in various areas of the state.

Children's Charity Fund
7061 S. Tamiami Trail
Sarasota, FL 34238
(800) 6HELPUS

This organization may fund assistive technology, including computers. Families may call for an application. After all information is submitted, applications are considered on an individual basis, and the process takes a few days.

Educational Resources
1550 Executive Drive
Elgin, Illinois 60123
(800) 624-2926

They have a catalog through which software can be purchased.

American Printing House for the Blind
1839 Frankfort Avenue
P.O. Box 6085
Louisville, KY 40206-0085
(800) 223-1839

This company has many books available on tape, including literature for all age levels.

Assistive Technology Training and Information Center
P.O. BOX 2441
Vincennes, IN 47591
(812) 886-0575

C.I.T.E. (Consumer Information and Technology Training Exchange)
215 E. New Hampshire
Orlando, FL 32804
(407) 898-2483

Center for Accessible Technology
2547 8th Street, 12-A
Berkeley, CA 94710-2572
(510) 841-3224

Team of Advocates for Specula Kids
100 West Cerritos Avenue
Anaheim, CA 92805-6546
(714) 533-8275

Massachusetts Special Technology Access Center
12 Mudge Way 1–6
Bedford, MA 01730-2138
(617) 275-2446

Carolina Computer Access Center
700 E. Second Street
Charlotte, NC 28202-2826
(704) 342-3004

The Computer Center for Citizens with Disabilities
c/o Utah Center for Assistive Technology
2056 South 1100 East
Salt Lake City, UT 84106
(801) 485-9152

Materials and Equipment

SPECIAL EDUCATION PROGRAMS AND PRODUCTS

Educational Resources
1550 Executive Drive
Elgin, IL 60123
(800) 624-2926
  They have a catalog through which software can be purchased.

American Printing House for the Blind
1839 Frankfort Avenue
P.O. Box 6085
Louisville, KY 40206-0085
(800) 223-1839
  This company has many books available on tape, including literature for all age levels.

Books On Tape Inc,
P.O. Box 7900
Newport Beach, CA 92658
(800) 88-BOOKS *or* (800) 223-1839
e-mail: botcs@booksontape.com
http://www.booksontape.com

Library for the Blind and Dyslexic
Princeton, NJ
(609) 452-0606

Logo Reading System
by Marcia L. Braden
219 E. StreetVrain
Colorado Springs, CO 80903

The Logo Reading System uses well-known logos, traditional flash cards, sort cards with placements, phrase cards, and matching/fine-motor worksheets.

Logo Math System
by Marcia L. Braden
219 E. St.Vrain
Colorado Springs, CO 80903
The Logo Math System uses a board game and familiar logos to teach math concepts.

SRA (Science Research Associates, Inc)
155 N. Wacker Drive
Chicago, IL 60606
Corrective Reading Comprehension develops the reasoning process (analogues, deductions, inductions, classification), vocabulary, and writing skills students need. Reasoning is taught, not just practiced, in carefully written lessons that foster an experience of success and self-worth.

Merrill Reading Series
Merrill Publishing Co.
P.O. Box 508
Columbus, OH 43216-0508
The Merrill Linguistic Reading Program motivates students to become independent readers and encourages them to learn, to know, to think, and to discover. The program offers readings in important areas such as science, health, history, mathematics and literature.

Appletree-Dormac, Inc.
P.O. Box 270459
San Diego, CA 92128-0983
Appletree is an acronym for "A Patterned Program of Linguistic Expansion Through Reinforced Experiences and Evaluations." It is a language system that provides sequential procedures for construction and development of the sentence structures that are the foundation of verbal language. The program has six workbooks, a teacher's manual, and a pre–post-test booklet.

Capture the Meaning
CC Publications
P.O. Box 23699
Tigard, OR 97223-0108
Here is an exciting new program that really teaches comprehension. Effective and easy to use, "Capture the Meaning: Strategies for Reading Comprehension" focuses on strategies for building comprehension. This 10-unit, 35-lesson program consists of teacher-guided instruction and practice, independent practice that includes individual and group activities, and tests—all designed to reinforce and build reading comprehension skills.

Reading Attainment System, 1987
Educational Design, Inc.
47 W. 13th Street
New York, NY 10011
This program is specially designed to supply practice for students who fail when basal texts reach the 3–5 grade reading levels. This system supplies that practice and produces fluency and confidence in students for whom ordinary methods of remediation have failed. Reading skill, vocabulary skills, and thinking skills are offered in three different sets of multiquestion exercises.

Pro Ed Publishers
8700 Shoal Creek Boulevard
Austin, TX 78757
(800) 897-3202
Lindamood Phoneme Sequencing Program for Reading, Spelling, and Speech (LIPS)

Gander Publishing Company
553 Thain Way
Palo Alto, CA 94306
(415) 858-0971; fax: (415) 858-0971
Lindamood-Bell, "Visualizing & Verbalizing"

Handwriting Without Tears, by Janice Z. Olsen
Distributed by Fred Sammons, Inc.
P.O. Box 32
Brookefield, IL 60513
(800) 323-7305; (312) 971-0610

Educator's Publishing Service
31 Smith Place
Cambridge, MA 02138-1089
(800) 225-5750
Orton Gillingham for reading and spelling

Innovative Learning Concepts, Inc.
6760 Corporate Drive
Colorado Springs, CO 80919
(800) 888-9191
Touch Math: Multisensory program for basic arithmetic and computation

Stop, Relax and Think
Child's Work, Child's Play
Center for Applied Psychology
(800) 962-1411
The *Stop, Relax and Think* game is a psychoeducational tool for helping children learn and practice techniques for self-control. It is designed for two to four players between ages 6 and 12.

Touch Math
Innovative Learning Concepts, Inc.,
6760 Corporate Drive
Colorado Springs, CO 80919-1999
   For more information and a comprehensive catalog, telephone (800) 888-9191.
   Touch Math emphasizes multisensory learning to introduce math to all elementary
   school students, including students with learning disabilities.

OT Supplies—Weighted Vests
Achievement Products
P.O. Box 9033
Canton OH 94711
(800) 373-4699; fax: (330) 453-0222
   or
Southpaw Enterprises, Inc.
109 Webb Street
Dayton OH, 45403-1144
(800) 228-1698

Slantboard and Raised Line Paper
K&L Resources, Inc.
P.O. Box 2612
Springfield, VA 22152
(703) 455-1503
   Paper: Flaghouse catalog 250 sheets: $42; 800-793-7900

Fast Forward
A Division of the Scientific Learning Corporation
417 Montgomery Street, Suite 500
San Francisco, CA 94104
(415) 296-1470
http://www.scientificlearning.com

Picture Exchange Communication System (PECS)
(888) PECS INC; (888) 732-7462
http://www.pecs.com

Lindamood-Bell Learning
Corporate Headquarters
416 Higuera Street
San Luis Obispo, CA 93401
(805) 541-3836; fax: (805) 541-8756
   The basic program's goal is to develop phonemic awareness and concept imagery.
   Recognized as being effective in the treatment of dyslexia, ADD, and learning disabil-
   ities in general.

How to Participate in Your Child's IEP
Coordinating Council for Handicapped Children
20E Jackson Boulevard, Room 900
Chicago, IL
Publication no. 312-939-3513

Attainment Company
For Children and Adults with Special Needs
P.O. Box 930160
Verona, WI 53593-0160
For a free catalog, telephone (800) 327-4269; fax: (800) 942-3865
http://www.attainment-inc.com

Money Math Program $135
Teaches real-life shopping skills using sales flyers and reproducible worksheets. Includes Money Math Grocery Store, Drug Store, and Super Store.

Edmark Reading Programs $475
A step-by-step program that teaches students with developmental disabilities to read. With two levels, students learn to recognize whole words, match them to pictures, and read them in sentences following a structured lesson.

SRA Reading Mastery Programs (Grade Levels 1–6)
Customer Service Rep: Erica
220 East Danieldale
De Soto, TX 75115
(800) 843-8855
A program designed to build a foundation of effective reading strategies. It begins with basic decoding skills such as letter sounds and blending and progresses to reading comprehension with skills such as inferring, predicting, and concluding. Skills are broken down into easily mastered subskills, and students receive instance feedback on their performance. The program concludes with works of literature designed to provide an appreciation and understanding of literary strategies.

Zaner-Bloser Handwriting Program   Grades K–6, $7.37 each; Grades 7–8, $6.37 each
Zaner-Bloser
2200 West Fifth Avenue
P.O. Box 16764
Columbus, OH 43216-6764
(800) 421-3018
A practice-based program designed to improve children's handwriting from kindergarten to 8th grade. The textbook material is age-group appropriate and works on skills such as spacing, size, and slant.

PRODUCT INFORMATION FOR PRAGMATIC LANGUAGE TRAINING

Academic Communication Associates
Publications Division, Dept. 83-C

4149 Avenida de la Plata
P.O. Box 586249
Oceanside, CA 92058

Knowing What to Say!
Talking on Purpose!
Conversation Express
Situation Communication (SITCOM)
Pragmatic Language Intervention Resource

Communication Skills Builders
3830 E. Bellevue/P.O. Box 42050-E93
Tucson, AZ 85733
Building Functional Social Skills, Group Activities for Adults

INTERACT, A Social Skills Game
A Sourcebook of Pragmatic Activities (Revised)
A Sourcebook of Adolescent Pragmatic Activities
Pragmatic Activities for Language Intervention
Tackling Teen Topics
Pragmatic-Language Trivia Junior

DLM
1 DLM Park
Allen, TX 75002

CONVERSATIONS; Language Intervention for Adolescents
Talk About It
STARTLINE, Social Education/Communication

LinguiSystems
3100 4th Avenue
P.O. Box 747
East Moline, IL 61244

Life Skills Workshop
On My Own with Language
Communication Workshop
RAPP (Resource of Activities for Peer Pragmatics)
Room 14, A Social Language Program
FriendZee, A Social Skills Game

PRO-ED
8700 Shoal Creek Boulevard
Austin, TX 78758

PALS: Pragmatic Activites in Language and Speech
BEING ME A Social/Sexual Training Program
Teaching the Moderately and Severely Handicapped, Vol. II: Communication and
    Socialization (2nd Ed.)
The Walker Social Skills Curriculum

The ACCEPTS Program: A Curriculum for Children's Effective Peer and Teacher Skills

The ACCESS Program: Adolescent Curriculum for Communication and Effective Social Skills

Peer Interaction Skills

Talking, Listening, Communicating

The Psychological Corporation
555 Academic Court
San Antonio, TX 78204

Conversation Connections: A Whole Language Preschool Program
Let's Talk: For Children (LTC)
Let's Talk: For Intermediate Level
Let's Talk: For Developing Prosocial Communication Skills

The Reverside Publishing Co
8420 Bryn Mawr Avenue
Chicago, IL 60631

SMALL TALK: Creating Conversation with Young Children

Thinking Publications
1713 Westgate Road
P.O. Box 163
Eau Claire, WI 54702

Scripting: Social Communication for Adolescents
Skillstreaming the Adolescent
Skillstreaming the Elementary School Child
Skillstreaming in Early Childhood
Daily Communication
Communicate (game)
Communicate Junior (game)
Social Skill Strategies
SOCIAL STAR, General Interaction Skills

TRAINING INSTITUTES OR CENTERS

All Kinds of Minds
P.O. Box 3580
Chapel Hill, NC 27515
telephone: (919) 933-8082
fax: (919) 967-3590
e-mail: AKOMinds@aol.com
http://www.allkindsofminds.org

Center for Literacy and Disability Studies
Division of Speech Pathology and Audiology

P.O. Box 3888
Duke University Medical Center
Durham, NC 27710
telephone: (800) 735-8262
fax: (919) 681-5738

BOOKS

Brackley, D. F., King-Sears, M. E., Tessier-Switlick, D. (1997) Teaching students in inclusive settings: From theory to practice. Allyn & Bacon, Boston.

Levine, M. (1994) Educational care: A system for understanding and helping children with learning problems at home and in school. New York: Simon & Schuster.

Meltzer, L. J., et al. (1996) Strategies for success: Classroom teaching techniques for students with learning problems. Austin, TX: Pro Ed.

Johnson, R. M. (1981) The picture communication symbols books. Solona Beach, CA: Mayer-Johnson Press.

The series of three symbols books can be obtained through the Mayer-Johnson Co. Call for a complete listing of products at (619) 550-0084 or fax at (619) 550-0449; e-mail: mayerj@aol.com; www.mayer-johnson.com

P.O. Box 1579
Solona Beach, CA 92075-7579

MISCELLANEOUS

Baby Go to Sleep Tape
(800) 537-7748
P.O. Box 550
Colorado Springs, CO 80901

How Is My Engine Running Program
telephone: (505) 897-3478
fax: (505) 899-4071
book: $36
24-page introductory booklet: $7.50
Audio tape: $15

Williams, M. S., and Shellenberger, S. (1996) "How is my engine running?": A leader's guide for self-regulation. Therapy Works.

Enuresis (Bed Wetting) and Toilet Training

ENURESIS OR BED WETTING ALARMS (APPROXIMATELY $50–$60)

The Potty Pager: A vibrating alarm from Ideas For Living in Boulder, CO
(800) 497-6573.

Nytone Alarm: A clip-on wet alarm from Nytone Medical Products in Salt Lake City, UT
(801) 973-4090.

Wet-Stop Alarm with Velcro fasteners: From Dalco Labs in Santa Cruz, CA
(800) 346-4488.

TOILET TRAINING VIDEOS

Learning through Entertainment: developed and distributed by Video Distributors, Duke University
(800) 23-potty.

READINGS ON TOILET TRAINING

Arzin, N. H., and Foxx, R. M. (1974), Toilet training in less than one day. New York: Pocketbook.
Baker, B. L., Brightman, A. J., Blacher, J. B., Heifetz, J., Hinshaw, S. P., and Murphy, D. M. (1989) Steps to independence: A skills training guide for parents and teachers of children with special needs. 2nd ed. Baltimore: Brookes.
Clark, L. (1985) SOS! Help for parents. Bowling Green: Parents Press.

Crepeau-Hobson, F., and O'Connor, R. (1996) Toilet training a child with fragile X syndrome. In Hagerman, R. J., and Cronister, A. (eds.). Fragile X syndrome: Diagnosis, treatment and research. 2nd ed. Johns Hopkins University Press, Baltimore MD, pp. 470–2.

Foxx, R. M., and Arzin, N. M. (1973) Toilet training persons with developmental disabilities: A rapid program for day and nighttime independent toiletting. Champagne: Research Press.

Linde, T. F., and Kopp, T. (1973) Training retarded babies and preschoolers. Springfield, IL: Thompson.

Luxen, M., and Christopherson, E. (1994) Behavioral training in early childhood: Research, practice and implications. Journal of Developmental and Behavioral Pediatrics 15: 370–8.

Mack, A. (1978) Toilet learning: The picture book technique for children and parents. Boston: Little, Brown.

Moffatt, M. E. K. (1997) Nocturnal enuresis: A review of the efficacy of treatments and practical advice for clinicians. Journal of Developmental and Behavioral Pediatrics 18 (1): 49–56.

Smith, R. (1993) Children with mental retardation: A parents guide. Rockville, MD: Woodbine House.

Wilson, R. (1995) Genetic habit-training program. Autistic Behavior 10:1–8.

OTHER RESOURCES

National Kidney Foundation
30 East 33rd Street
New York, NY 10016
(800) 622-9010; (888) WAKE-DRY (toll free); (212) 889-2210
fax: 212-779-0068
http://www.kidney.org
   All callers receive the NKF brochure entitled "When Bed-Wetting Becomes a Problem" and are offered the opportunity to listen to a 4-minute prerecorded message on bed-wetting.

General Family Support—
Internet Resources

The Family Village

http://www.familyvillage.wisc.edu

This site was organized by the Waisman Center of the University of Wisconsin-Madison. The Family Village integrates resources and communication opportunities on the Internet for people with disabilities, their families, and those who support and serve them. Selections include: Library (information re disabilities), Coffee Shop (connections with other families), Hospital (links re health care concerns), Shopping Mall (assistive technology suppliers), and others.

Family Voices

http://www.ichp.edu/mchb/fv

Family Voices is a national grassroots network of families and friends speaking on behalf of children with special health care needs. Selections include: About Family Voices, ACCESS-MCH/Family Voices, PIC Project, To Join Family Voices, Voices Newsletter, Español, Search.

National Parent Network on Disabilities (NPND)

http://www.npnd.org

NPND was established to provide a presence and national voice for parents of children, youth, and adults with special needs. NPND shares information and resources in order to promote and support the power of parents to influence and affect policy issues concerning the needs of people with disabilities and their families. The selections include news releases, the Friday Fax (weekly newsletter from the Department of Health and Human Services), conferences, federal issues, links to Federal Government sites, and information on IDEA.

PACER Center

http://www.pacer.org

PACER stands for Parent Advocacy Coalition for Educational Rights. Selections include: Publications (including order forms), Who We Are, PACER Center Articles,

Events, Legislative Information (including alerts), Frequently Asked Questions, Projects, National Information (links to other organizations).

PEP: Parents, Educators, and Publishers
http://www.microweb.com/pepsite/index.html

The PEP site is intended as an informational resource for parents, educators, and children's software publishers. The creators of this site have developed its content in response to the interests and needs of these three audiences. Selections include: Children's Software Revue, Educational Software Publishers, Computer Camps, Shopper Resources, and Cool School Sites.

INDEX